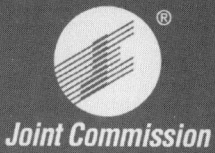

Hospital Accreditation Standards

2005 | HAS

Accreditation Policies

Standards

Elements of Performance

Scoring

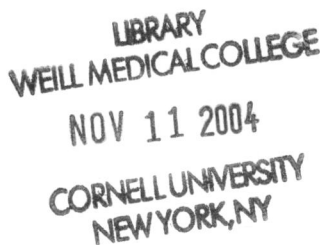

Joint Commission Mission

The mission of the Joint Commission on Accreditation of Healthcare Organizations is to continuously improve the safety and quality of care provided to the public through the provision of health care accreditation and related services that support performance improvement in health care organizations.

© 2005 by the Joint Commission on Accreditation of Healthcare Organizations

Joint Commission Resources, Inc. (JCR), a not-for-profit affiliate of the Joint Commission on Accreditation of Healthcare Organizations (Joint Commission), has been designated by the Joint Commission to publish publications and multimedia products. JCR reproduces and distributes these materials under license from the Joint Commission.

JCR educational programs and publications support, but are separate from, the accreditation activities of the Joint Commission. Attendees at JCR educational programs and purchasers of JCR publications receive no special consideration or treatment in, or confidential information about, the accreditation process.

All rights reserved. No part of this publication may be reproduced in any form or by any means without written permission from the publisher.

Printed in the U.S.A. 5 4 3 2 1

Requests for permission to make copies of any part of this work should be mailed to
Permissions Editor
Department of Publications
Joint Commission Resources
One Renaissance Boulevard
Oakbrook Terrace, Illinois 60181
permissions@jcrinc.com

ISBN: 0-86688-880-2
ISSN: 1522-1083

For more information about the Joint Commission on Accreditation of Healthcare Organizations, please visit http://www.jcaho.org.

Contents

How to Use This Book HB-1

The New Joint Commission Accreditation Process ACC-1

Accreditation Policies and Procedures APP-1

Sentinel Events SE-1

National Patient Safety Goals NPSG-1

Accreditation Participation Requirements...APR-1

Standards, Rationales, Elements of Performance, and Scoring

Section 1: Patient-Focused Functions
Ethics, Rights, and Responsibilities (RI) RI-1
Provision of Care, Treatment, and Services (PC) PC-1
Medication Management (MM) MM-1
Surveillance, Prevention, and Control of Infection (IC) IC-1

Section 2: Organization Functions
Improving Organization Performance (PI) PI-1
Leadership (LD)...LD-1
Management of the Environment of Care (EC) EC-1
Management of Human Resources (HR) HR-1
Management of Information (IM) IM-1

Section 3: Structures with Functions
Medical Staff (MS) MS-1
Nursing (NR) NR-1

Crosswalks of Standards..CW-1

Glossary GL-1

Index IX-1

How to Use This Book

The "How to Use This Book" chapter is designed to help hospitals understand both the purpose and the content of this publication. Further, this chapter highlights new and updated initiatives about the evolving accreditation process and orients readers to the structure of the book.

The *2005 Hospital Accreditation Standards* (*HAS*) is designed to facilitate a hospital's continuous operational improvement, as well as the self-assessment of its performance against Joint Commission hospital standards. The *HAS* includes information a hospital needs for continuous operational improvement: standards, rationales, elements of performance (EPs), scoring, and accreditation policies and procedures. The standards are provided in a new, user-friendly format that fosters a better understanding of each standard, its rationale (when applicable), and its EPs. Additional chapters that support ongoing accreditation efforts provide guidance on how to use the standards-related information found throughout the book.

What Is the Purpose of the *HAS*?

The *HAS* is designed to provide hospitals with information about the accreditation process. The *HAS* includes more than the latest standards and compliance information; it also includes material that supports a hospital's continuous operational improvement and its accreditation efforts.

The *HAS* also provides a better understanding of the connection between safety and quality-focused standards and day-to-day activities and the accreditation process. In essence, the book is a one-stop resource for hospital accreditation and continuous standards compliance.

What's New in the *HAS*?

The New Joint Commission Accreditation Process (Shared Visions–New Pathways®)

The Joint Commission implemented its new accreditation process initiative (Shared Visions–New Pathways®), in January 2004. This initiative stemmed from the Joint Commission's critical look at its services, which included significant input from health care organizations, to dramatically redesign and improve the value of the accreditation process. The new accreditation process represents a paradigm shift away from a focus on survey preparation to one of continuous operational improvement.

Specifically, this initiative does the following:
- Focuses the survey to a greater extent on the actual delivery of care, treatment, and services
- Increases the value of and the satisfaction with accreditation among accredited hospitals and their staff

2005 Hospital Accreditation Standards

HB

- Shifts the accreditation-related focus from survey preparation and scores to continuous operational improvement
- Makes the accreditation process more continuous
- Increases the public's confidence that hospitals continuously comply with standards that emphasize patient safety and health care quality

See "The New Joint Commission Accreditation Process" chapter for more detailed information about this initiative.

Changes to the *HAS* are made in response to suggestions from accredited hospitals and relate to important issues that clearly support high-quality care, treatment, and services. Since 2004, many chapters have been revised and improved to include additional information requested by customers. Table 1, page HB-3, summarizes the major revisions that have occurred during 2004.

Table 2, pages HB-8–HB-20, identifies changes to scoring category and MOS designations that became effective July 1, 2004.

What Does This Book Include?

The "New Joint Commission Accreditation Process" chapter explains the Joint Commission's new accreditation process. This chapter includes a description of the components of the new accreditation process, a sample time line, and the new decision categories for hospitals.

The "Accreditation Policies and Procedures" chapter includes current information on accreditation policies and procedures relevant to all health care organizations. This chapter, which has been updated to reflect the new accreditation process, details the types of surveys and provides in-depth discussions of, for example, the Joint Commission's Information Accuracy and Truthfulness Policy and its Public Information Policy. This chapter contains updated information about the accreditation and appeals procedures. Specific links to the "Accreditation Participation Requirements" (APR) chapter are provided to facilitate understanding of the policies that appear in both chapters.

The "Sentinel Events" chapter contains background information on the Joint Commission's Sentinel Event Policy, including the definition of a sentinel event, the goals of the Policy, which adverse events constitute sentinel events, sentinel event–related standards, definitions of what occurrences are reviewable under the Policy, and the various activities that surround the Policy.

The new "National Patient Safety Goals" chapter details the Joint Commission's 2005 National Patient Safety Goals for hospitals.

"Accreditation Participation Requirements" addresses the ongoing requirements for continued participation in the accreditation process and includes requirements related to the integration of the periodic performance review (PPR) into the accreditation process. These requirements are scorable.

The central portion of the manual is divided into three sections—Patient-focused Functions, Organization Functions, and Structures with Functions. The three sections

How to Use This Book

Table 1. Summary of Major Revisions to the *HAS* During 2004

Chapter	Summary of Major Revisions to *HAS*
How to Use This Book	• Clarification to explanation on how to score EPs • New table identifying scoring category and MOS designation changes effective July 1, 2004 • Revised and updated chapter, with summary of changes, for 2005
The New Joint Commission Accreditation Process (Formerly Shared Visions–New Pathways: The New JCAHO Accreditation Process)	• Revised chapter for 2005 • Decision rules for 2005
Accreditation Policies and Procedures	• Revision to accreditation decision resulting from Early Survey Policy Option 2 • Revised chapter for 2005
Sentinel Events	• Revised chapter for 2005
National Patient Safety Goals	• **New chapter** detailing the Joint Commission's 2005 National Patient Safety Goals for hospitals
Accreditation Participation Requirements	• Revised APR 14 addressing PPR options • New Accreditation Participation Requirement 23 to address implementation of Universal Protocol for Preventing Wrong Site, Wrong Procedure, Wrong Person™ • Revised APR 14 to include Option 3 of Periodic Performance Review • Revised scoring for EPs 1 and 2 in APR 19 • Revised chapter for 2005
Ethics, Rights, and Responsibilities (RI)	• Clarification to explanation on how to score EPs • Changes to MOS designations

continued on next page

Table 1. Summary of Major Revisions to the *HAS* During 2004 *(continued)*

Chapter	Summary of Major Revisions to *HAS*
Provision of Care, Treatment, and Services (PC)	• Clarification to explanation on how to score EPs • Expanded definition of "sufficient qualified individuals" and monitoring vital signs • Revised EP 1 in standard PC.13.20 to address staff performing and monitoring anesthesia and sedation • Revised EP 7 in standard PC.13.20 to address assessing anticipated needs of patients • Clarification to EP 3 in standard PC.2.120 to identify who completes a nursing assessment • Scoring category for EP 9 in standard PC.13.20 changed to A • Changes to MOS designations • Clarification to EP 5 in standard PC.5.60 • Clarification to standard language and new rationale for PC.8.10 • Waived testing standards: Revised standards and EPs for PC.16.10; revised EPs for PC.16.30; addition to rationale for PC.16.40; and new and revised EPs for PC.16.50
Medication Management (MM)	• Clarification to explanation on how to score EPs • Clarification to EP 3 in standard MM.2.10 to address ambiguous language • Clarification to EP 4 in standard MM.4.30 to address ambiguous language • Changes to MOS designations
Surveillance, Prevention, and Control of Infection (IC)	• Clarification to explanation on how to score EPs • New standards for 2005 • Changes to MOS designations • New EP 4 added to standard IC.3.10; this EP is not applicable to hospitals

continued on next page

Table 1. Summary of Major Revisions to the *HAS* During 2004 *(continued)*

Chapter	Summary of Major Revisions to *HAS*
	• New standard, EPs, and scoring information for IC.6.10 addressing infection control and emergency management activities
Improving Organization Performance (PI)	• Clarification to explanation on how to score EPs • Changes to MOS designations
Leadership (LD)	• Clarification to explanation on how to score EPs • New EP 12 in standard LD.1.20 to address system for resolving conflicts • EP 26 moved to standard LD.3.10 from EP 3 in standard LD.3.20 to clarify requirement • Clarification to EP 2 in standard LD.3.70 to be consistent with requirements in the "Medical Staff" chapter • New standard LD.3.11 addressing managing patient flow; standard LD.3.11 renumbered to LD.3.15 • Revised EP 1 in standard LD.3.110 addressing a hospital's agreement with an organ procurement organization • Changes to MOS designations
Management of the Environment of Care (EC)	• Clarification to explanation on how to score EPs • Clarification to EP 15 in standard EC.4.10 to address health care organizations' collaboration on emergency planning • New EP 5 in standard EC.5.20 to address organization's progress on corrective actions in Statement of Conditions™ • Changes to MOS designations

continued on next page

Table 1. Summary of Major Revisions to the *HAS* During 2004 *(continued)*

Chapter	Summary of Major Revisions to *HAS*
	• New EP 14, with scoring information, addressing labeling controls for partial or complete emergency shutdown added to standard EC.7.10; subsequent EPs renumbered • New EP 12 with scoring information in EC.8.10 addressing emergency access provision
Management of Human Resources (HR)	• Clarification to explanation on how to score EPs • Changes to MOS designations • EP 9 in standard HR.2.10 moved to EP 8 in standard HR.3.10; subsequent EPs renumbered • In standard HR.3.10, EP 7 clarified to address use of qualified individuals; EP 9 (formerly EP 8) clarified to address assessment of individuals • New EP 4, with scoring information, addressing documentation of performance evaluations added to standard HR.3.20
Management of Information (IM)	• Clarification to explanation on how to score EPs • Changes to MOS designations • EP 3 in standard IM.2.10 deleted; subsequent EPs renumbered • New EP 6, with scoring information, addressing retention of data and information added to standard IM.3.10; subsequent EPs renumbered • EP 1 in standard IM.4.10 divided into EPs 1 through 5; subsequent EPs renumbered • In standard IM.6.10: New EP 11, scoring information, and note addressing medical record delinquency rate; revised EP 12 addressing medical record reviews; new EP 13 with scoring information addressing criteria for medical record review; subsequent EPs renumbered

continued on next page

Table 1. Summary of Major Revisions to the *HAS* During 2004 *(continued)*

Chapter	Summary of Major Revisions to *HAS*
	• EP 1 divided into EPs 1, 2, and 3 in standard IM.6.20; no new requirements • Revised EP 2 in standard IM.6.30 addressing procedure reports • Revised EP 3 in standard IM.6.30 addressing progress notes
Medical Staff (MS)	• Clarification to explanation on how to score EPs • Note added to clarify Medicare Conditions of Participation requirement related to a single medical staff • Clarification to EP 4 in standard MS.4.20 to address setting-specific privileges • Revised language for standard MS.4.70 and EP 2 to address use of practitioner-specific data • Clarification to EPs 4, 5, and 6 in standard MS.4.100 to address temporary privileges • Clarification to EP 11 in standard MS.4.20 addressing description of a provisional period of initial appointment • Changes to MOS designations
Nursing (NR)	• Clarification to explanation on how to score EPs • Changes to MOS designations
Crosswalks of Standards (formerly Crosswalk of 2003 Standards to 2004 Standards)	• Revised entries for 2003 standards TX.2.4, TX.2.4.1, TX.6.3, TX.6.4, TX.6.5, LD.1.9, HR.4.1, HR.4.3, and HR.4.5) • New crosswalk for 2005 IC chapter • Chapter renamed
Glossary	• Revised definitions for 2005

© Joint Commission 2005.

2005 Hospital Accreditation Standards

Table 2. Scoring Category and Measure of Success (MOS) Designation Changes

This table identifies whether the scoring category and/or the measure of success (MOS) designation has changed for an element of performance (EP) effective July 1, 2004. Column 1 identifies a standard and EP for which the scoring category and/or MOS has changed; if a standard and EP aren't listed, then there were no changes. Column 2 indicates what the previous scoring category designation was. Column 3 indicates what the new scoring category designation is. Column 4 indicates whether an MOS designation has been added, removed, or remains the same. If nothing is listed in Column 4, then the EP does not require an MOS.

Standard and Element of Performance	Previous Scoring Category	New Scoring Category	MOS Designation
Ethics, Rights, and Responsibilities (RI)			
RI.1.10, EP 3	B	B	Removed
RI.1.10, EP 4	A	B	Removed
RI.1.10, EP 5	C	C	Added
RI.1.10, EP 6	A	B	Removed
RI.1.10, EP 7	A	C	Remains
RI.1.20, EP 1	B	A	
RI.1.30, EP 2	A	C	Added
RI.2.10, EP 2	C	C	Added
RI.2.10, EP 3	C	C	Added
RI.2.10, EP 4	C	C	Added
RI.2.60, EP 1	B	C	Added
RI.2.120, EP 3	C	C	Added
RI.2.140, EP 1	B	B	Removed
RI.2.140, EP 2	C	B	Removed
RI.2.140, EP 3	C	B	Removed
Provision of Care, Treatment, and Services (PC)			
PC.1.10 EP 1	A	B	
PC.2.20 EP 1	A	B	
PC.2.20 EP 2	A	B	
PC.2.20 EP 3	B	A	
PC.2.120 EP 6	B	A	Removed
PC.2.120 EP 7	C	A	Removed
PC.2.130 EP 3	A	A	Removed
PC.3.10 EP 2	B	B	Removed
PC.3.10 EP 4	C	B	Removed
PC.3.10 EP 5	C	B	Removed
PC.3.10 EP 6	A	A	Removed
PC.3.10 EP 7	A	A	Removed
PC.3.120 EP 2	C	B	Removed
PC.3.120 EP 3	C	B	Removed
PC.3.120 EP 3	C	B	Removed
PC.3.130 EP 1	C	A	Removed
PC.3.130 EP 2	C	B	Removed
PC.3.130 EP 3	C	B	Removed

continued on next page

Table 2. Scoring Category and Measure of Success (MOS) Designation Changes *(continued)*

Standard and Element of Performance	Previous Scoring Category	New Scoring Category	MOS Designation
PC.3.130 EP 4	C	B	Removed
PC.3.130 EP 6	C	B	Removed
PC.4.10 EP 1	C	B	Removed
PC.4.10 EP 2	C	B	Removed
PC.4.10 EP 6	C	B	Removed
PC.4.10 EP 14	C	B	Removed
PC.4.10 EP 17	C	B	Removed
PC.5.50 EP 1	C	B	Removed
PC.5.60 EP 1	B	B	Removed
PC.5.60 EP 5	C	B	Removed
PC.6.10 EP 1	C	B	Removed
PC.6.10 EP 3	C	B	Removed
PC.6.30 EP 1	C	B	Removed
PC.6.30 EP 2	C	B	Removed
PC.6.30 EP 3	C	B	Removed
PC.6.30 EP 4	C	B	Removed
PC.6.50 EP 2	B	B	Removed
PC.7.10 EP 1	C	B	Removed
PC.7.10 EP 2	B	C	Remains
PC.7.10 EP 6	B	A	
PC.7.10 EP 11	B	C	Remains
PC.8.60 EP 7	C	B	Removed
PC.8.70 EP 1	C	B	Removed
PC.9.30 EP 1	A	B	
PC.9.30 EP 2	A	A	Removed
PC.9.30 EP 3	A	A	Removed
PC.9.30 EP 4	A	A	Removed
PC.11.20 EP 1	B	B	Removed
PC.11.40 EP 2	C	A	Removed
PC.11.40 EP 3	C	A	Removed
PC.11.40 EP 4	C	A	Removed
PC.11.40 EP 5	C	A	Removed
PC.11.40 EP 6	C	A	Removed
PC.11.40 EP 7	C	A	Removed
PC.11.50 EP 1	A	A	Removed
PC.11.60 EP 1	A	B	
PC.11.60 EP 3	A	A	Removed
PC.11.70 EP 2	C	A	Removed
PC.12.10 EP 1	B	A	
PC.12.20 EP 1	A	A	Removed

continued on next page

Table 2. Scoring Category and Measure of Success (MOS) Designation Changes *(continued)*

Standard and Element of Performance	Previous Scoring Category	New Scoring Category	MOS Designation
PC.12.20 EP 2	B	B	Removed
PC.12.20 EP 3	B	B	Removed
PC.12.20 EP 4	B	B	Removed
PC.12.20 EP 5	B	B	Removed
PC.12.20 EP 6	B	B	Removed
PC.12.30 EP 1	C	A	Remains
PC.12.30 EP 3	C	A	Removed
PC.12.30 EP 4	C	A	Removed
PC.12.30 EP 5	C	A	Removed
PC.12.30 EP 6	C	A	Removed
PC.12.30 EP 7	C	A	Removed
PC.12.30 EP 11	B	B	Removed
PC.12.30 EP 12	B	B	Removed
PC.12.40 EP 9	C	A	Removed
PC.12.40 EP 10	A	A	Removed
PC.12.50 EP 1	C	A	Removed
PC.12.60 EP 3	A	A	Removed
PC.12.70 EP 1	A	A	Removed
PC.12.70 EP 2	A	A	Removed
PC.12.70 EP 3	C	A	Removed
PC.12.90 EP 1	A	A	Removed
PC.12.90 EP 2	C	A	Removed
PC.12.90 EP 3	A	A	Removed
PC.12.90 EP 4	A	A	Removed
PC.12.100 EP 1	A	A	Removed
PC.12.100 EP 2	A	A	Removed
PC.12.110 EP 1	C	B	Removed
PC.12.110 EP 5	A	A	Removed
PC.12.110 EP 6	A	A	Removed
PC.12.120 EP 1	B	A	Removed
PC.12.120 EP 2	B	A	Removed
PC.12.130 EP 2	C	B	Removed
PC.12.140 EP 1	C	A	Removed
PC.12.140 EP 3	A	A	Removed
PC.12.160 EP 1	B	B	Removed
PC.12.160 EP 3	C	B	Removed
PC.12.160 EP 4	B	B	Removed
PC.12.170 EP 4	B	B	Removed
PC.12.180 EP 2	B	A	Removed
PC.12.180 EP 3	B	C	Remains

continued on next page

Table 2. Scoring Category and Measure of Success (MOS) Designation Changes *(continued)*

Standard and Element of Performance	Previous Scoring Category	New Scoring Category	MOS Designation
PC.12.180 EP 4	B	B	Removed
PC.12.180 EP 5	B	B	Removed
PC.12.180 EP 6	B	B	Removed
PC.12.180 EP 7	B	B	Removed
PC.12.180 EP 8	B	B	Removed
PC.13.20 EP 1	B	B	Removed
PC.13.20 EP 2	A	A	Removed
PC.13.20 EP 4	A	B	Removed
PC.13.20 EP 5	A	B	Removed
PC.13.20 EP 6	A	B	Removed
PC.13.20 EP 9	A	A	Removed
PC.13.20 EP 10	C	A	Removed
PC.13.20 EP 11	C	A	Removed
PC.13.20 EP 12	C	A	Removed
PC.13.30 EP 1	A	A	Removed
PC.13.40 EP 1	C	A	Removed
PC.13.40 EP 3	C	B	Removed
PC.13.40 EP 4	C	B	Removed
PC.13.50 EP 1	A	B	
PC.13.50 EP 3	A	A	Removed
PC.13.50 EP 4	C	A	Removed
PC.13.60 EP 1	A	B	
PC.13.60 EP 2	C	B	Removed
PC.13.70 EP 1	B	C	Remains
PC.13.70 EP 2	B	B	Removed
PC.13.70 EP 3	A	A	Removed
PC.13.70 EP 4	B	B	Removed
PC.13.70 EP 5	B	B	Removed
PC.13.70 EP 6	A	A	Removed
PC.13.70 EP 8	B	B	Removed
PC.13.70 EP 9	A	B	Removed
PC.13.70 EP 10	A	C	Remains
PC.13.70 EP 12	C	A	Removed
PC.16.20 EP 2	B	B	Removed
PC.16.40 EP 2	A	B	
PC.16.40 EP 3	B	C	Remains
PC.16.40 EP 4	A	A	Removed
PC.16.50 EP 1	A	B	
PC.16.60 EP 3	C	B	Removed
PC.16.60 EP 4	C	B	Removed

continued on next page

Table 2. Scoring Category and Measure of Success (MOS) Designation Changes *(continued)*

Standard and Element of Performance	Previous Scoring Category	New Scoring Category	MOS Designation
Medication Management (MM)			
MM.1.10 EP 1	A	B	
MM.1.10 EP 2	B	A	
MM.2.10 EP 2	B	A	
MM.2.10 EP 4	B	B	Removed
MM.2.10 EP 5	B	B	Removed
MM.2.10 EP 6	A	B	
MM.2.20 EP 2	B	A	Remains
MM.2.20 EP 3	B	A	Removed
MM.2.20 EP 4	B	A	Removed
MM.2.20 EP 5	B	A	Removed
MM.2.20 EP 6	B	B	Removed
MM.2.20 EP 7	B	A	Removed
MM.2.20 EP 9	A	A	Added
MM.2.20 EP 10	B	B	Removed
MM.2.30 EP 6	C	A	Remains
MM.2.30 EP 7	C	B	Removed
MM.3.20 EP 7	A	B	
MM.3.20 EP 10	C	B	Removed
MM.4.10 EP 1	B	C	Remains
MM.4.10 EP 3	B	A	Removed
MM.4.10 EP 4	B	C	Remains
MM.4.10 EP 5	B	B	Removed
MM.4.10 EP 6	B	B	Removed
MM.4.20 EP 1	B	B	Removed
MM.4.20 EP 2	B	C	Remains
MM.4.20 EP 3	B	C	Remains
MM.4.20 EP 4	B	C	Remains
MM.4.30 EP 1	B	B	Removed
MM.4.30 EP 2	B	B	Removed
MM.4.30 EP 3	B	A	Removed
MM.4.30 EP 4	B	A	Removed
MM.4.40 EP 1	B	B	Removed
MM.4.40 EP 2	B	B	Removed
MM.4.40 EP 3	B	C	Remains
MM.4.40 EP 4	B	C	Remains
MM.4.40 EP 5	B	B	Removed
MM.4.50 EP 3	C	B	Removed
MM.4.70 EP 1	A	A	Removed
MM.4.70 EP 2	A	A	Removed

continued on next page

Table 2. Scoring Category and Measure of Success (MOS) Designation Changes *(continued)*

Standard and Element of Performance	Previous Scoring Category	New Scoring Category	MOS Designation
MM.4.70 EP 3	A	A	Removed
MM.4.80 EP 4	B	C	Remains
MM.6.20 EP 3	C	C	Added
MM.7.10 EP 1	B	A	
MM.7.40 EP 1	B	B	Removed
MM.8.10 EP 1	B	B	Removed
MM.8.10 EP 2	B	B	Removed
MM.8.10 EP 3	B	B	Removed
Surveillance, Prevention, and Control of Infection (IC)*			
IC.4.10 EP 2	C	A	Removed
IC.4.10 EP 3	C	B	Removed
IC.4.10 EP 6	C	C	Added
IC.4.10 EP 7	C	C	Added
IC.7.10 EP 1	B	A	
Improving Organization Performance (PI)			
PI.1.10 EP 1	B	B	Removed
PI.1.10 EP 2	B	A	Removed
PI.1.10 EP 3	B	B	Removed
PI.1.10 EP 4	A	A	Removed
PI.1.10 EP 5	A	A	Removed
PI.1.10 EP 6	A	A	Removed
PI.1.10 EP 7	A	A	Removed
PI.1.10 EP 8	A	A	Removed
PI.1.10 EP 10	A	A	Removed
PI.1.10 EP 12	A	A	Removed
PI.1.10 EP 13	B	B	Removed
PI.1.10 EP 14	B	B	Removed
PI.1.10 EP 15	B	B	Removed
PI.1.10 EP 16	B	B	Removed
PI.1.10 EP 17	B	B	Removed
PI.1.10 EP 18	B	B	Removed
PI.2.10 EP 1	B	B	Removed
PI.2.10 EP 2	B	B	Removed
PI.2.10 EP 3	B	B	Removed
PI.2.10 EP 4	B	B	Removed
PI.2.10 EP 5	B	B	Removed
PI.2.20 EP 1	B	B	Removed
PI.2.20 EP 2	B	B	Removed
PI.2.20 EP 3	B	B	Removed
PI.2.20 EP 4	A	A	Removed

continued on next page

---

* Changes are for the 2005 version of the IC chapter

Table 2. Scoring Category and Measure of Success (MOS) Designation Changes *(continued)*

Standard and Element of Performance	Previous Scoring Category	New Scoring Category	MOS Designation
PI.2.20 EP 5	A	A	Removed
PI.2.20 EP 6	A	A	Removed
PI.2.20 EP 7	A	A	Removed
PI.2.20 EP 8	A	A	Removed
PI.2.20 EP 9	A	A	Removed
PI.2.20 EP 10	A	A	Removed
PI.2.30 EP 2	A	A	Removed
PI.2.30 EP 3	B	B	Removed
PI.2.30 EP 4	B	B	Removed
PI.2.30 EP 5	B	B	Removed
PI.3.10 EP 1	B	B	Removed
PI.3.10 EP 2	B	B	Removed
PI.3.10 EP 3	B	B	Removed
PI.3.10 EP 4	B	B	Removed
PI.3.10 EP 5	B	B	Removed
PI.3.20 EP 4	B	B	Removed
PI.3.20 EP 5	B	B	Removed
PI.3.20 EP 6	B	B	Removed
PI.3.20 EP 7	B	B	Removed
PI.3.20 EP 8	B	B	Removed
PI.3.20 EP 9	B	B	Removed
Leadership (LD)			
LD.1.10 EP 3	A	A	Removed
LD.1.20 EP 1	A	A	Removed
LD.1.20 EP 2	A	A	Removed
LD.1.20 EP 3	B	B	Removed
LD.1.20 EP 4	A	A	Removed
LD.1.20 EP 5	A	A	Removed
LD.1.20 EP 6	B	B	Removed
LD.2.10 EP 2	A	A	Removed
LD.2.10 EP 4	B	B	Removed
LD.2.20 EP 1	B	B	Removed
LD.2.20 EP 2	B	B	Removed
LD.2.20 EP 5	B	B	Removed
LD.3.10 EP 3	A	A	Removed
LD.3.10 EP 26	B	B	Removed
LD.3.15 EP 7	A	A	Removed
LD.3.15 EP 8	B	B	Removed
LD.3.15 EP 9	A	B	
LD.3.20 EP 1	C	B	Removed

continued on next page

Table 2. Scoring Category and Measure of Success (MOS) Designation Changes *(continued)*

Standard and Element of Performance	Previous Scoring Category	New Scoring Category	MOS Designation
LD.3.20 EP 2	B	B	Removed
LD.3.30 LD 1	A	A	Removed
LD.3.30 LD 2	A	A	Removed
LD.3.50 EP 1	B	A	
LD.3.50 EP 2	B	A	Removed
LD.3.50 EP 4	B	A	
LD.3.50 EP 5	A	B	
LD.3.50 EP 6	B	B	Removed
LD.3.50 EP 7	B	A	
LD.3.60 EP 1	C	B	Removed
LD.3.60 EP 2	C	B	Removed
LD.3.60 EP 3	C	B	Removed
LD.3.70 EP 1	B	B	Removed
LD.3.70 EP 2	B	B	Removed
LD.3.80 EP 1	C	B	Removed
LD.3.80 EP 2	C	B	Removed
LD.3.80 EP 3	C	B	Removed
LD.3.80 EP 4	C	B	Removed
LD.3.90 EP 1	B	B	Removed
LD.3.110 EP 14	C	A	Removed
LD.3.120 EP 1	B	B	Removed
LD.3.120 EP 2	C	B	Removed
LD.3.130 EP 1	A	A	Removed
LD.3.140 EP 1	B	B	Removed
LD.3.140 EP 2	B	B	Removed
LD.3.150 EP 1	B	B	Removed
LD.3.150 EP 2	B	B	Removed
LD.3.150 EP 3	B	B	Removed
LD.3.150 EP 4	B	B	Removed
LD.3.150 EP 5	B	B	Removed
LD.4.20 EP 1	B	B	Removed
LD.4.20 EP 2	B	B	Removed
LD.4.20 EP 3	B	B	Removed
LD.4.20 EP 4	B	B	Removed
LD.4.20 EP 5	B	B	Removed
LD.4.20 EP 6	B	B	Removed
LD.4.50 EP 3	C	B	
LD.4.60 EP 4	A	B	
LD.4.70 EP 1	C	B	
LD.4.70 EP 2	C	B	
LD.4.70 EP 3	C	B	

continued on next page

Table 2. Scoring Category and Measure of Success (MOS) Designation Changes *(continued)*

Standard and Element of Performance	Previous Scoring Category	New Scoring Category	MOS Designation
Management of the Environment of Care (EC)			
EC.1.10 EP 4	B	B	Removed
EC.1.10 EP 6	C	C	Added
EC.1.10 EP 9	C	B	Removed
EC.1.20 EP 2	A	C	Remains
EC.1.20 EP 3 (EP 4 in 2004)	C	C	Added
EC.1.30 EP 4	C	B	Removed
EC.1.30 EP 6	C	B	Removed
EC.1.30 EP 7	C	B	Removed
EC.2.10 EP 3	B	B	Removed
EC.2.10 EP 5	C	B	Removed
EC.2.10 EP 7	A	B	
EC.2.10 EP 8	A	B	
EC.2.10 EP 9	C	B	
EC.2.10 EP 10	C	B	
EC.3.10 EP 2	C	B	Removed
EC.3.10 EP 7 (EP 4 in 2004)	C	B	Removed
EC.3.10 EP 8 (EP 5 in 2004)	C	B	Removed
EC.3.10 EP 9 (EP 6 in 2004)	A	B	
EC.3.10 EP 10 (EP 7 in 2004)	C	A	Removed
EC.3.10 EP 11 (EP 8 in 2004)	C	C	Remains
EC.3.10 EP 12 (EP 9 in 2004)	C	C	Remains
EC.3.10 EP 13 (EP 10 in 2004)	C	B	Removed
EC.4.20 EP 2	C	A	
EC.5.10 EP 2	C	B	Removed
EC.5.10 EP 3	C	B	Removed
EC.5.10 EP 5	C	B	
EC.5.30 EP 4	C	C	Added
EC.5.30 EP 5	C	B	Removed
EC.5.40 EP 3	A	A	Removed
EC.5.40 EP 9	A	A	Removed
EC.5.40 EP 10	A	A	Removed
EC.5.50 EP 3	A	A	Removed
EC.7.10 EP 8	C	B	

continued on next page

Table 2. Scoring Category and Measure of Success (MOS) Designation Changes *(continued)*

Standard and Element of Performance	Previous Scoring Category	New Scoring Category	MOS Designation
EC.7.10 EP 11	C	B	
EC.7.10 EP 12	B	A	
EC.7.10 EP 13	C	B	
EC.7.10 EP 15 (EP 14 in 2004)	C	B	Removed
EC.7.10 EP 16 (EP 15 in 2004)	A	A	Removed
EC.7.20 EP 2	C	C	Added
EC.7.20 EP 4	C	C	Added
EC.7.30 EP 2	A	A	Removed
EC.7.30 EP 3	A	A	Removed
EC.7.30 EP 4	A	A	Removed
EC.7.50 EP 1	A	A	Removed
EC.7.50 EP 2	A	A	Removed
EC.7.50 EP 3	A	A	Removed
EC.8.10 EP 2	C	B	Removed
EC.8.10 EP 3	C	B	Removed
EC.8.10 EP 5	C	B	Removed
EC.8.10 EP 7	C	B	Removed
EC.8.10 EP 11	A	A	Removed
EC.8.30 EP 1	C	B	
EC.8.30 EP 2	C	B	Removed
EC.8.30 EP 3	C	B	
EC.8.30 EP 4	C	B	Removed
EC.9.10 EP 1	B	B	Removed
EC.9.10 EP 2	B	B	Removed
EC.9.10 EP 3	A	B	
EC.9.10 EP 10 (EP 9 in 2004)	C	B	Removed
EC.9.20 EP 1	C	B	Removed
EC.9.20 EP 3	C	B	
EC.9.20 EP 4	C	B	
EC.9.20 EP 5	C	B	
EC.9.20 EP 6	C	B	
EC.9.20 EP 8	C	A	
EC.9.20 EP 9	C	B	
EC.9.30 EP 1	C	B	Removed
EC.9.30 EP 2	C	B	Removed
EC.9.30 EP 3	C	B	Removed
EC.9.30 EP 4	C	B	Removed
EC.9.30 EP 5	C	B	Removed

continued on next page

2005 Hospital Accreditation Standards

Table 2. Scoring Category and Measure of Success (MOS) Designation Changes *(continued)*

Standard and Element of Performance	Previous Scoring Category	New Scoring Category	MOS Designation
Management of Human Resources (HR)			
HR.1.10 EP 1	B	B	Removed
HR.1.20 EP 1	B	B	Removed
HR.1.20 EP 2	B	B	Removed
HR.1.20 EP 18	A	A	Removed
HR.1.20 EP 19	A	A	Removed
HR.1.30 EP 1	B	A	Removed
HR.1.30 EP 4	B	B	Removed
HR.1.30 EP 5	B	B	Removed
HR.1.30 EP 6	B	B	Removed
HR.1.30 EP 7	B	B	Removed
HR.1.30 EP 8	A	A	Removed
HR.2.30 EP 1	C	B	Removed
HR.3.10 EP 1	A	B	Removed
HR.3.10 EP 2	A	B	Removed
HR.3.10 EP 3	A	B	Removed
HR.3.10 EP 4	A	B	Removed
HR.3.10 EP 5	A	B	Removed
HR.3.10 EP 6	B	B	Removed
Management of Information (IM)			
IM.1.10 EP 1	C	B	
IM.1.10 EP 2	C	B	
IM.2.10 EP 1	B	B	Removed
IM.2.10 EP 2	B	B	Removed
IM.2.10 EP 3	C	B	Removed
IM.2.10 EP 4	C	B	Removed
IM.2.10 EP 6	C	B	Removed
IM.2.10 EP 8	C	B	Removed
IM.2.20 EP 2	B	B	Removed
IM.2.20 EP 7	C	B	Removed
IM.3.10 EP 2	A	A	Added
IM.3.10 EP 5	B	A	
IM.5.10 EP 2	A	B	
IM.5.10 EP 3	A	B	
IM.6.10 EP 8	A	B	
IM.6.10 EP 10	C	A	Removed
IM.6.10 EP 11	C	B	Removed
IM.6.10 EP 18 (EP 14 in 2004)	B	C	Added
IM.6.30 EP 7	B	C	Added

continued on next page

Table 2. Scoring Category and Measure of Success (MOS) Designation Changes *(continued)*

Standard and Element of Performance	Previous Scoring Category	New Scoring Category	MOS Designation
IM.6.40 EP 1	B	C	Added
IM.6.40 EP 2	B	C	Added
IM.6.50 EP 1	C	A	Removed
Medical Staff (MS)			
MS.1.10 EP 4	B	B	Removed
MS.1.10 EP 5	A	A	Removed
MS.1.40 EP 4	A	A	Removed
MS.1.40 EP 5	C	C	Added
MS.1.40 EP 7	B	B	Removed
MS.1.40 EP 8	A	A	Removed
MS.1.40 EP 9	B	B	Removed
MS.1.40 EP 10	A	A	Removed
MS.1.40 EP 11	A	A	Removed
MS.1.40 EP 12	B	B	Removed
MS.2.10 EP 4	B	B	Removed
MS.2.10 EP 5	B	B	Removed
MS.2.10 EP 7	B	B	Removed
MS.2.20 EP 1	A	A	Removed
MS.2.20 EP 2	C	C	
MS.2.20 EP 3	B	B	Removed
MS.2.30 EP 6	B	B	Removed
MS.2.30 EP 8	A	A	Removed
MS.3.10 EP 1	B	B	Removed
MS.3.10 EP 2	B	B	Removed
MS.3.10 EP 3	B	B	Removed
MS.3.10 EP 4	B	B	Removed
MS.3.10 EP 5	B	B	Removed
MS.3.10 EP 6	B	B	Removed
MS.3.10 EP 7	B	B	Removed
MS.3.10 EP 8	B	B	Removed
MS.3.10 EP 9	B	B	Removed
MS.3.10 EP 10	B	B	Removed
MS.3.10 EP 11	B	B	Removed
MS.3.20 EP 1	B	B	Removed
MS.3.20 EP 2	B	B	Removed
MS.3.20 EP 3	B	B	Removed
MS.3.20 EP 4	B	B	Removed
MS.3.20 EP 5	B	B	Removed
MS.4.10 EP 2	C	B	
MS.4.20 EP 4	A	A	Removed

continued on next page

Table 2. Scoring Category and Measure of Success (MOS) Designation Changes *(continued)*

Standard and Element of Performance	Previous Scoring Category	New Scoring Category	MOS Designation
MS.4.20 EP 6	B	B	Removed
MS.4.20 EP 8	A	C	Remains
MS.4.20 EP 10	C	A	Removed
MS.4.20 EP 15	A	A	Removed
MS.4.40 EP 1	A	A	Removed
MS.4.40 EP 3	B	B	Removed
MS.4.40 EP 5	A	A	Removed
MS.4.50 EP 1	B	B	Removed
MS.4.100 EP 3	B	A	Removed
MS.4.100 EP 4	A	A	Removed
MS.4.100 EP 5	A	A	Removed
MS.4.100 EP 6	A	A	Removed
MS.4.110 EP 5	A	A	Removed
MS.4.110 EP 6	A	A	Removed
MS.4.110 EP 8	B	B	Remove
MS.4.120 EP 1	A	A	Removed
MS.4.130 EP 1	B	B	Removed
MS.4.130 EP 2	B	B	Removed
MS.5.10 EP 2	A	A	Removed
MS.5.10 EP 3	A	A	Removed
MS.5.10 EP 4	A	B	Removed
Nursing (NR)			
NR.1.10 EP 2	B	A	
NR.1.10 EP 5	A	B	
NR.3.10 EP 1	C	A	Removed
NR.3.10 EP 2	C	A	Removed
NR.3.10 EP 3	C	A	Removed

© JCAHO 2004

contain the 11 functional chapters of the safety and quality-focused standards, rationales, EPs, and scoring that apply to hospitals.

Section 1 includes patient functions directly related to the provision of care, treatment, and services. Patient-focused standards appear in the following four functional chapters:
1. "Ethics, Rights, and Responsibilities" (RI)
2. "Provision of Care, Treatment, and Services" (PC), a new chapter including requirements from the former "Assessment of Patients" (PE), "Care of Patients" (TX), "Education" (PF), and "Continuum of Care" (CC) chapters
3. "Medication Management" (MM), a new chapter including medication requirements that previously appeared in the "Care of Patients" (TX) chapter

How to Use This Book

4. "Surveillance, Prevention, and Control of Infection" (IC), which has been moved from the organization function section because of its direct relationship to patient care, treatment, and services

Section 2 contains organization functions that, although not directly experienced by the patient, are vital to the hospital's ability to provide high-quality care, treatment, and services. Organization standards appear in the following five functional chapters:
1. "Improving Organization Performance" (PI)
2. "Leadership" (LD), which now includes requirements previously included in the "Governance" (GO) and "Management" (MA) chapters
3. "Management of the Environment of Care" (EC)
4. "Management of Human Resources" (HR)
5. "Management of Information" (IM)

Section 3 contains standards for structures with functions. Standards appear in the following chapters:
1. "Medical Staff" (MS)
2. "Nursing" (NR)

Functions include the processes and activities common to all health care organizations that cut across and are performed in all areas of a hospital. The standards in the 11 functional chapters have been adapted to hospitals and focus on processes, activities, and outcomes related to both patient and the hospital itself.

Immediately following the functional chapters is the new "Crosswalk of Standards" chapter, which identifies where previous standards requirements appear in the reformatted standards chapters. The crosswalks list the current standards and the corresponding reformatted standards, if applicable, and identify what changes have occurred between the previous standards and the current standards.

The Glossary provides definitions of many terms used throughout the book. In addition, the first page of every functional chapter includes a special box with key terms to recognize. These terms are highlighted so readers know to access the Glossary for the Joint Commission definition and use of these terms. Please note that not all terms defined in the Glossary appear in these boxes, only those terms for which readers are encouraged to look up the unique Joint Commission definitions.

A comprehensive Index appears at the end of the book.

What Do the Reformatted Functional Chapters Include?

One goal of the new Joint Commission accreditation decision initiative is to ensure and enhance the relevance of the Joint Commission standards to critical patient safety and health care quality issues.

Through the Standards Review Task Force, the Joint Commission has streamlined standards and reduced documentation burdens to do the following:

- Ensure the relevance of standards to safety and quality
- Reduce redundancy
- Improve the clarity of standards
- Reduce the associated paperwork and the documentation of compliance burden

As a result of this review, the standards are displayed in a new format, which includes the following:
- Each chapter has an Overview that provides background and explanatory information.
- Standards are statements that define the performance expectations and/or structures or processes that must be in place for a hospital to provide safe, high-quality care, treatment, and services.

Accreditation decisions are based on simple counts of the standards that are determined to be "not compliant."
- A rationale is background, justification, or additional information about a standard. A rationale is included for those standards needing additional text describing the purpose of the standard. In some cases, the rationale for a standard is self-evident. Therefore, not every standard has a written rationale.
- EPs are statements that detail the specific performance expectations and/or structures or processes that must be in place in order for an organization to provide high-quality care, treatment, and services.

Note: *For more information about how to score each EP, please refer to the "Understanding the Parts of This Chapter" section at the beginning of each functional chapter.*

What are Some Tips for Success?

The following tips are intended as helpful suggestions for using this book to successfully achieve continuous compliance with the standards:
- Make the *HAS* available to staff by keeping a complete copy or multiple copies of the manual in a resource center. Let staff and others know that the book is available and how they can access it.
- Read all parts of each chapter in this book.
- Keep a record of calls to the Joint Commission's Standards Interpretation Group (630/792-5900), including both questions and answers, for future reference and to avoid duplicate calls by other staff members.
- Focus on the concepts described and the points made in all standards and EPs. Concentrate on incorporating the frameworks and concepts of standards and EPs into day-to-day work, rather than on viewing the concepts as rules that must be followed just for Joint Commission survey purposes.
- Keep up with *HAS* changes as they occur instead of waiting until your survey is near. Read *Joint Commission Perspectives*®, the official monthly Joint Commission newsletter, to find new scoring, standard interpretations, and other useful information as the year progresses.
- View changes to requirements under the "JCAHO Requirements" page on the *Perspectives* Web site for free access to standards and policy revisions and

requirements that are specific to your organization. Look for the JCAHO Requirements page at http://www.jcrinc.com/2815.
- Subscribe to the *CAMH* Subscription Update Service to receive new materials and revisions to the *CAMH* on a quarterly basis.
- Check the Joint Commission's Web site (http://www.jcaho.org) for any revisions to hospital standards.
- Go to http://www.jcaho.org/accredited+organizations/standards+faqs.htm for Standards' Frequently Asked Questions. You can also use the online form for submitting standards questions to the Joint Commission at http://www.jcaho.org/onlineform/onlineform.asp.
- Keep a year's track record of evidence of implementation on hand. Data from the preceding 12 months will be reviewed and assessed during the on-site accreditation survey.
- Develop a team responsible for creating innovative ways to achieve and maintain continuous operational improvement and standards compliance, such as the following:
  ○ Question of the week or month
  ○ Standards-related posters
  ○ Column in a weekly all-staff newsletter

Where Should I Go if I Still Have Questions?

If you still have questions about how to use this book, *see* Table 3 (page HB-24), "Whom Do I Call?" which includes Joint Commission staff to whom specific questions can be directed.

Table 3. Whom Do I Call?

The following is a list of information resources at the Joint Commission and Joint Commission Resources.

The Joint Commission's **main** telephone number is **630/792-5000**. The Joint Commission's business hours are 8:30 A.M. to 5:00 P.M. central standard time, Monday through Friday.

Written correspondence should be sent to
Joint Commission on Accreditation of Healthcare Organizations
One Renaissance Boulevard
Oakbrook Terrace, IL 60181
ATTN: _____
[Area Indicated (such as Account Representative or Accreditation Operations)]

The Joint Commission's **main fax number** is **630/792-5005**. If you experience difficulties in transmission, please call 630/792-5541.

Call your **account representative** at **630/792-3007** for information about hospitals or with questions about the following:
- Request for survey for hospitals
- Scheduling of surveys
- Survey agenda or survey process
- Status of a survey report
- Content of a survey report
- Focused surveys

Call the **Standards Interpretation Group** at **630/792-5900** for information and questions about:
- Interpretation of hospital standards
- How to comply with hospital standards
- Credentialing

The **Customer Service** telephone number is **630/792-5800**. Joint Commission customer service representatives are available from 8:00 A.M. to 5:00 P.M. central standard time, Monday through Friday. Call Joint Commission's Customer Service with questions about:
- General information on Joint Commission services, mission, or history
- How to apply for a survey for the first time
- Ernest A. Codman Award program and for applications
- Your organization's accreditation status or history
- Obtaining a list of accredited organizations
- Checking the current accreditation status of an organization
- Quality reports
- Help in accessing information on Joint Commission's Web site

The Joint Commission's **Web site** address is http://www.jcaho.org. For an extensive e-mail or telephone list of contacts, click on **"Contact Us"** located near the top of the Joint Commission's home page. Throughout the online directory you will see e-mail addresses listed in parentheses. In general, e-mail addresses consist of the first letter of the person's first name and the entire last name @jcaho.org. In most cases, to reach the appropriate person and department by telephone, dial 630/792- and the extension number listed.

continued on next page

Table 3. Whom Do I Call?

Joint Commission Resources **main** telephone number is **630/268-7400**. Joint Commission Resources' business hours are 8:30 A.M. to 5:00 P.M. central standard time, Monday through Friday. Visit the **Web site** at http://www.jcrinc.com for information, questions, or to order the following:
- Continuous Service Readiness
- Custom education
- Domestic consulting services
- Educational seminars
- International accreditation services
- Publications

Joint Commission Resources' **Customer Service** telephone number for publications orders and education program registrations is **877/223-6866**. Customer service representatives are available from 8:00 A.M. to 8:00 P.M. central standard time, Monday through Friday. Call Customer Services for the following:
- Obtaining a free catalog for Joint Commission Resources Publications or Education
- Orders for Joint Commission Resources publications and registration for education seminars
- Multimedia education products
- Publications or education related to specific care programs (such as Disease Management)
- Call **630/792-5429** with request for permission to reprint any Joint Commission Resources publication

Call **Joint Commission Satellite Network (JCSN)** at **800/711-6549** for information and questions about how to sign up for the series of education programs broadcast across the United States.

The New Joint Commission Accreditation Process

Overview

The Joint Commission's new accreditation process focuses on systems critical to the safety and the quality of care, treatment, and services. It represents a shift from a focus on survey preparation to a focus on continuous operational improvement by encouraging hospitals to incorporate the standards as a guide for routine operations.

Under this new accreditation process, the survey is the on-site evaluation piece of a continuous process. The new accreditation process encourages hospitals to continuously use the standards to achieve and maintain excellent operational systems. Initiatives like the Periodic Performance Review (PPR) (discussed on page ACC-5) and the sharing of Priority Focus Process (PFP) information (discussed on page ACC-7) will facilitate this.

This chapter explains the following:
- Implementation and time line
- Revised standards and scoring format
- Periodic Performance Review
- Priority Focus Process
- Priority focus areas
- Clinical/service groups
- Tracer methodology and changes in the on-site survey process
- Evidence of Standards Compliance and measures of success

Implementation and Time Line

The time line in Figure 1 on page ACC-2 shows how components of the new accreditation process play out across a time continuum. The graphic displays the three-year accreditation cycle in terms of how it is experienced by a hospital from full on-site survey in July 2002 to its next full on-site survey in July 2005.*

Key Milestones in the Time Line[†]
- Approximately 15 months after your last on-site survey, Joint Commission will electronically send PPR access,[‡] the output of the PFP (*see* pages ACC-7–ACC-8 for more information), and instructions to your hospital on how to proceed.

---

* Organizations that were surveyed in July 2002 were the first to submit their PPR at the midpoint in their accreditation cycle. These organizations will undergo another full on-site survey in July 2005.

[†] In 2004, the Joint Commission continues to conduct voluntary unannounced surveys on a limited basis, opening up the option to all types of accredited organizations, and then transitioning to a completely unannounced survey process in 2006. *See* page APP-5 of the "Accreditation Policies and Procedures" chapter for more information on random unannounced surveys.

[‡] The Joint Commission will be transitioning to a completely unannounced survey process in 2006. While these key milestones will all still be a part of the accreditation process, their time lines will be adjusted to "fit" into an unannounced survey model.

2005 Hospital Accreditation Standards

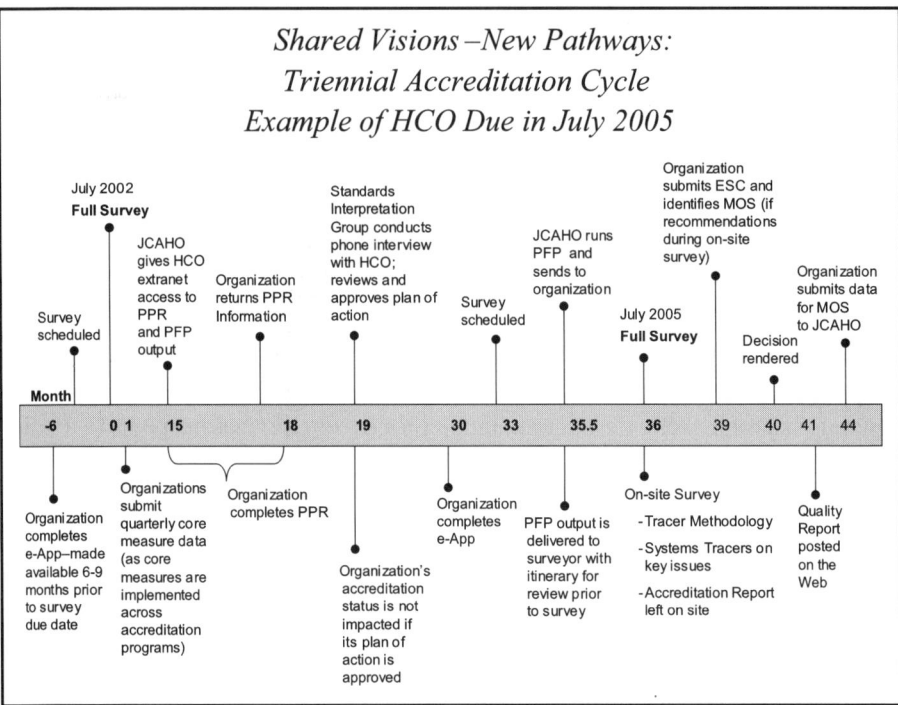

Figure 1. *This time line depicts the events experienced by an organization through a three-year accreditation cycle from 6 months before one survey (–6) to 39 months later, or 3 months after its next full survey. JCAHO events appear above the time line and health care organization (HCO) events appear below the time line.**

- Your hospital has 3 months to complete its PPR, during which time staff will evaluate compliance with standards using elements of performance (EPs) *(see* the section "Revised Standards and Scoring Format" on pages ACC-3–ACC-5 for more information). For standards identified as "not compliant," your hospital will develop a plan of action with measures of success (MOS), if required. At the 18-month point in the accreditation cycle, you will submit via a secure extranet Web space your PPR containing plan(s) of action to Joint Commission.
- Approximately 30 days after your plan of action has been submitted, Joint Commission staff will review plans of action over the telephone† and indicate whether the corrective actions, MOS, and the time frames are acceptable. Your accreditation decision is not affected if you conduct a PPR.
- Nine months before your next triennial on-site survey, your hospital will complete an electronic application for accreditation.

---

* **Note:** *Beginning in 2005, you will have continual access to the continuous PPR tool, but you will receive access to the "official" PPR tool for submission at the 15- through 18-month point in your accreditation cycle. There will be an annual update to the continuous PPR beginning in 2006. See pages ACC-5–ACC-7 for more information on the PPR options.*

† Joint Commission staff will phone your hospital to set up a time for this telephone call.

- Two weeks before your survey, Joint Commission will provide the most current output of the PFP for your hospital. (For more information on this process, please *see* the PFP component on page ACC-7.) The surveyor(s) scheduled to conduct your survey will also receive the PFP output for your hospital. This information will help the surveyor(s) develop a survey process that focuses on issues that are unique to your hospital.
- Triennial on-site survey occurs. The surveyor(s) will visit various units/programs or services using tracer methodology. (For more information on this process, please see the tracer methodology component on pages ACC-18–ACC-20.) During the survey, the surveyor(s) will also look for evidence that your plan of action from the PPR has been implemented.
- After evaluating your hospital's performance, the survey team will review the results of its individual findings. Before the closing conference, the survey team will enter its findings into laptop computers, thus producing a report of survey findings. After the report has been rendered, the team leader will meet with your hospital's chief executive officer (CEO) to provide him or her with a copy of the report. It is up to the CEO to decide whether the report will be distributed at the exit conference; however, the survey team will use the contents of the report during its exit conference. (For more information on this process, please see the "Accreditation Policies and Procedures" chapter on pages APP-30–APP-31.)
- Approximately 48 hours after your survey has taken place, Joint Commission will post your report of survey findings on a secure automated area of the extranet site that is password protected for each organization. If the surveyor(s) find requirements for improvement in your hospital, you have 90 days (45 days beginning July 1, 2005) following the posting of your organization's Accreditation Report on the Jayco extranet to submit an Evidence of Standards Compliance (ESC). During the 90-day/45-day period, your hospital's prior accreditation decision will remain in effect.
- If, at the end of the 90-day/45-day period, your hospital successfully addresses its requirements for improvement, it will be moved to an accreditation decision of "Accredited." After the 90-day/45-day time frame, either the ESC report is received and approved or your hospital is moved to an accreditation decision of "Provisional Accreditation." Your Quality Report will be made available to the public on Joint Commission's Quality Check®.

Revised Standards and Scoring Format

As part of the Joint Commission's new accreditation process initiative (Shared Visions–New Pathways®), the Joint Commission conducted a major review of the standards. During this process, all standards were reviewed and subsequently streamlined to enhance the focus on key quality and safety issues. The revisions achieve the following:
- Reduce redundancy
- Improve the clarity of standards language
- Reduce the associated paperwork and documentation of compliance burden

The standards chapters have been reformatted significantly. Please refer to the section "Understanding the Parts of This Chapter" at the beginning of each functional chapter and to pages HB-21–HB-23 in the "How to Use This Book" chapter for a detailed explanation.

For a complete crosswalk of previous standards from the *2004 Hospital Accreditation Standards* (*HAS*) to the current *HAS*, please *see* pages CW-1–CW-51.

Scoring was also revised. The revised framework provides for the scoring of the standards as compliant or not compliant. The accreditation decision will be based on a simple count of the standards that are judged not compliant. The EPs for each standard will be scored on the following scale:

- 0 Insufficient compliance
- 1 Partial compliance
- 2 Satisfactory compliance
- NA Not applicable

The determination as to whether a hospital is compliant with a given standard is based on the scoring of that standard's EPs. An EP is a specific performance expectation related to a standard that details the specific structures or processes that must be in place for a hospital to provide quality care, treatment, and services.

Two components are scored for each EP: (1) compliance with the requirement itself and (2) compliance with the track record* for that requirement. Scoring has been simplified, and track record achievements (which have always been part of the scoring) have been appropriately modified.

For more information on scoring, please refer to the "Understanding the Parts of This Chapter" at the beginning of each standards chapter as well as in the "How to Use This Book" chapter.

In addition to the requirements specifically stated in the EPs, EPs are also scored in accordance with the following track record achievements:

Score	Initial Survey[†]	Full Survey
2	4 months or more	12 months or more
1	2 to 3 months	6 to 11 months
0	Fewer than 2 months	Fewer than 6 months

---

* **Track record** The amount of time that an organization has been in compliance with a standard, element of performance, or other requirement.

[†] **Initial survey** An accreditation survey of a health care organization not previously accredited by the Joint Commission, or an accreditation survey of an organization performed without reference to any prior survey findings.

The New Joint Commission Accreditation Process

If during an on-site survey, your hospital has been found to be not compliant with one or more standards, you must submit an ESC* for each standard that is not compliant. The ESC must address compliance at the EP level; when an EP within a non-compliant standard requires an MOS,† your hospital must demonstrate achievement with the MOS when completing the ESC.‡

See the "How to Use This Book" chapter for detailed information on sample sizes.

Revised Accreditation Process
Presurvey Activities
Periodic Performance Review

The Joint Commission's new accreditation process is designed to shift the focus from survey preparation and passing the triennial exam to continuous standards compliance and operational improvement in the provision of safe, high-quality care, treatment, and services. One component of the accreditation process that supports this paradigm shift is the Periodic Performance Review (PPR), a compliance assessment at the midpoint of your hospital's accreditation cycle. The PPR is an Accreditation Participation Requirement (APR) for ambulatory care, behavioral health care, home care, hospitals, and long term care organizations.

The PPR helps your hospital review applicable standards, assess compliance, develop and implement plans of action, and identify measures by which you will gauge your success in carrying out those plans. By participating in the PPR, your hospital will be better able to incorporate Joint Commission standards into routine operations, which in turn will help to ensure the provision of safe, high-quality care on an ongoing basis.

Beginning January 1, 2005, your hospital will have continuous access to the PPR tool through the password-protected "Jayco"™ extranet site. At the 15-month point of the accreditation cycle, your hospital will be notified that it must submit to the Joint Commission no later than the 18-month point of your accreditation cycle your selection and completion of the full PPR, option 1, option 2, or option 3. Table 1 outlines some of the activities in each of these options.

---

* **Evidence of Standards Compliance (ESC)** A report submitted by a surveyed organization within 45 days (90 days between January 1, 2004 and June 30, 2005) of its survey, which details the action(s) that it took to bring itself into compliance with a standard or clarifies why the organization believes that was in compliance with the standard for which it received a requirement for improvement. An ESC must address compliance at the element of performance (EP) level and include a measure of success (MOS) (*see* definition) for all appropriate EP corrections.

† **Measure of success (MOS)** A numerical or quantifiable measure usually related to an audit that determines if an action was effective and sustained due four months after Evidence of Standards Compliance (*see* definition) approval.

‡ **Note:** *Not every EP requires an MOS. EPs that do require an MOS are clearly marked in the standards chapters in this book. Organizations are required to demonstrate achievement with an MOS only for EPs within a noncompliant standard that require an MOS. Organizations* do not *need to demonstrate achievement with an MOS for any EP within a compliant standard.*

Table 1. Current PPR Options

Full PPR

- Organization uses the automated PPR tool to assess and score compliance with elements of performance (EPs) for each applicable standard
- Organization creates a plan of action* addressing each EP scored partial or insufficient compliance within any standards found not compliant
- Organization identifies a measure of success (MOS), if required, for each EP scored partial or insufficient compliance within any standards scored not compliant
- Organization submits PPR data to Joint Commission
- Organization and Joint Commission's Standards Interpretation Group (SIG) hold a conference call within 30 days after PPR submission to discuss standards scored not compliant, plan(s) of action, and MOS
- SIG reviews and approves plan(s) of action during conference call
- Surveyors review any required MOS at triennial survey

Option 1

- Organization uses PPR tool to affirm that, for substantive reasons, legal counsel advises organization not to participate in the full PPR
- Organizations cannot use PPR tool to score compliance, but can print and view standards and EPs to conduct its assessment on paper
- Organization affirms that it has completed an assessment of its compliance with applicable EPs and developed plans of action and MOS, as necessary, but does not submit data to Joint Commission
- Organization can submit standards-related issues in the PPR tool for telephone discussion with SIG, if desired, and receive design approval
- Surveyors review any required MOS at triennial survey

Option 2

- Organization uses PPR tool to affirm that, for substantive reasons, legal counsel advises organization not to participate in full PPR
- Decision triggers scheduling of on-site survey at the midpoint of accreditation cycle
- Survey will be approximately one-third the length of the triennial survey; a fee will be charged
- Survey will be conducted primarily using tracer methodology and Priority Focus Process (PFP) output; all standards are subject to review
- Surveyor leaves written report of findings with organization
- Organization creates a plan of action and any required MOS for each standard scored not compliant and submits data to Joint Commission via the PPR tool within 30 days of survey
- Organization and SIG hold a conference call to discuss any standards scored not compliant, plan(s) of action, and MOS

---

* A plan of action details the action(s) an organization will take to come into compliance with each standard identified as not compliant.

Table 1. Current PPR Options *(continued)*

- SIG reviews and approves plan(s) of action during conference call
- Surveyors will review any required MOS at triennial survey

Option 3

- Organization must attest that after careful consideration with legal counsel, it has decided not to participate in the full Periodic Performance Review and instead intends to undergo a limited survey at the midpoint in its accreditation cycle.
- Organization is subject to an on-site survey (like option 2).
- Survey will be approximately one-third the length of the triennial survey; a fee will be charged
- Survey will be conducted primarily using tracer methodology and Priority Focus Process (PFP) output; all standards are subject to review
- Unlike option 2, however, option 3 stipulates that no report of findings will be submitted to the Joint Commission and that the surveyor delivers the results orally at the closing conference of the on-site survey.
- Additionally, there is no review of the PPR survey findings during the organization's next triennial survey.
- Following the survey, the organization may elect to participate in a conference call to discuss standards-related issues with Joint Commission staff. At the time of the organization's triennial survey, the surveyors will receive no information relating to the organization's option 3 survey findings.

Plans of Action

A plan of action is a detailed description of how a hospital plans to bring into compliance any standard identified as "not compliant" in the PPR (plans of action are not required for standards where some EPs are marked "partial compliance" but where the standard does not meet the level of "not compliant"). The plan of action should include the planned action to be taken and target dates. If the EP has an MOS, you must also describe the MOS or how you plan to gauge your successful implementation of your plans of action.

The PPR will only affect an organization's accreditation decision if the organization fails to participate in the PPR process, whether the full or one of the three options, or through the PPR process, an immediate threat to life situation* is identified.

If you need more information while completing your PPR, please contact your account representative.

Priority Focus Process

An important component of the Joint Commission's accreditation process is the Priority Focus Process (PFP), which guides surveyors in planning and conducting your on-site survey. The PFP uses an automated tool, which takes available data from a

---

* *See* page APP-30 of this book for more information.

variety of sources—including electronic applications (e-Apps) for accreditation, previous survey findings, complaint data, ORYX core measure data (for hospitals only), and publicly available external data (such as MedPAR or OASIS)—and integrates them to identify clinical/service groups (CSGs) and priority focus areas (PFAs) for your hospital. The PFP converts this data into information that focuses survey activities, increases consistency in the accreditation process, and customizes the accreditation process to make it specific to your hospital.

Surveyors will receive enhanced information and insight about a hospital before the on-site survey. The PFP integrates various presurvey data (listed below) on each hospital and recommends the PFAs ("priority focus areas" and "clinical/service groups") for the on-site survey. This information will guide tracer activities (*see* pages ACC-18–ACC-20 for more information on the tracer methodology). However, the PFP does not preclude any area from being surveyed.

From these sources, the PFP identifies PFAs for each hospital on which surveyors initially will focus during the initial part of the on-site survey. Surveyors will use the PFP in the following ways:

- Two weeks before the triennial survey, the surveyor(s) assigned to your hospital will have access to your hospital's PFP information via the surveyor extranet
- Surveyors will review the PFP information for hospital-specific PFAs as well as for hospital-specific clinical/service groups
- As part of the planning process, surveyors will begin to assess and plan their tracer activities
- During the on-site survey, the surveyors will use the hospital's active patient list to select tracer patients

The PFP will also be used for a hospital undergoing its initial survey. The only difference with this type of hospital (versus a hospital that has already gone through a survey) is in the available data inputs that feed the PFP. Hospitals undergoing initial survey will not have previous requirements for improvement (referred to as "type I recommendations" before January 1, 2004) or ORYX data available to feed into the PFP. For initial surveys, Joint Commission will only be able to feed electronic application (e-App) data, external data (as applicable), and Office of Quality Monitoring (OQM) data into the PFP.

After these data are transformed to become the PFP information, the process for initial surveys is no different from any other type of survey. The data will be aggregated in the same manner to determine the PFAs and clinical/service groups for the hospital.

Priority Focus Areas

Priority focus areas (PFAs) are processes, systems, or structures in a health care organization that significantly impact safety and/or the quality of care provided. The list of PFAs was developed from information provided by the Joint Commission's Office of Quality Monitoring, expert literature, and expert opinions. Joint Commission categorized the different processes, systems, and structures leading to improved health care in 14 PFAs. The PFAs evolved from this process of identifying common patterns useful toward building positive health care outcomes and safe, quality health care.

The PFAs provide a consistent yet customized approach to providing an initial focus for the on-site survey process, and they may assist the health care organization at the time of its PPR.

The PFAs are the following:
1. Assessment and Care/Services
2. Communication
3. Credentialed Practitioners
4. Equipment Use
5. Infection Control
6. Information Management
7. Medication Management
8. Organizational Structure
9. Orientation & Training
10. Patient Safety
11. Physical Environment
12. Quality Improvement Expertise/Activities
13. Rights & Ethics
14. Staffing

PFAs guide the surveyor throughout a portion of the survey—namely, the tracer portion. Outside of formal conferences/interviews, much of the survey will consist of reviewing systems issues in the form of tracer methodology (for more information, please *see* the Tracer Methodology section on page ACC-18). The CSGs affect tracer selection more than the PFAs do. Once a patient is selected for a tracer activity, the surveyor will put more focus on the prioritized list of PFAs for your hospital.

Definitions for each PFA follow.

Assessment and Care/Services Assessment and Care/Services for patients comprise the execution of a series of processes including, as relevant: assessment; planning care, treatment, and/or services; provision of care; ongoing reassessment of care; and discharge planning, referral for continuing care, or discontinuation of services. Assessment and Care/Services are fluid in nature to accommodate a patient's needs while in a care setting. While some elements of Assessment and Care/Services may occur only once, other aspects may be repeated or revisited as the patient's needs or care delivery priorities change. Successful implementation of improvements in Assessment and Care/Services rely on the full support of leadership.

Subprocesses of Assessment and Care/Services include the following:
- Assessment
- Reassessment
- Planning care, treatment, and services
- Provision of care, treatment, and services
- Discharge planning or discontinuation of services

Communication Communication is the process by which information is exchanged between individuals, departments, or organizations. Effective communication successfully permeates every aspect of a health care organization, from the provision of care to performance improvement, resulting in a marked improvement in the quality of care delivery and functioning.

Subprocesses of Communication include the following:
- Provider and/or staff-patient communication
- Patient and family education
- Staff communication and collaboration
- Information dissemination
- Multidisciplinary teamwork

Credentialed Practitioners Credentialed Practitioners are health care professionals whose qualifications to provide patient care services have been verified and assessed, resulting in the granting of clinical privileges. They typically are not employed staff at the health care organization. The category varies from organization to organization and from state to state. It includes licensed independent practitioners and, in some settings, nurse practitioners, advanced practice registered nurses, and physician assistants who are permitted to provide patient care services under the direction of a sponsoring physician. Licensed independent practitioners are permitted by law and the health care organization to provide care and services without clinical supervision or direction within the scope of their license and consistent with individually granted clinical privileges.

Equipment Use Equipment Use incorporates the selection, delivery, setup, and maintenance of equipment and supplies to meet patient and staff needs. It generally includes movable equipment, as well as management of supplies that staff members use (for example, gloves, syringes). (Equipment Use does not include fixed equipment such as built-in oxygen and gas lines and central air conditioning systems; this is included in the Physical Environment focus area.) Equipment Use includes planning and selecting; maintaining, testing, and inspecting; educating and providing instructions; delivery and setup; and risk prevention related to equipment and/or supplies.

Subprocesses of Equipment Use include the following:
- Selection
- Maintenance strategies
- Periodic evaluation
- Orientation and training

Infection Control Infection Control includes the surveillance/identification, prevention, and control of infections among patients, employees, physicians, and other licensed independent practitioners, contract service workers, volunteers, students, and visitors. This is a systemwide, integrated process that is applied to all programs, services, and settings.

Subprocesses of Infection Control include the following:
- Surveillance/identification
- Prevention and control
- Reporting
- Measurement

The New Joint Commission Accreditation Process

Information Management Information Management is the interdisciplinary field concerning the timely and accurate creation, collection, storage, retrieval, transmission, analysis, control, dissemination, and use of data or information, both within an organization and externally, as allowed by law and regulation. In addition to written and verbal information, supporting information technology and information services are also included in Information Management.

Subprocesses of Information Management include the following:
- Planning
- Procurement
- Implementation
- Collection
- Recording
- Protection
- Aggregation
- Interpretation
- Storage and retrieval
- Data integrity
- Information dissemination

Medication Management Medication Management encompasses the systems and processes an organization uses to provide medication to individuals served by the organization. This is usually a multidisciplinary, coordinated effort of health care staff, implementing, evaluating, and constantly improving the processes of selecting, procuring, storing, ordering, transcribing, preparing, dispensing, administering (including self-administering), and monitoring the effects of medications throughout the patients' continuum of care. In addition, Medication Management involves educating patients and, as appropriate, their families, about the medication, its administration and use, and potential side effects.

Subprocesses of Medication Management include the following:
- Selection
- Procurement
- Storage
- Prescribing or ordering
- Preparing
- Dispensing
- Administration
- Monitoring

Organizational Structure The Organizational Structure is the framework for an organization to carry out its vision and mission. The implementation is accomplished through corporate bylaws and governing body policies, organization management, compliance, planning, integration and coordination, and performance improvement. Included are the organization's governance; business ethics, contracted organizations, and management requirements.

Subprocesses of Organizational Structure include the following:
- Management requirements

- Corporate by-laws and governing body plans
- Organization management
- Compliance
- Planning
- Business ethics
- Contracted services

Orientation & Training Orientation is the process of educating newly hired staff in health care organizations to organizationwide, departmental, and job-specific competencies before they provide patient care services. "Newly hired staff" includes, but is not limited to, regular staff employees, contracted staff, agency (temporary) staff, float staff, volunteer staff, students, housekeeping, and maintenance staff.

Training refers to the development and implementation of programs that foster staff development and continued learning, address skill deficiencies, and thereby help to ensure staff retention. More specifically, it entails providing opportunities for staff to develop enhanced skills related to revised processes that may have been addressed during orientation, new patient care techniques, or expanded job responsibilities. Whereas orientation is a one-time process, training is a continuous one.

Subprocesses of Orientation & Training include the following:
- Organizationwide orientation
- Departmental orientation
- Job-specific orientation
- Training and continuing or ongoing education

Patient Safety Effective Patient Safety entails proactively identifying the potential and actual risks to safety, identifying the underlying cause(s) of the potential, and making the necessary improvements so risk is reduced. It also entails establishing processes to respond to sentinel events, identifying cause through root cause analysis, and making necessary improvements. This involves a systems-based approach that examines all activities within an organization that contribute to the maintenance and improvement of patient safety, such as performance improvement and risk management to ensure the activities work together, not independently, to improve care and safety. The systems-based approach is driven by organization leadership, anchored in the organization's mission, vision, and strategic plan, endorsed and actively supported by medical staff and nursing leadership, implemented by directors, integrated and coordinated throughout the organization's staff, and continuously re-engineered using proven, proactive performance improvement modalities. In addition, effective reduction of errors and other factors that contribute to unintended adverse outcomes in an organization requires an environment in which patients, their families, and organization staff and leaders can identify and manage actual and potential risks to safety.

Subprocesses of Patient Safety include the following:
- Planning and designing services
- Directing services

- Integrating and coordinating services
- Error reduction and prevention
- The use of Sentinel Event Alerts
- Joint Commission's National Patient Safety Goals
- Clinical practice guidelines
- Active patient involvement in their care

Physical Environment The Physical Environment refers to safe, accessible, functional, supportive, and effective Physical Environment for patients, staff members, workers, and other individuals, by managing physical design; construction and redesign; maintenance and testing; planning and improvement; and risk prevention, defined in terms of utilities, fire protection, security, privacy, storage, and hazardous materials and waste. The Physical Environment may include the home in the case of home care and foster care.

Subprocesses of Physical Environment include the following:
- Physical design
- Construction and redesign
- Maintenance and testing
- Planning and improvement
- Risk prevention

Quality Improvement Expertise/Activities Quality Improvement identifies the collaborative and interdisciplinary approach to the continuous study and improvement of the processes of providing health care services to meet the needs of consumers and others. Quality Improvement depends on understanding and revising processes on the basis of data and knowledge about the processes themselves. Quality Improvement involves identifying, measuring, implementing, monitoring, analyzing, planning, and maintaining processes to ensure they function effectively. Examples of Quality Improvement Activities include designing a new service, flowcharting a clinical process, collecting and analyzing data about performance measures or patient outcomes, comparing the organization's performance to that of other organizations, selecting areas for priority attention, and experimenting with new ways of carrying out a function.

Subprocesses of Quality Improvement Expertise/Activities include the following:
- Identifying issues and establishing priorities
- Developing measures
- Collecting data to evaluate status on outcomes, processes, or structures
- Analyzing and interpreting data
- Making and implementing recommendations
- Monitoring and sustaining performance improvement

Rights & Ethics Rights & Ethics include patient rights and organizational ethics as they pertain to patient care. Rights & Ethics addresses issues such as patient privacy, confidentiality and protection of health information, advance directives (as appropriate), organ procurement, use of restraints, informed consent for various procedures, and the right to participate in care decisions.

Subprocesses of Rights & Ethics include the following:
- Patient rights
- Organizational ethics pertaining to patient care
- Organizational responsibility
- Consideration of patient
- Care sensitivity
- Informing patients and/or family

Staffing Effective Staffing entails providing the optimal number of competent personnel with the appropriate skill mix to meet the needs of a health care organization's patients based on that organization's mission, values, and vision. As such, it involves defining competencies and expectations for all staff (the competency of licensed independent practitioners and medical staff are addressed in the Credentialed Practitioners priority focus area for all accreditation programs); Staffing includes assessing those defined competencies and allocating human resources necessary for patient safety and improved patient outcomes.

Subprocesses of Staffing include the following:
- Competency
- Skill mix
- Number of staff

Clinical/Service Groups

Clinical/service groups (CSGs) categorize patients and/or services into distinct populations for which data can be collected. The Joint Commission created the list of CSGs based on data gathered from e-Apps from each accreditation program and on publicly available data from external sources. The list then underwent a thorough review to make sure that all categories were actually representative of populations served or services provided by the organizations surveyed by the individual accreditation programs. Joint Commission surveyors use a hospital's CSGs combined with other hospital-specific data to get a better understanding of the hospital's systems and the patients it serves. Tracer patients are selected according to CSGs.

Clinical/Service Groups for Hospitals
- Cardiac surgery
- Cardiology*
- Dentistry
- Dermatology
- Endocrinology
- Gastroenterology
- General medicine
- General surgery
- Gynecology
- Hematology
- HIV infection
- Neonatology*

---

* ORYX core measure areas

- Nephrology
- Neurology
- Neurosurgery
- Normal newborns
- Obstetrics*
- Oncology
- Ophthalmology
- Orthopedic
- Otolaryngology
- Pediatrics*
- Psychiatry
- Pulmonary*
- Rehabilitation
- Rheumatology
- Substance abuse
- Thoracic surgery
- Trauma
- Urology
- Vascular surgery
- Other

On-Site Survey Activities
Survey Agenda
The on-site survey process shifts the focus from survey preparation and scores to continuous operational improvement in support of safe, high-quality care, treatment, and services.

The survey agenda will include the following elements (in no particular order):[†]
- *Opening Conference and Orientation to the Organization.* The opening session will be an opportunity for introductions and for an orientation to the structure and content of the survey. At this time, your hospital will briefly explain its structures, mission, vision, and relationship with the community.
- *Surveyor Planning Session.* During this session, the surveyor(s) will review data and information about the hospital, including plans of action generated from the PPR, and plan the survey agenda. The surveyor(s) will also select initial tracer patients.
- *Leadership Session.* Surveyors will discuss the following with leaders:
  - Information gathering and baseline assessment of leadership-level, system issues—system standards, management oversight and direction, and other leadership responsibilities
  - Leadership's approach to the PPR and methods used to address areas needing improvement

---

* ORYX core measure areas

[†] Please *see* the *Survey Activity Guide*, available by calling your Account Representative, for more detailed information on the survey process.

- Ongoing initiatives to improve delivery of health care
- Safety program and National Patient Safety Goals
- Oversight by trustees or board

- *Individual Tracer Activity.* During the tracer activity, the surveyor will do the following:
  - Follow the course of a type of care, treatment, and service provided to the patient by the hospital
  - Assess the interrelationships among disciplines and departments (where applicable) and the important functions in the care, treatment, and services provided
  - Evaluate the performance of processes relevant to the care, treatment, and service needs of the patient, with particular focus on the integration and coordination of distinct but related processes
  - Identify vulnerabilities in the care processes
- *Special Issue Resolution.* This session provides an opportunity for surveyors to follow up on potential findings that could not be resolved in other survey activities.
- *Daily Briefing.* During the daily briefing, the surveyor will do the following:
  - Facilitate leadership's understanding of the survey process and the findings that contribute to the accreditation decision
  - Report on findings from the previous day's survey activities
  - Emphasize patterns or trends of significant concern that could lead to non-compliance determinations
  - Highlight any positive findings or exemplary performance
  - Allow the hospital to provide information that may have been missed during the previous survey day
  - Review the agenda for the survey day ahead and make any necessary adjustments based on hospital needs or the need for more intensive assessment of an issue
- *Competence Assessment Process.* This process will help the hospital and the surveyor to do the following:
  - Identify the competence-assessment, process-related strengths and vulnerabilities of staff and, as applicable, licensed independent practitioners
  - Begin the assessment or determine the degree of compliance with relevant standards
  - Identify human resources issues requiring further exploration
- *Medical Staff Credentialing and Privileging.* This activity will help the hospital and the surveyor to identify specific issues related to the following:
  - Evaluation of the process the hospital uses to collect relevant data for decisions for appointment
  - Evaluation of consistent implementation of the credentialing and privileging process
  - Evaluation of processes for the granting and the appropriate delineation of privileges
  - Determination that practitioners practice within the limited scope of delineated privileges

- Link results of peer review and focused monitoring to the credentialing and privileging process
- Identify vulnerabilities in the credentialing, privileging, and appointment process
- *Environment of Care Session.* This session will help the hospital and the surveyor do the following:
  - Identify vulnerabilities and strengths in their processes
  - Begin to identify or determine the action(s) necessary to address any identified vulnerabilities
  - Begin the assessment or determine the hospital's actual degree of compliance with relevant standards
  - Identify EC processes requiring further evaluation of implementation
  - Identify issues requiring further exploration
- *System Tracer Sessions.* System tracers are interactive sessions with surveyors and hospital staff that explore the performance of important patient-related functions that cross the hospital. Surveyors and hospital staff will address critical risk points and provide education during the system tracer sessions. The following are the system tracers:
  - Medication Management
  - Infection Control
  - Data Use
- *CEO Exit Briefing and Organization Exit Conference.* During this conference, the surveyor(s) will do the following:
  - Report the outcome of the survey and present the Accreditation Report if desired by the CEO or administrator
  - Review the issues of standards compliance that have been identified during the survey
  - Allow the hospital a final on-site opportunity to question the survey findings or provide additional material regarding standards compliance
  - Gain agreement between the surveyor(s) and the hospital regarding the survey findings, when possible
  - Review required follow-up actions, as applicable
- *Life Safety Code® (LSC) Building Tour.* This session will help the organization and surveyor do the following:
  - Identify areas of concern in the organization's processes for designing buildings to *LSC* requirements
  - Identify areas of concern in the organization's processes for maintaining buildings to *LSC* requirements
  - Identify areas of concern in the organization's processes for identifying and resolving *LSC* problems
  - Determine the organization's degree of compliance with relevant *LSC* requirements
  - Identify or determine the action(s) necessary to address any identified *LSC* problems
- *Surveyor Team Meeting.* On surveys being conducted by more than one surveyor, scheduled team meetings provide an opportunity for surveyors to share

information and observations, plan for upcoming survey activities, and plan for communication and coordination with the organization.
- *Surveyor Report Preparation.* The surveyor(s) will use this time to compile, analyze, and organize the data he or she has collected throughout the survey into a report reflecting the organization's compliance with standards.

Tracer Methodology
Individual Tracer Activity
The tracer methodology is the cornerstone of the new survey process. The individual tracer activity is an evaluation method conducted during an on-site survey designed to "trace" the care experiences that a patient had while at the hospital. The tracer methodology is a way to analyze a hospital's systems of providing care, treatment, and services using actual patients as the framework for assessing standards compliance. Surveyors will use the following general criteria to select initial individual tracers:
- Patients in top CSGs and PFAs for that organization
- Patients who cross programs, for example, long term care residents who present at a hospital or some care patients received from a hospital in complex organizations
- Patients related to system tracer topics (*see* the section "System Tracer Activity" on page ACC-19), such as infection control or medication management
- Patients receiving complex services, such as surgery or treatment in an intensive care unit*

The typical patients selected for initial tracer activity will be those identified in the hospital's PFP information as listed in the CSGs. Based on identified PFAs and CSGs, the surveyor will identify patient tracers and follow specific patients through the hospital's processes. A surveyor will not only examine the individual components of a system but will also evaluate how the components of a system interact with each other. In other words, a surveyor will look at the care, treatment, and services provided by each department/unit/program and service, as well as how departments/units/programs and services work together. Surveyors may start where the patient is currently located. They then can move to where the patient first entered the organization's systems, an area of care provided to the patient that may be a priority for that organization, or to any areas in which the patient received care, treatment, and services. The order will vary. Along the way, surveyors will speak with health care staff members who actually provided the care to that tracer patient—or, if that staff member is not available, will speak with another staff member who provides the same type of care.

Based on the surveyor's findings, he or she may select similar patients to trace. The tracer methodology permits surveyors to "pull the threads" if there is a reason to believe that an issue needs further exploration.

---

* Please *see* the *Survey Activity Guide*, available by calling your Account Representative, for more detailed information on other program-specific criteria for tracer selection.

System Tracer Activity

System tracers differ from individual tracers in that during individual tracers, the surveyor follows a specific patient through his or her course of care, evaluating all aspects of care. System tracers follow the flow of one specific system or process across the organization. During the system tracer sessions, surveyors evaluate the system/process including, the integration of related processes, and the coordination and communication among disciplines and departments in those processes.

A system tracer includes an interactive session (involving a surveyor and relevant staff members). Points of discussion in the interactive session include the following:
- The flow of the process across your hospital, including identification and management of risk points, integration of key activities, and communication among staff/units involved in the process
- Strengths in the process and possible actions to be taken in areas needing improvement
- Issues requiring further exploration in other survey activities
- A baseline assessment of standards compliance
- Education by the surveyor, as appropriate

The three topics evaluated with system tracers are data use, infection control, and medication management, although the number of system tracers varies based on survey length.

Data Use The data use system tracer focuses on how your hospital collects, analyzes, interprets, and uses data to improve patient safety and care.

Infection Control The infection control system tracer explores your hospital's infection control processes. The goals of this session are to assess your hospital's compliance with the relevant infection control standards, identify infection control issues that require further exploration, and determine actions that may be necessary to address any identified risks and improve patient safety.

Medication Management The medication management system tracer explores your hospital's medication management processes, while focusing on subprocesses and potential risk points (such as hand-off points). This tracer activity helps the surveyors evaluate the continuity of medication management from procurement of medications through the monitoring of their effects on patients.

The Role of Staff in Tracer Methodology

To help the surveyor or survey team in the tracer methodology, staff will be instructed to provide the surveyor or survey team with a list of active patients including the patients' names, current locations in the hospital, and diagnoses, as appropriate. Surveyors may request assistance from hospital staff for selection of appropriate tracer patients. As surveyors move around a hospital, they will ask to speak with the staff members who have been involved in the tracer patient's care, treatment, and services. If those staff members are not available, they will ask to speak to another staff member who would perform the same function(s) as the member who has cared for or is caring for the tracer patient. Although it is preferable to speak with the direct caregiver, it is not mandatory because the questions that will be asked are questions that any caregiver should be able to answer in providing care to the patient being traced.

Accreditation Policies and Procedures

Overview
This chapter provides information on the Joint Commission's accreditation policies and procedures relevant to all health care organizations interested in Joint Commission accreditation, whether they are applying for the first time or on a renewal basis. These policies and procedures apply to all organizations either currently accredited by, or seeking accreditation by, the Joint Commission.

This chapter includes information about the continuous accreditation process and specific components that occur at various stages, including information hospitals need to know about the Periodic Performance Review (PPR), the on-site survey, and the Evidence of Standards Compliance (ESC) process. The time line on page ACC-2 of "The New Joint Commission Accreditation Process" chapter identifies all the stages of the continuous accreditation process and their timing in that process.

The chapter is organized into major sections reflecting the elements of the accreditation process. You will be able to locate the policies and procedures applicable to your organization according to where your organization is in the accreditation process or cycle. An organization must follow the policies and procedures described in this chapter in order to participate and continue to participate in the accreditation process. Failure to follow the policies and procedures described in this chapter can result in denial or withdrawal of accreditation.

Note: *The "Accreditation Participation Requirements" chapter includes specific requirements for accreditation participation. The requirements are existing policies within this "Accreditation Policies and Procedures" chapter and are currently effective for accreditation purposes. Cross-references to the accreditation participation requirements can be found in the applicable sections of this chapter.*

General Information
This section provides information relevant to an organization either applying for initial Joint Commission accreditation or seeking continued accreditation. Because this material is revised on a regular basis, all organizations are encouraged to review it.

Organizations Eligible for Accreditation
General Eligibility Requirements
Any health care organization may apply for Joint Commission accreditation under the standards in this book* if all the following requirements are met:

---

* The Joint Commission will work with the organization to determine which standards from other accreditation programs are applicable.

- The organization is in the United States or its territories or, if outside the United States, is operated by the U.S. government, under a charter of the U.S. Congress, meeting the following criteria:
  - The nature of the health care practices in the applicant organization is compatible with the intents of Joint Commission standards and their elements of performance (EPs)
  - With the use of interpreters provided by the organization, as necessary, the surveyor(s) can effectively communicate with substantially all of the organization's management and clinical personnel and at least half of the organization's patients, and can understand medical records and documents that relate to the organization's performance
  - U.S. citizens make up at least 10% of the organization's patient population
  or
  - A U.S. government agency contracts with the organization to provide services to U.S. citizens
  or
  - U.S. citizens preferentially use the organization in that country
- The organization assesses and improves the quality of its services. This process includes a review of care by clinicians, when appropriate.
- The organization identifies the services it provides, indicating which services it provides directly, under contract, or through some other arrangement
- The organization provides services addressed by the Joint Commission's standards

Scope of Accreditation Surveys
General Survey Categories
The Joint Commission surveys and accredits health care organizations using standards from one or more of the following manuals:
- *Accreditation Manual for Assisted Living*
- *Accreditation Manual for Critical Access Hospitals*
- *Accreditation Manual for Office-Based Surgery Practices*
- *Accreditation Manual for Preferred Provider Organizations*
- *Comprehensive Accreditation Manual for Ambulatory Care*
- *Comprehensive Accreditation Manual for Behavioral Health Care*
- *Comprehensive Accreditation Manual for Home Care* (includes standards for home health, personal/support care, hospice, home medical equipment, and pharmacies)
- *Comprehensive Accreditation Manual for Hospitals: The Official Handbook*
- *Comprehensive Accreditation Manual for Integrated Delivery Systems*
- *Comprehensive Accreditation Manual for Long Term Care* (includes standards for subacute care programs)
- *Comprehensive Accreditation Manual for Laboratory and Point-of-Care Testing*
- *Comprehensive Accreditation Manual for Managed Care Organizations*

In addition to standards, the Joint Commission also surveys organizations using the standards' EPs, performance measurement data (when applicable), and Accreditation Participation Requirements (APRs), including the Joint Commission National

Patient Safety Goals (*see* the "National Patient Safety Goals" chapter). Used in conjunction with the standards, these items help assess an organization's performance.

Single Accreditation Awards

The Joint Commission survey, assuming satisfactory compliance, provides one accreditation award for all of the organization's services, programs, and related organizations. Included in each organization's survey and accreditation decision are all services, programs, and related organizations that are organizationally and functionally integrated. If, after accreditation is rendered to an organization, the organization's structure changes whereby one or more of its services, programs, or related organizations are no longer part of the organization that was originally surveyed, the service, program, or related organization is no longer included in the organization's accreditation.

Tailored Survey Policy

The Joint Commission survey, assuming satisfactory compliance, provides one accreditation award for all the organization's services, programs, and related organizations. Another service, program, or related entity (that is, component), whether providing services or through a contractual arrangement, will be included in the survey of the applicant organization under the following circumstances:
- There are Joint Commission standards applicable to the component
- The component is overseen and managed by the applicant organization through organizational and functional integration

Note: *Any service, program, or related entity that is a component of an accreditation-eligible organization may independently seek accreditation if it can meet Joint Commission survey eligibility requirements.*

Organizational and functional integration refers to the degree to which the component is overseen and managed by the applicant organization. An *applicant organization* refers both to an organization seeking accreditation and to an organization that is currently accredited. A *component* is a service, program, or related entity that delivers care or services and is eligible for survey under one of the Joint Commission's accreditation programs. These include the following:
- General, psychiatric, pediatric, critical access, surgical specialty, and rehabilitation hospitals
- Home care organizations, including those that provide home health services, personal care and support services, home infusion and other pharmacy services, long term care pharmacies and infusion centers, durable medical equipment services, and hospice services
- Nursing homes and other long term care facilities, including subacute care programs and dementia programs
- Assisted living residences that provide or coordinate personal services, 24-hour supervision and assistance (scheduled and unscheduled) activities, and health-related services
- Behavioral health care organizations, including those that provide mental health services, substance abuse treatment services, foster care services, and services

for persons with developmental disabilities for individuals of various ages in various organized service settings
- Ambulatory care providers, including outpatient surgery facilities and office-based surgery, rehabilitation centers, sleep labs, imaging centers, group practices, and others
- Clinical laboratories

Organizational integration exists when the applicant organization's governing body, either directly or ultimately, controls budgetary and resource allocation decisions for the component or, where individual corporate entities are involved, there is greater than 50% common governing board membership for the applicant organization and on the board of the component.

Functional integration exists when the entity meets at least three of the following eight criteria:
1. The applicant organization and the component do the following:
   - Use the same process for determining membership of licensed independent practitioners in practitioner panels or medical or professional staff and/or
   - Have a common organized medical or professional staff for the applicant organization and the component
2. The applicant organization's human resources function hires and assigns staff at the component and has the authority to do the following:
   - Terminate staff at the component
   - Transfer or rotate staff between the applicant organization and the component
   - Conduct performance appraisals of the staff who work in the component
3. The applicant organization's policies and procedures are applicable to the component with few or no exceptions
4. The applicant organization manages significant operations of the component; that is, the component has little or no management authority or autonomy independent of the applicant organization
5. The component's patient records are integrated in the applicant organization's patient record system
6. The applicant organization applies its performance improvement program to the component and has authority to implement actions intended to improve performance at the component
7. The applicant organization bills for services provided by the component under the name of the applicant organization
8. The applicant organization and/or the component portrays to the public that the component is part of the organization through the use of common names or logos; references on letterheads, brochures, telephone-book listings, or Web sites; or representations in other published materials

The Joint Commission evaluates all health care services provided by the organization for which the Joint Commission has standards and makes one accreditation decision and survey report. An organization must be prepared to provide evidence of its compliance with each applicable standard. To gain accreditation, an organization must demonstrate overall compliance with the standards and their EPs.

Complex Organization Survey Process

The complex organization survey process is applied to organizations that are governed by the Tailored Survey Policy (see pages APP-3–APP-4). The Joint Commission will conduct a complex organization survey based on the services provided by the organization, as reported in its application for accreditation. Because a complex organization survey process will involve standards in more than one of the manuals listed in this chapter, the Joint Commission provides the organization with a copy of each of the manuals to be used in the survey before it is conducted.

Organizations that have acquired a new component will be given a 12-month grace period from the time the component is acquired before the performance of that component will be factored into the organization's overall accreditation decision. The newly acquired component will usually be surveyed within six months of its acquisition as an extension survey; however, the accreditation decision rendered from the extension survey will be in effect for the component only for 12 months following the acquisition before impacting the organization's overall accreditation decision.

Contracted Services

The Joint Commission evaluates the organization's assessment of the quality of services provided under contractual arrangements. The Joint Commission reserves the right to evaluate, as part of its survey, services provided by another organization or provider. It may survey performance issues between the contracted organization and the applicant organization, regardless of the accreditation decision of the contracted organization. The Joint Commission also surveys services provided on site under contract.

Inclusion of Physician Practices

Physician practices are included in an accreditation survey, provided that one or both of the following criteria are met:
- The physician practice is included in the hospital's Medicare cost report as a provider-based (that is, not freestanding) practice
or
- The physician is employed by the hospital, and the hospital or the physician practice positively portrays to the public that the physician practice is part of the hospital

Unannounced Surveys

Historically, Joint Commission regular, triennial surveys have been conducted in an announced fashion. Beginning in 2004 and through 2005, the Joint Commission will conduct unannounced triennial surveys on an optional and limited basis. The Joint Commission plans to transition to all unannounced surveys by 2006.

For organizations that elect to undergo an unannounced survey in 2004 or 2005, the following policies are applicable:
- The survey can be scheduled anywhere between January and December in the year that the organization is due for survey
- The organization will be invoiced immediately after the survey
- The organization will be removed from the pool of organizations eligible for a random unannounced survey throughout its accreditation cycle
- Because the date of an organization's survey cannot be announced and, therefore, a Public Information Interview (PII) will most often not be able to be scheduled during the organization's survey, the policy no longer applies. In place of the PII policy, the organization is required to fulfill the new APR for continuous public involvement. This APR is effective in 2006 for all programs and immediately for the organizations that voluntarily undergo unannounced surveys. Through this APR, the organization will be required to demonstrate how it communicates with its public to provide information on how an individual can contact the Joint Commission with any patient safety or quality-of-care concerns.

All other policies and procedures in this chapter will apply to organizations undergoing an unannounced regular survey.

Multiorganization Option

The Joint Commission offers multiorganization systems that own or lease at least two organizations the option of a modified survey process. This option has the following three components:
1. A corporate orientation
2. A consecutive survey of participating organizations with the same survey team leader
3. A corporate summation

A system may choose to have either a corporate orientation, a corporate summation, or both. The orientation session provides an opportunity for corporate staff to orient the survey team to the structure and practices of the system. The survey team will also survey centralized corporate services, documentation, and policies and procedures applicable to Joint Commission standards. The corporate summation provides an overall analysis of the system's strengths and weaknesses. It also provides consultation and education related to accreditation survey findings across the system. There is one fee for both the corporate orientation and corporate summation.

Continuity in the composition of the survey team will be maintained by the survey team leader(s). The remaining members of the survey team will rotate in and out of the system's scheduled route. The survey team leader will compile the information necessary to support the corporate summation.

In order to allow for consecutive surveys of a system's participating organizations, the Joint Commission can advance or extend the survey due dates of participating organizations by up to six months. Any participating organization that requires an extension of due date greater than six months must undergo an extension survey.

Successful completion of the extension survey will extend the organization's accreditation survey due date for up to one year from its original survey due date.

Through the multiorganization option, the Joint Commission accredits the individual health care organizations that are part of a multiorganization system, not the system itself. Therefore, each organization within a system will receive its own accreditation decision and report. The findings and decision for one organization within a system will have no bearing on those of another organization within the system.

Early Survey Policy

The sidebar on page APP-9 highlights Early Survey Policy Options 1 and 2 described below. An organization wishing to be accredited for the first time by the Joint Commission may choose one of two Early Survey Policy Options described here. Under both Option 1 and Option 2, organizations are required to undergo two surveys. However, the nature of the surveys and potential outcomes differ. The first survey under Option 1 is a more limited survey, while the first survey under Option 2 is a full accreditation survey. The Public Information Policy (pages APP-13–APP-17) applies to both Option 1 and Option 2.

Early Survey Policy Option 1 (Preliminary Accreditation)

A. Eligibility. This option is available to any organization that is currently not accredited except an organization that has been denied accreditation. Organizations must declare during the application process that they wish to be surveyed under this option.

B. The First Survey. When an organization chooses Option 1, the Joint Commission will conduct two on-site surveys. The Joint Commission can conduct the first survey as early as two months before the organization begins operating, provided the organization meets the following criteria:
- It is licensed or has a provisional license, according to applicable law and regulation
- The building in which the services will be offered or from which the services will be coordinated is identified, constructed, and equipped to support such services
- It has identified its chief executive officer (CEO) or administrator; its director of clinical or medical services; its nurse executive, if applicable
- It has identified the date it will begin operations

Generally, the first survey uses a limited set of standards and assesses only the organization's physical facilities, policies and procedures, plans, and related structural considerations. For this reason, the Early Survey Policy Option 1 has not been recognized by the Centers for Medicare & Medicaid Services (CMS) to meet the requirements for Medicare certification.

C. Preliminary Accreditation. The Joint Commission grants Preliminary Accreditation to an organization in satisfactory compliance with a subset of the standards and their EPs assessed in the first survey under Option 1. An organization not in satisfactory compliance must reapply and begin the accreditation process again. An organization that meets the decision rules for Conditional Accreditation will also be granted a Preliminary Accreditation decision.

The Preliminary Accreditation decision will include assignment of an additional survey against the full set of applicable standards within six months of the first survey. The survey will assess evidence of compliance with the standards for at least four months.

For an organization operating when the survey is conducted, the effective date for its Preliminary Accreditation decision is the day after the survey was conducted. For an organization not in operation, the effective date is the day after it begins operating. If the organization is not in operation at the time of survey, the organization must confirm in writing the date it begins operating.

A Preliminary Accreditation decision remains until the organization has completed a second, full survey or until the Joint Commission has withdrawn the Preliminary Accreditation. The Joint Commission may withdraw Preliminary Accreditation in the following situations:
- When an organization that was not providing services at the time of the first survey does not begin services when expected
- If an organization does not meet the survey eligibility criteria (see page APP-1)
- If an organization fails to accept the date of the second survey or
- If an organization is found not in satisfactory compliance with the applicable standards and their EPs

In these cases, the organization must begin the accreditation process again.

D. The Second Survey. The second survey is a full accreditation survey. The Joint Commission conducts this survey at the following times:
- Approximately six months after the first survey
- At least four months after the organization has begun operating

The organization's accreditation status, based on survey results, will change to one of the following:
- Accredited
- Provisional Accreditation
- Conditional Accreditation
- Preliminary Denial of Accreditation
- Denial of Accreditation

The effective date of the accreditation decision is the day after the second survey. The organization's three-year accreditation cycle begins the day after the second survey was conducted, unless the Joint Commission reached a decision to deny accreditation. Submission of ESC may be required based on the survey findings of the second survey under this option.

Early Survey Policy Option 2

A. Eligibility. Option 2 is available only to an organization that has the following:
- Never been surveyed by the Joint Commission or has been unaccredited by the Joint Commission for the previous two years

Early Survey Policy Options

Early Survey Policy Option 1
First Survey
- Conducted up to two months before opening
  - Licensed
  - Building identified, constructed, and equipped
  - CEO or administrator, director of clinical or medical services (medical director) identified
  - Identified opening date
- Limited set of standards (physical plant, policies and procedures)
- Outcome: Preliminary Accreditation

Second Survey
- Six months after first survey
- Full survey
- Outcome: Change in Preliminary Accreditation decision to Accredited, Provisional Accreditation, Conditional Accreditation, or Preliminary Denial of Accreditation. The effective date of the accreditation decision is the day after the *second* survey.

Early Survey Policy Option 2
First Survey
- Conducted when an organization
  - Has been in operation (licensed) at least one month
  - Has cared for at least ten patients
  - Has one patient in active treatment at time of survey
- Full survey; no track record
- Outcome: Accredited, Conditional Accreditation, or Preliminary Denial of Accreditation

Second Survey
- A full, follow-up survey four months after first survey
- Addresses track record and standards compliance issues
- Outcome: Accredited or Provisional Accreditation, Conditional Accreditation, or Preliminary Denial of Accreditation. The effective date of the accreditation decision is the day after the *first* survey.

Note: *For all surveys, the organization will incur a fee. Contact the Department of Planning and Financial Affairs at 630/792-5115 for more information.*

- Been in actual operation for at least one month
- Cared for at least 10 patients by the time of the first survey with at least one patient in active treatment at the time of survey
- Not been denied participation in the Medicare program as a result of a survey conducted by or action taken by CMS or the state on behalf of CMS

B. The First Survey. When an organization chooses Early Survey Policy Option 2, the Joint Commission will conduct an initial full accreditation survey. If the organization demonstrates satisfactory compliance with standards and their EPs in the first survey, it will be granted an Accredited decision, including a requirement for a second survey to assess for sufficient track record of compliance. This accreditation decision reflects the preliminary nature of the assessed performance. The effective date of the accreditation decision is the day after the first survey.

C. The Second Survey. The organization will undergo a full follow-up survey in four months to address track record requirements that could not be assessed during the first survey due to the limited time of operation. The full scope of applicable standards will be reviewed with particular attention being paid to the issue of sustained performance since the first survey. Organizations surveyed under the Early Survey Policy will also be required to complete an ESC after the first and second surveys, as appropriate.

Initial Surveys

Organizations that are seeking Joint Commission accreditation for the first time or have been unaccredited by the Joint Commission during the previous two years are eligible for an initial survey. The full scope of applicable standards will be reviewed during the survey. The scoring of the standards will be based on a 4-month track record of compliance (prior to survey), rather than the 12-month track record of compliance required for triennial surveys.

Organizations seeking first-time accreditation are required to contract with a performance measurement system and submit ORYX core and non-core measure data to the Joint Commission beginning with patient discharges effective the first day of the first calendar quarter following survey. Hospitals with an average daily census of 10 or less and critical access hospitals are not required to contract with a measurement system and submit performance measurement data to the Joint Commission. This also covers any merged organization that requires an initial full survey. An organization that has been denied participation in the Medicare program as a result of a survey or an action taken by CMS or the state on behalf of CMS may not obtain organization deemed status as a result of an initial survey.

Information Accuracy and Truthfulness Policy

The accuracy and veracity of relevant information, whether actually used in the accreditation process or not, are essential to the integrity of the Joint Commission's accreditation process. Information provided at any time by the organization must be accurate and truthful.* Such information may do the following:
- Be provided verbally or in writing
- Be obtained through direct observation or interview by Joint Commission surveyors
- Be derived from documents supplied by the organization to the Joint Commission including, but not limited to, an organization's root cause analysis in response to a sentinel event, an organization's request for accreditation, or a plan of correction submitted as part of the Conditional Accreditation process
- Involve data or documents transmitted electronically to the Joint Commission, including, but not limited to, data or documents provided as part of the electronic application process
  or
- Involve an attestation that an organization has not knowingly used Joint Commission full-time, part-time, or intermittent surveyors to provide any accreditation-related consulting services after January 1, 2004. Examples of such services include, but are not limited to the following:
  o Helping an organization to meet Joint Commission standards

---

* See APR 10 on pages APR-6–APR-7 in the "Accreditation Participation Requirements" chapter.

- Helping an organization in the PPR process
- Conducting mock surveys for an organization

or

- Providing consultation to an organization to address Priority Focus Process (PFP) information

Falsification, as the term is used in this policy, applies to both commissions and omissions in sharing information with the Joint Commission.

Policy Requirements

The Joint Commission's Information Accuracy and Truthfulness Policy includes the following:

1. An organization must never provide the Joint Commission with falsified information relevant to the accreditation process. The Joint Commission construes any efforts to do so as a violation of the organization's obligation to engage in the accreditation process in good faith.
2. Falsification is defined for this policy as the fabrication, in whole or in part, and through commission or omission, of any information provided by an applicant or accredited organization to the Joint Commission. This includes, but is not limited to, any redrafting, reformatting, or content deletion of documents.
3. The organization may submit additional material that summarizes or otherwise explains original information submitted to the Joint Commission. These materials must be properly identified, dated, and accompanied by the original documents.
4. The Joint Commission conducts an evaluation when it has cause to believe that an accredited organization may have provided falsified information to the Joint Commission relevant to the accreditation process. Except as otherwise authorized by the president of the Joint Commission, the evaluation includes an unannounced on-site survey. This survey uses special protocols designed to address the alleged information falsification. It assesses the degree of actual organization compliance with the standards and their elements of performance that are the subject of the allegation, if appropriate.
5. The Joint Commission immediately takes action to deny accreditation or remove the accreditation award from an accredited organization whenever the Joint Commission is reasonably persuaded that the organization has provided falsified information. If nonmanagerial employees or contractors have undertaken the falsification and the organization's leadership takes no immediate action upon becoming aware of the falsification, or at least one individual in a supervisory or managerial position directs or participates in the falsification, the Joint Commission will act to declare Preliminary Denial of Accreditation or to remove the accreditation award from an accredited organization.
6. The Joint Commission notifies responsible federal and state government agencies of any organization subject to such action.
7. If an organization is denied accreditation because it provided falsified information, the Joint Commission prohibits it from participating in the accreditation process for a period of one year. The president of the Joint Commission, for good cause only, may waive all or a portion of this waiting period.

Good Faith Participation in Accreditation

The Joint Commission requires each organization seeking accreditation or reaccreditation to engage in the accreditation process in good faith. The Joint Commission may deny accreditation to any organization failing to participate in good faith in the accreditation process.

Certain categories of issues interfering with good faith participation can be described as follows:
- *Deceiving the Joint Commission.* Compliance with the Information Accuracy and Truthfulness Policy requires a commitment on the part of the accredited organization not to deceive the Joint Commission in any aspect of the accreditation process. The Joint Commission believes that appropriate preparation for an accreditation survey is a fully acceptable and positive practice, which helps improve the quality and safety of individual care. It is rare that such preparation would overstep the bounds of good faith activity to reach the level of deception. For example, to hire additional caregiving staff shortly before a survey for the express purpose of their presence during the survey, with the intent to terminate the employment of such caregivers promptly after survey, is an act of such deception.
- *Deceiving the Public.* Accredited organizations are not acting in good faith if they mislead the public about the meaning and limitations of accreditation. Also, accredited organizations must not inaccurately suggest to the public that their accreditation award applies to any unaccredited affiliated or otherwise related activities.
- *Reprisals.* The Joint Commission invites open communication from any accredited organization's staff and recipients of care and services about any standards compliance or other issues relating to the accreditation process. An organization's good faith participation in the accreditation process would be questioned if the organization does the following:
  - Attempts to discourage such communication, for example, by taking disciplinary steps against an employee solely because that employee provides information to the Joint Commission
  - Threatens those who communicate with the Joint Commission with a defamation lawsuit based solely on what was said to the Joint Commission or
  - Allows the treatment or access to services of any individual or staff to be adversely impacted by his or her or a family member's communication with the Joint Commission.
- *Standards Compliance.* If an organization's conduct reflects a lack of commitment to standards compliance, issues of good faith may be raised. For example, an intentional refusal to attempt to comply with a standard could suggest a cavalier view of the accreditation process.

The "good faith participation" requirement applies continuously throughout the accreditation cycle.

Public Information Policy*

The Joint Commission is committed to making relevant and accurate information about surveyed health care organizations available to interested parties. Information regarding a health care organization's quality and safety of care helps organizations improve their services. This information may also help educate consumers and health care purchasers in making informed choices about health care. At the same time, it is important that confidentiality be maintained for certain information to encourage candor in the accreditation process.

Quality Reports

The Quality Report provides summary information about the provision of quality and safety at an accredited organization. Quality Reports are created at the organization level and are designed to provide national and state information that can be compared against other accredited organizations and nonaccredited organizations.

Joint Commission Quality Reports for each accredited organization include the following information:
- The date of the most recent triennial survey
- The accreditation decision based on the most recent triennial survey
- An organization's current accreditation decision
- The current decision of any component or program whose accreditation decision is different from that of the organization as a whole
- The date of the most recent evaluation activity for the organization, if any
- Standards areas with requirements for improvement
- Subsequent satisfaction of requirements for improvement and the date(s) of resolution for specific standards areas
- Subsequent new requirements for improvement and the date(s) assigned
- Services included in the accreditation survey
- Joint Commission policies or rules that lead to a Preliminary Denial of Accreditation or Denial of Accreditation
- Disease-specific care certification(s) and the effective date of each certification
- The receipt of Special Quality Recognition Awards, as recognized by the Joint Commission's Board of Commissioners (for example, the Ernest A. Codman Awards, Magnet Status)
- Achievement of National Patient Safety Goals
- Performance against National Quality Improvement Goals
- Performance in relation to Patient Experience of Care Measures

Each accredited organization is afforded the opportunity to prepare a commentary of up to two pages regarding its Quality Report. The commentary accompanies any organization Quality Reports distributed by the Joint Commission, whether via hard copy or the Joint Commission's Web site.

Each Quality Report released by the Joint Commission will also include appropriate background information.

---

* This policy meets the requirements of the Health Insurance Portability and Accountability Act of 1996.

The Joint Commission may also make available information contained in Quality Reports to other third-party providers of information. An organization's Quality Report may be obtained via the Customer Service Department or through Quality Check®, a directory on the Joint Commission's Web site (http://www.jcaho.org).

Performance measurement data will be included in Quality Reports when all the following conditions are met:
- Accredited organizations are reporting data on standardized core measures
- Performance measurement data have been integrated into the accreditation process
- Sufficient data to assure statistical significance are available
- Appropriate reporting formats have been developed and approved by the Board of Commissioners

In addition, released data must satisfy the following requirements:
- The data are accompanied by an explanation of the following:
  o Source or derivation
  o Accuracy, reliability, and validity
  o Appropriate uses
  o Limitations and potential misuses

Information That Is Publicly Disclosed on Request

In addition to information provided in Quality Reports, the following information may be obtained by writing or calling the Joint Commission:
- The organization's accreditation history
- Survey fees paid by an accredited organization
- The organization's scheduled survey date(s) once the organization has been notified of the dates
- Applicable standards used for an accreditation survey
- For a complex survey, the organizational component(s) contributing to a Conditional Accreditation or Denial of Accreditation decision
- Requirements for improvements for which the Joint Commission had no or insufficient evidence of resolution when an organization withdrew from accreditation
- The standards areas for which the Joint Commission had no or insufficient evidence of resolution of requirements for improvement when an organization withdrew from accreditation
- As applicable, confirmation of the occurrence of a sentinel event at an accredited organization and the Joint Commission's intent to apply its Sentinel Event Policy to this occurrence

Release of Complaint-Related Information on Request

The Joint Commission addresses all complaints that pertain to patient safety or quality-of-care issues within the scope of Joint Commission standards. Complaints may be forwarded by CMS or other federal or state agencies having oversight responsibilities for health care organizations, or may be received directly from consumers, payers, or health care professionals.

The Joint Commission has a toll-free hotline to provide patients, their families, caregivers, and others with an opportunity to share concerns regarding quality-of-care issues at accredited health care organizations. The toll-free number is 800/994-6610 and is available 24 hours a day, seven days a week; however, staff members are available weekdays between 8:30 A.M. and 5:00 P.M. central standard time to answer calls.

Upon request from any party, the Joint Commission releases the following aggregate information relating to complaints about an accredited organization for the three-year period prior to receipt of the request:
- The number of standards-related written complaints filed against an accredited organization that have met criteria for review
- The applicable standards areas involved in a specific complaint review
- The standards areas in which requirements for improvement were issued as a result of complaint evaluation activities
- When an unannounced or unscheduled survey is based on information derived from a complaint or public sources, the standards areas related to the complaint

The Joint Commission also provides the following information as appropriate to complainants regarding their complaints:
- Any determination that the complaint is not related to Joint Commission standards
- If the complaint is related to standards, the course of action to be taken regarding the complaint
- Whether the Joint Commission has decided to take action regarding an organization's accreditation decision following completion of the complaint investigation
- Any change in an organization's accreditation decision following completion of the complaint investigation

Release of Aggregate Performance Data
The Joint Commission reserves the right to publish or release aggregate performance data.

Data Release to Government Agencies*
The Joint Commission makes available to federal, state, local, or other government certification or licensing agencies specific accreditation-related information under the following circumstances:
- When the Joint Commission identifies a serious situation in an organization that may jeopardize the health or safety of patients or the public and immediately takes action to deny accreditation

---

* Section 92, PL 96-499, the Omnibus Budget Reconciliation Act of 1980, requires that Medicare providers include, in all their contracts for services costing $10,000 or more in any 12-month period, a clause allowing the Secretary of the U.S. Department of Health and Human Services (DHHS), the U.S. Comptroller General, or their representatives to examine the contract and the contractor's books and records. The Joint Commission herein stipulates that if its charges to any such provider amount to $10,000 or more in any 12-month period, the contract or any agreement on which such charges are based and any of the Joint Commission's books, documents, and records that may be necessary to verify the extent and nature of Joint Commission costs will be available to the Secretary of DHHS, the Comptroller General, or any of their duly authorized representatives for four years after the survey. The same conditions will apply to any related subcontracts the Joint Commission has if the payments under such subcontracts amount to $10,000 or more in any 12-month period.

- Upon request, when the request involves otherwise publicly available information

Additional information is made available when an organization is certified for participation in a federal or state program or licensed to operate by a state agency on the basis of its accreditation. The Joint Commission so advises the organization's chief executive officer and provides timely notice to local, state, and federal authorities having jurisdiction. The information available to government agencies includes the following:
- The official accreditation decision and any subsequent change in this decision or any designation, such as Accreditation Watch.
- Complaint information requested by CMS or state agencies in accordance with deemed status or other recognition requirements, including the following:
  - Action taken on the complaint
  - The standards area(s) in which a requirement for improvement was issued as a result of the complaint evaluation
  - The status of the case
- Specific information when an organization is assigned a Conditional Accreditation, Preliminary Denial of Accreditation, or Denial of Accreditation decision, which includes the following:
  - All final requirements for improvement
  - A statement, if any, from the organization regarding its views on the validity of the Joint Commission survey findings
  - A copy of the approved plan of correction and the results of the plan of correction follow-up survey
- Notification of upcoming triennial or focused surveys and retrospective dates of other surveys conducted, such as random unannounced, other announced, or unannounced for-cause surveys
- A copy of the Accreditation Report is included for the following:
  - CMS upon request respecting deemed status determinations
  - State agencies that have entered into specific information-sharing agreements that permit provider-authorized release of such reports to the state agency

Joint Commission Right to Clarify

The Joint Commission reserves the right to clarify information, even if the information involved would otherwise be considered confidential, when an organization disseminates inaccurate information regarding its accreditation.

Confidential Information

The Joint Commission keeps confidential the following information received or developed during the accreditation process:
- The Accreditation Report unless its submission is required by a government agency (see "Data Release to Government Agencies")
- Information learned from the organization before, during, or following the accreditation survey, which is used to determine compliance with specific accreditation standards

- An organization's root cause analysis and related action plan prepared in response to a sentinel event or in response to other circumstances specified by the Joint Commission
- All other materials that may contribute to the accreditation decision
- Written staff analyses and Accreditation Committee minutes and agenda materials
- The algorithms used in the PFP
- The PFP information used in an organization's survey
- An organization's PPR and related plan of action and measures of success (MOS)

This policy applies to all organizations with an accreditation history, subject to any requirements of any applicable laws.

Survey Fees

The Joint Commission determines survey fees annually as needed to meet the cost of its operations. Surveyed organizations are charged for all surveys with the exception of random unannounced surveys. The Joint Commission bases an organization's survey fees on several factors, including the volume and type of services provided, and the sites to be included in the organization's accreditation. Contact the Pricing Unit at the Joint Commission at 630/792-5115 for a fee schedule or more information on survey fees.

The survey fee is not finalized until the Joint Commission has received and reviewed the organization's application. The Joint Commission sends an invoice when it schedules an organization for survey. It asks the organization to pay the fees according to specified terms. The Joint Commission charges an organization the fee rate in effect at the time of survey. For an initial survey, an organization must send a nonrefundable processing fee with the application for accreditation (e-App). The Joint Commission credits this payment toward the organization's total fee.

The Joint Commission offers organizations two payment options. An organization can do one of the following:
- Pay the full survey fee upon receipt of the invoice, which is sent approximately 30 calendar days before the survey is scheduled
- Pay 50% of the fee upon receipt of the invoice and the remaining 50% within 60 calendar days after completion of the survey

An organization that did not pay its survey fee in full prior to issuance of the accreditation decision and report must remit the outstanding balance within 60 calendar days from receipt of the report. Failure to provide timely payment may result in the loss of accreditation. The Joint Commission notifies an organization with significant standards compliance problems of either a Conditional Accreditation or a Preliminary Denial of Accreditation decision as soon as possible, whether or not payment has been received.

Organizations participating in optional, voluntary unannounced triennial surveys in 2004 and 2005 will be invoiced after their survey takes place.

Before the Survey

This section provides information on the steps leading to a full accreditation survey. These include the application process, the assignment of an account representative, the PPR process, the PFP, survey scheduling, the assignment of a survey team, policies regarding survey scheduling, postponements and delays, the notification of the public about a forthcoming Joint Commission survey, and the conduct of a PII. The accreditation time line included on page ACC-2 is also a good reference for viewing the accreditation process as a whole. In accordance with the requirements of the Health Insurance Portability and Accountability Act of 1996 (HIPAA), a health care organization and the Joint Commission must have a signed Business Associate agreement before the organization's survey can begin.

An Organization's Extranet Site

A key feature of the Shared Visions–New Pathways® initiative is increased use of technology in the accreditation process. The use of technology better enables the Joint Commission and accredited organizations to communicate accreditation-related information in a more efficient and timely manner.

In order to fully use technology in the accreditation process, each organization will have a secured Web site on the Joint Commission's extranet—access to the site can only be accomplished through the use of the organization's password. This site will permit organizations to complete their e-App and PPR electronically. In addition, approximately 48 hours following an organization's survey, the organization's Accreditation Report and its ESC report will be posted on the organization's Web site. Only the accredited organization will have access to this site when it is ready for the organization to complete.

Periodic Performance Review

The Periodic Performance Review (PPR) process is a key component in a more continuous accreditation process. It is designed to help organizations incorporate Joint Commission standards as part of routine operations and ongoing quality improvement efforts. As such, organizations will have access to their PPR tool on a continuous basis throughout their accreditation cycle. The PPR tool will permit organizations to evaluate compliance with all applicable Joint Commission standards and EPs. However, approximately 15 months into its accreditation cycle, the Joint Commission will notify that the organization needs to complete its PPR process and submit it to the Joint Commission by the 18th month in its accreditation cycle.* For every noncompliant standard, the organization must identify a plan of action at the EP level identifying how it plans to come into compliance with the requirement(s). This plan must include an MOS, if applicable, for each EP within a standard identified as not compliant that requires an MOS (not all EPs require an MOS, and organizations need to demonstrate achievement with an MOS only for an EP that is within a noncompliant standard and which requires an MOS). The MOS is

---

* Beginning in 2005, organizations will have continual access to the continuous PPR tool. There will be an annual update to the continuous PPR beginning in 2006. *See* pages ACC-5–ACC-7 for more information on the PPR.

a numerical or other quantitative measure usually related to an audit that can help determine whether a planned action was effective and sustained.

The evaluation and plan of action must be completed electronically on the organization's secure site on the Joint Commission's extranet and transmitted to the Joint Commission within three months. Following receipt of the evaluation and plan of action, staff from the Joint Commission's Standards Interpretation Group will schedule a telephone call with the organization to discuss and agree upon an acceptable plan of action. The time line for the PPR is such that the organization should have sufficient time (at least 6 months) to implement the actions identified in the plan of action and demonstrate a 12-month track record prior to the organization's regular on-site survey. (The PPR process will not be applicable to organizations undergoing an initial survey.) Beginning in 2006, organizations will be required to submit to the Joint Commission an update to their PPR on an annual basis. (*See* APR chapter, page APR-8, for the full text of the PPR and its options.)

Application for Accreditation

An organization begins the accreditation process by completing an application. An electronic version of the application for accreditation can be completed via the organization's extranet site. When an organization is due to complete its application, the Joint Commission will electronically notify the organization how to access its application electronically. Likewise, when an organization notifies the Joint Commission that it wishes to become accredited, the Joint Commission will provide the organization with information explaining how to access and complete its application on its extranet site.

Organizations using this electronic application will type data directly in the application and, once complete, will submit the application to the Joint Commission electronically. The application provides essential information about an organization, including ownership, demographics, and types and volume of services provided.

The application does the following:
- Describes the organization seeking accreditation
- Requires the organization to provide the Joint Commission with all official records and reports of public or publicly recognized licensing (for example, a state license), examining, reviewing, or planning bodies*
- Authorizes the Joint Commission to obtain any records and reports not possessed by the organization
- When accepted, establishes the terms of the relationship between the organization and the Joint Commission

For an organization that chooses not to complete its application via its extranet site, the organization may request a print copy of the application by contacting its account representative. If you do not know who your account representative is, please call 630/792-3007.

---

* *See* APR 1 on page APR-2 in the "Accreditation Participation Requirements" chapter.

Except for unannounced surveys, the Joint Commission will notify the organization of the scheduled survey at least four weeks before the survey date. For information on receiving applications for resurvey, see "Continuing Accreditation" on page APP-37.

Accuracy of the Application Information

The Joint Commission schedules surveys based on information provided in the organization's e-App. With the information provided, the Joint Commission determines the number of days required for a survey and the composition of the survey team.

Inaccurate or incomplete information in the e-App may necessitate an additional survey, which could delay the Joint Commission's survey report and accreditation decision. The organization may also incur additional survey charges.

Handling Changes Affecting the Application Information*

At any time during the accreditation process, if an organization undergoes a change that modifies the information reported in its e-App, the organization must notify the Joint Commission in writing within 30 calendar days after such change is made. Information that must be reported includes the following:
- A change in ownership
- A change in location
- A significant increase or decrease in the volume of services
- The addition of a new type of health service or site of care
- The acquisition of a new component
- The deletion of an existing health service or site of care
or
- The deletion of an existing component

The Joint Commission may schedule an additional survey for a later date if its surveyor or survey team arrives at the organization and discovers that a change was not reported. The Joint Commission may also survey any unreported services and sites addressed by its standards. The Joint Commission will make the final accreditation decision for the organization only after surveying all or an appropriate sample of all services and sites provided by the organization for which the Joint Commission has standards. Information reported in the e-App is subject to the Joint Commission's policy on information accuracy and truthfulness (see page APP-10).

Role of the Account Representative

The Joint Commission assigns an account representative to each organization after receipt of the e-App. This person serves as the primary contact between the organization and the Joint Commission. He or she coordinates survey planning and covers policies, procedures, accreditation issues or services, and inquiries throughout the accreditation process. If your organization does not know who your account representative is, please call 630/792-3007.

---

* See APR 2 on page APR-2 in the "Accreditation Participation Requirements" chapter.

Accreditation Policies and Procedures

Survey Scheduling and Postponements

Note: *This section is not applicable to organizations that choose to have their survey conducted unannounced.*

Schedules for Surveys

The Joint Commission schedules surveys systematically and efficiently to keep survey fees to a minimum. Resurveys are scheduled within 45 calendar days before or after the organization's triennial due date. An organization's first full accreditation survey, an initial survey, must be scheduled within six months from the time the Joint Commission receives the organization's application.

Survey Postponement Policy

A postponement is an organization's request to alter an already scheduled survey date. An organization should direct a request for a postponement to its account representative. A request to postpone a survey may be granted if one or more of the following criteria are met:

- A natural disaster or other major unforeseen event has occurred that has totally or substantially disrupted operations
- The organization is involved in a major strike, has ceased admitting patients, and is transferring patients to other facilities or organizations
- Patients and/or the organization is being moved to a new building on the day or days of the survey
  or
- The Joint Commission has provided fewer than four weeks' advance notice to the organization (by telephone or in writing) of the survey date(s)

Note: *If a survey postponement is requested because of a natural disaster, strike, or movement to a new building, an on-site extension survey may be required if the organization is continuing to provide patient care services.*

An organization undergoing its first Joint Commission survey will be asked to specify on its application the month in which it wishes to be surveyed. Following the scheduling of the survey, the organization will be permitted to postpone its survey only if it meets the above criteria.

Fees for Postponements

In rare circumstances, the Joint Commission may, at its discretion, approve a request to postpone a survey for an organization not meeting any of the criteria described above. In such cases, the organization may be charged a fee to defray costs and may be required to undergo an extension survey. Please contact your account representative or the Pricing Unit at 630/792-5115.

Timeliness of Application and Deposits

The Joint Commission requires an organization to submit a new e-App if the organization does not accept a scheduled survey within six months. This ensures that the organization's information is current.

A nonrefundable, nontransferable survey deposit is required for initial surveys only. The Joint Commission applies the deposit to the organization's survey fee if a survey is conducted.

Forfeiture of Survey Deposit

An organization scheduled for an initial survey will forfeit its survey deposit if its survey is not conducted within six months of submission of its application. The organization must then reapply and submit a new survey deposit to begin the accreditation process again.

The Survey Agenda

The Joint Commission's account representative works with the organization to develop a tentative survey agenda based on survey task assignments required as part of the survey. A generic agenda template will be sent to all organizations with a similar number of required survey days and similar survey teams. The draft of the tentative agenda is reviewed and revisions made, as appropriate.

Notifying the Public about a Joint Commission Survey

The Joint Commission evaluates all relevant information about an organization's compliance with applicable standards and intent statements. It therefore requires an organization to inform the public of a scheduled full survey and invite them to provide the surveyor or survey team with relevant information.* The organization must provide an opportunity for members of the public to participate in a Public Information Interview (PII) during a full survey, including the second survey under Early Survey Policy Option 1 and both surveys under Early Survey Policy Option 2 (*see* pages APP-7–APP-8). A full survey refers to the survey of all components of an organization under all applicable standards and intent statements. The public includes, but is not limited to the following:
- Patients and their families
- Patient advocates and advocacy groups
- Members of the community for whom services are provided
- Staff

Public Posting

The organization is responsible for making the PII process widely known and effective as a source of compliance information in the accreditation process. The Joint Commission requires an organization scheduled for full survey to post or make announcements of the following:
- The survey date
- The opportunity for a PII
- How to request an interview

In the event that all organization components are not surveyed at the same time, the requirement to announce the upcoming full survey applies at the time the pri-

---

* *See* APR 8 on page APR-5 in the "Accreditation Participation Requirements" chapter.

Accreditation Policies and Procedures

mary program is surveyed. For example, if an organization with ambulatory, long term care, and home care components is scheduled for a tailored survey in which the organization is the primary program and each component's survey is scheduled for a different date, the notice of survey is to be posted consistent with the organization's survey dates.

To maximize participation, postings or announcements must be made throughout the organization, including components being surveyed at a different time, in a form consistent with one provided by the Joint Commission. *See* Figure 1, page APP-24, for an example of a Public Notice form. This example may be used by the organization, or the organization may design its own Public Notice form that conveys the same information as this example. An organization should post notices in staff eating areas, break rooms, on bulletin boards near major entrances, and in treatment areas. In addition, the organization must provide each staff person with a written announcement of the survey if such postings are not likely to be seen by all staff.

Advance Notice

The Joint Commission requires an organization scheduled for survey to post public notices at least 30 calendar days before the scheduled date. An organization receiving the scheduled date fewer than 30 calendar days before the survey date should post public notices promptly. Notices must remain posted until the survey is completed.

Informing the Public to Notify the Joint Commission Regarding Safety and Quality of Care Concerns

The organization must take reasonable steps to inform its community of the opportunity for public information interviews during the full survey at least 30 calendar days before the survey. Steps include the following:

- Informing all advocacy groups (such as organized patient groups and unions) that have substantively communicated with the organization in the previous 12 months
- Reaching other members of the community through means such as a public service announcement on radio or television, a classified advertisement in a local newspaper, postings on the organization's Web site, or a notice in a community newsletter or other publication*
- Informing individuals who inquire about the survey of the survey date(s) and opportunity to participate

An organization opting to have its survey conducted on an unannounced basis will not be required to comply with the requirements of this policy. Rather, the organization will be required, by a new APR, to demonstrate how it informs its public(s) that they should notify the Joint Commission if they have issues concerning safety and quality of care in that organization on a continuous basis. The organization can demonstrate its compliance with this APR, by distributing information about the Joint Commission through including contact information in pub-

---

* This type of notification must be published or broadcast at least once.

> **PUBLIC NOTICE**
>
> The Joint Commission on Accreditation of Healthcare Organizations will conduct an accreditation survey of _____ on _____.
> *(Insert the name of your organization)*   *(Insert your survey dates)*
>
> The purpose of the survey will be to evaluate the organization's compliance with nationally established Joint Commission standards. The survey results will be used to determine whether, and the conditions under which, accreditation should be awarded the organization.
>
> Joint Commission standards deal with organization quality, safety-of-care issues, and the safety of the environment in which care is provided. Anyone believing that he or she has pertinent and valid information about such matters may request a public information interview with the Joint Commission's field representatives at the time of the survey. Information presented at the interview will be carefully evaluated for relevance to the accreditation process. Requests for a public information interview must be made in writing and should be sent to the Joint Commission no later than five working days before the survey begins. The request must also indicate the nature of the information to be provided at the interview. Such requests should be addressed to
>
> **Division of Accreditation Operations
> Office of Quality Monitoring
> Joint Commission on Accreditation of Healthcare Organizations
> One Renaissance Boulevard
> Oakbrook Terrace, IL 60181**
>
> Or
> **Faxed to 630/792-5636**
>
> Or
> **E-mailed to complaint@jcaho.org**
>
> The Joint Commission's Office of Quality Monitoring will acknowledge in writing or by telephone requests received 10 days before the survey begins. An Account Representative will contact the individual requesting the public information interview prior to survey, indicating the location, date, and time of the interview and the name of the surveyor who will conduct the interview.
>
> This notice is posted in accordance with the Joint Commission's requirements and may not be removed before the survey is complete.
>
> **Date Posted:** _____

Figure 1. *This is a sample Public Notice form.*

lished materials such as admission brochures and/or posting this information on the organization's Web site.

Compliance with the Public Information Interview Policy

The surveyor(s) reviews the organization's compliance with the policy outlined above. The team indicates at the exit conference whether it believes the organization has complied with the policy and reports on this to the Joint Commission. Failure to comply with the PII policy ordinarily results in a recommendation, which needs to be addressed as part of the ESC process (see "Accreditation Decisions" on page APP-32). As a result, the Joint Commission may also conduct a postsurvey PII at the organization's expense, if requested.

In addition, the surveyor(s) conducting a postsurvey PII also conduct(s) whatever follow-up survey he or she (they) believes appropriate in view of the information obtained during the PII. An organization's subsequent failure to comply with the Joint Commission's PII policy may result in loss or denial of its accreditation.

Conduct of the Public Information Interview
Handling Requests*
Individuals requesting a PII are to forward their requests and the nature of the information they will provide in writing to the Joint Commission. The organization must explain this process in its communications. To ensure participation, individuals are encouraged to forward written requests as soon as possible, and no later than five calendar days before the scheduled survey.

Sometimes an individual may make a written request for a PII directly to the organization. When this occurs, the organization must promptly forward it to the Office of Quality Monitoring at the Joint Commission. An organization receiving oral requests should instruct individuals to make the request in writing and mail them to the Joint Commission. The organization should provide individuals needing assistance in doing this with the necessary support.

Scheduling Interviews
The organization must provide potential PII participants with sufficient advance notice. The Joint Commission acknowledges all PII requests to the individual participants. Before the survey, the Joint Commission schedules a time-limited PII to be conducted during the survey. The Joint Commission is responsible for notifying the individuals requesting PIIs of the interview's exact date, time, and place. The organization must try to alleviate any potential concerns about reprisals to individuals who participate in the interview process.

Interview Eligibility
Individuals whose written requests arrive late or who simply appear at the stated time, requesting the opportunity to be heard without a prior written request, are heard by a Joint Commission surveyor if time permits. Otherwise, the surveyor informs them that it is not possible to honor their requests and then offers them the opportunity to provide a subsequent written statement.

Individuals contacting the Joint Commission and stating an interest in supplying information anonymously are informed that they may provide written complaints through the Joint Commission's Office of Quality Monitoring at 800/994-6610. The Joint Commission will maintain confidentiality, as requested.

---

* See APR 9 on page APR-6 in the "Accreditation Participation Requirements" chapter.

The Interview Process

The Joint Commission's survey team conducts the PII. A representative of the organization may attend, unless the individual requesting the PII asks that no representative from the organization be present. The Joint Commission will honor such requests. The interview will be conducted on the organization's premises, whether a representative from the organization is present or not.

The organization is expected to provide reasonable accommodations for all PIIs.

An interview consists of the orderly receipt of information, orally or in writing, within a set time limit. The interview is not a debate between an organization's representative and an interviewee. Surveyors may, however, ask clarifying questions.

In addition, surveyors will not debate with or convey conclusions to any interviewee. Rather, the Joint Commission considers the information gathered in the interview by the surveyor along with the surveyor's findings and recommendations during the survey process.

The On-Site Survey

This section includes information relevant to an organization that has applied for an accreditation survey and is ready for the survey process. It provides an overview of the survey process, including use of the PFP.

Priority Focus Process

The PFP guides the overall survey process, including planning and the on-site survey, by providing enhanced insight into and information about each organization before its survey. This focuses survey activities on organization-specific issues that are most relevant to safety and quality of care (referred to as priority focus areas [PFAs]). The PFP can be considered as a process for standardizing the PFAs for review during survey.

As part of the PFP, an automated tool called the Priority Focus Tool (PFT) takes data gathered before the survey about an organization and, through the use of algorithms or sets of rules, transforms the data into information that guides the survey process. Examples of sources for the data may include but are not limited to the following:
- Data from an organization's application
- Complaint and sentinel event information
- Performance measurement data, when applicable
- An organization's previous survey results
- Data collected from external sources, such as Medicare Provider Analysis and Review (MedPar*) data

For additional information on the PFP process, *see* "The New Joint Commission Accreditation Process" chapter.

---

* MedPar data is data that are collected by the Centers for Medicare & Medicaid Services (CMS) from hospitals in order for hospitals to receive reimbursement for performed services and procedures.

Accreditation Policies and Procedures

The Survey Process in Brief
Overview
During an accreditation survey, the Joint Commission evaluates an organization's performance of functions and processes aimed at continuously improving patient outcomes. The survey process focuses on assessing performance of important patient-centered and organization functions that support the safety and quality of patient care and may include the conduct of a PII. This assessment is accomplished through evaluating an organization's compliance with the applicable standards in this manual based on the following:
- Tracing the care delivered to patients
- Verbal and written information provided to the Joint Commission
- On-site observations and interviews by Joint Commission surveyors
- Documents provided by the organization

In addition, throughout the survey, MOS identified by an organization as part of its PPR process will be validated.

The Joint Commission's accreditation process seeks to help organizations identify and correct problems and improve the safety and quality of care and services provided. In addition to evaluating continuous compliance with standards and their EPs, significant time is spent on education.

Joint Commission will begin conducting surveys on an unannounced basis in 2004 for organizations that volunteer. Unannounced surveys will be optional and conducted on a limited basis throughout 2004 and 2005. Beginning in 2006, all accreditation resurveys will be unannounced. Initial surveys will remain announced.

Surveys are designed to be individualized to each organization, to be consistent, and to support the organization's efforts to improve performance. The length of the survey is determined by the Joint Commission based on information supplied in the application describing organization size and scope of services. In addition, Joint Commission surveyors may conduct some survey activities during evening, night, and weekend shifts ("off-shift") for full surveys of three or more days and a sample of two-day surveys in health care organizations that provide 24-hour care. These off-shift visits will not occur before the opening conference at the start of the survey.

Survey Agenda
The survey agenda will contain the following elements:

Opening Conference. The opening session of the survey process will be an opportunity for organization leaders and key staff to meet with the surveyor(s) and make any last-minute adjustments to the survey schedule or elements.

Leadership Conference. During the conference, surveyors will discuss with leaders (including nursing, performance improvement, and safety leadership) their roles in performance improvement and other key issues of organization operations, such as patient safety, review of National Patient Safety Goals, and PFP output related to CSGs and clinical focus areas. Some organizations may experience two Leadership Conferences, as necessary.

Validating the Organization's Implementation of Its Plan of Action Generated as Part of the PPR Process. The organization will have already submitted this plan as part of the PPR process to the Joint Commission for review and approval and will have worked with Joint Commission Standards Interpretation Group staff on areas for improvement. As part of conducting an organization's full survey, surveyors will review MOS information and verify that the organization has implemented the plan of action.

Visits to Care and Service Areas Guided by the PFP Using the Tracer Methodology. These two elements of Joint Commission's survey process, PFP and tracer, allow surveyors to analyze the functioning of organization systems.

Tracer Methodology. One element driving this revised accreditation process is analysis of the organization's systems of providing care and services using actual patients as the framework for assessing compliance with selected standards. This process, called *tracer methodology*, works with PFP to trace patients, using PFAs as a starting point, within the health care organization's systems. For more information on tracer methodology, *see* "The New Joint Commission Accreditation Process" chapter.

Systems Tracer Session. During this session, high priority safety and quality of care issues on a systemwide basis will be evaluated throughout the organization.

Daily Briefings. During this session, organization staff will be briefed on the previous day's survey findings and any significant patterns or trends that are becoming evident in the survey.

Closing Conference. The closing or exit conference will be devoted to a discussion of the surveyor's findings. At the completion of the survey, the surveyors will provide the organization's accreditation report before leaving the organization.

Survey Team Composition

Accreditation surveys may be conducted by a survey team rather than an individual surveyor. The composition of an organization's survey team is also based on the information provided in its e-App. In most instances, an organization survey team is composed of one to five surveyors, including physicians, nurses, administrators, or other specialties as needed. All surveyors assess and provide consultation regarding all functions addressed by the standards.

In addition, depending on the organization's service configuration, there may be additional surveyors assigned to survey specialized areas, such as long term care, home care, and behavioral health care. The findings of additional surveyors are integrated into the organization's accreditation decision and survey report.

Survey Team Leadership

If more than one surveyor is required, one of the surveyors on each organization survey team is designated as the "team leader." The team leader is responsible for integration, coordination, and communication of on-site survey activities. In addition to direct participation as an active member of the survey team, the team leader serves as the primary point of on-site contact between the organization and the Joint Commission. Among other responsibilities, the team leader leads the opening conference and the daily and exit briefings.

Scoring Compliance and Track Record Achievements

Accredited organizations are expected to remain in continuous compliance with the standards and their EPs throughout their accreditation cycle. Standards will be judged "compliant" or "not compliant." EPs will be scored on the following scale:

- **0** Insufficient compliance
- **1** Partial compliance
- **2** Satisfactory compliance
- **NA** Not applicable

For a complete discussion on the scoring methodology, *see* "The New Joint Commission Accreditation Process" chapter.

For practical purposes in conducting the survey, surveyors will ordinarily limit their evaluation of the organization's track record of compliance, which is 12 months for a triennial survey and four months prior to an initial survey.

Surveyors may evaluate compliance over a shorter or longer time frame depending on circumstances encountered during the survey. For example, the required time frame for full compliance with applicable standards and EPs for new services will not exceed the time the service has been in operation. In another example, certain activities that are conducted infrequently, such as biennial credentialing, may require evaluation over a longer interval to ensure an adequate sample size for valid assessment. For a triennial survey, an organization's track record will generally impact the scoring of standards according to the following:

Score 0 Fewer than 6 consecutive months before survey
Score 1 6 to 11 consecutive months before survey
Score 2 12 consecutive months before survey

During initial surveys, an organization's track record will generally impact the scoring of standards according to the following:

Score 0 Fewer than 2 consecutive months before survey
Score 1 2 to 3 consecutive months before survey
Score 2 4 consecutive months before survey

Feedback Sessions

Final scores about compliance are not reached until all required patient care settings have been visited and all survey activities have been conducted. However, surveyors will communicate their observations at daily briefings, as requested by the organization. If the organization has additional information that would demonstrate compliance with a standard that the surveyor has indicated may be a recommendation, the organization should supply that information to the surveyor(s) as soon as possible.

Final On-Site Survey Activities

At the leadership closing conference, the survey team will present survey findings and a written Accreditation Report.

Immediate Threat to Life

The Joint Commission may consider for accreditation purposes a surveyor's finding that some aspect of an organization's operation is having or may potentially have a serious, adverse effect on patient health or safety, and that immediate action must be taken.

In these cases, surveyors will notify the organization's chief executive officer and Joint Commission's headquarters staff immediately if they identify any condition they believe poses a serious threat to public or patient health and safety. The president of the Joint Commission, or if the president is unavailable his or her designee, can then issue an expedited Preliminary Denial of Accreditation decision based on such notification. He or she will promptly inform the organization's chief executive officer and appropriate governmental authorities of this decision and the findings that led to this action. The Accreditation Committee of the Board of Commissioners will confirm or reverse the decision at its next meeting. The Accreditation Committee may take into consideration an organization's corrective actions or responses to a serious threat situation. The organization can provide information to demonstrate that the serious threat-to-life situation has been corrected prior to the Accreditation Committee's consideration of the Preliminary Denial of Accreditation decision.

In these situations, the corrective action will be considered when a single issue leads to the adverse finding and the organization demonstrates that it did the following:
- Took immediate action to completely remedy the situation
- Prepared a thorough and credible root cause analysis
- Adopted systems changes to prevent a future recurrence of the problem

Accreditation Reports

Following evaluation of the organization's performance of functions and processes, the survey team reviews the results of integrated individual findings. Then, with the use of laptop-based decision support software, the team produces the organization's Accreditation Report. The team leader meets with the organization's chief executive officer (CEO) prior to the closing conference and provides him or her with a copy of the report. The CEO determines whether or not the preliminary report is distributed at the closing conference. The survey team uses the report contents in making its closing conference presentations.

Within approximately 48 hours of a survey, the organization's report of survey findings will be posted on the organization's secured extranet site. The report will include, as appropriate, an organization's strengths, requirements for improvement, and supplemental findings.

If an organization does not receive any recommendations, then the organization's accreditation decision will be rendered at the same time that the organization's

Accreditation Report is available and will be effective the day after the completion of the survey. If an organization receives requirements for improvement, then the organization's accreditation decision will be rendered following the submission of an ESC report. The ESC report is due within 90 calendar days following the survey; however, the organization's accreditation decision will be retroactive to the day after the last day of the survey.* For organizations that receive a notification that they will be recommended for either Conditional Accreditation or Preliminary Denial of Accreditation, their accreditation decisions will be rendered by the Joint Commission's Accreditation Committee.

After the Survey

This section includes information relevant to an organization that recently has participated in an accreditation survey. Material includes information on the ESC process, the MOS process, the types of accreditation decisions, how to request review of Preliminary Denial of Accreditation decisions, how to appeal Denial of Accreditation decisions, and how to use and display an accreditation award.

Evidence of Standards Compliance Process

For every requirement for improvement cited in an organization's Accreditation Report, the organization must submit an Evidence of Standards Compliance (ESC). The ESC report will be available for completion on the organization's extranet site at the same time the organization's Accreditation Report is posted, which is approximately 48 hours of the organization's survey.

The ESC report must detail the action(s) that the organization took to bring itself into compliance with a standard or clarify why the organization believes that it is in compliance with the standard in which it received a requirement for improvement. An ESC must address compliance at the element of performance level and include an MOS, if applicable. An MOS is a numerical or quantifiable measure usually related to an audit that will determine if an action is effective and sustained. (*See* Measure(s) of Success Report on the next page.)

The ESC report is due within 90 calendar days[†] after an organization's survey. Following submission of the report, an organization will receive an accreditation decision. If an organization implements actions to address its requirements for improvement, the organization's accreditation decision will be Accredited. If an organization's ESC report does not address its requirements for improvement, then the organization's accreditation decision will be Provisional Accreditation.

Conditional Accreditation, Preliminary Denial of Accreditation, and the ESC Report

If an organization is notified that a recommendation will be made to the Joint Commission's Accreditation Committee for either Conditional Accreditation or

---

* Beginning July 1, 2005, the ESC will be due within 45 days of survey.

[†] 45 days beginning July 1, 2005.

Preliminary Denial of Accreditation, the organization will have an opportunity to provide information to clarify any of the recommendations cited in its Accreditation Report through its ESC report. This information will be provided to the Accreditation Committee.

Measure(s) of Success Report

An organization will be required to submit an MOS report within four months of submitting an acceptable ESC report. The MOS report will demonstrate whether each MOS identified in the organization's ESC report was reached.

Accreditation Decisions

An organization's accreditation decision becomes official following submission of its ESC report, which is retroactive to the day after the last day of the survey, or, in the case of Conditional Accreditation or Preliminary Denial of Accreditation, on the date the Accreditation Committee makes a decision. When an organization's accreditation decision becomes official, it is publicly disclosable. There are six possible accreditation decisions, as follows:
1. Accredited
2. Provisional Accreditation
3. Conditional Accreditation
4. Preliminary Denial of Accreditation
5. Denial of Accreditation
6. Preliminary Accreditation

Table 1 (page APP-33) provides a description of each category and the conditions that lead to it.

An organization's request to withdraw from the accreditation process after undergoing survey and before a final decision has been made does not terminate the decision-making process. The Joint Commission will issue a final accreditation decision.

Review and Appeal of Preliminary Denial of Accreditation or Denial of Accreditation Decisions

The appeal procedures are set forth in the Review and Appeal Procedure section of this chapter on pages APP-40–APP-50. Two additional procedures specific to Preliminary Denial of Accreditation and Denial of Accreditation decisions are listed here.

When an organization receives written notice from the Joint Commission that a recommendation of Preliminary Denial of Accreditation is proposed for submission to the Accreditation Committee, the organization has 10 business days from receipt of that notification to submit to the Joint Commission an ESC report, clarifying information that demonstrates that it was in fact in compliance with one or more standards in question at the time of survey. If after Joint Commission review of any submitted materials, the Preliminary Denial of Accreditation recommendation will still be made, the organization will have five business days from receipt of notification to submit a written response directly to the Accreditation Committee.

Table 1. Types of Joint Commission Accreditation Decisions

The Joint Commission has six accreditation decision categories. Each decision and the conditions that lead to it are described below.

Accreditation Decision Category	Conditions That Lead to This Type of Decision
Accredited	The organization is in compliance with all standards at the time of the on-site survey or has successfully addressed all requirements for improvement in an Evidence of Standards Compliance within 90 days following the survey (45 days beginning July 1, 2005).
Provisional Accreditation	
Conditional Accreditation	The organization fails to successfully address all requirements for improvement in an Evidence of Standards Compliance within 90 days following the survey (45 days beginning July 1, 2005).
Preliminary Denial of Accreditation	The organization is not in substantial compliance with the standards, as usually evidenced by a count of the number of standards identified as not compliant at the time of survey which is between two and three standard deviations above the mean number of noncompliant standards for organizations in that accreditation program. The organization must remedy identified problem areas through preparation and submission of an ESC and subsequently undergo an on-site, follow-up survey.
	There is justification to deny accreditation to the organization as usually evidenced by a count of the number of noncompliant standards at the time of survey which is at least three standard deviations above the mean number of standards identified as not compliant for organizations in that accreditation program. The decision is subject to appeal prior to the determination to deny accreditation; the appeal process may also result in a decision other than Denial of Accreditation.

continued on next page

Table 1. Types of Joint Commission Accreditation Decisions *(continued)*

Denial of Accreditation	The organization has been denied accreditation. All review and appeal opportunities have been exhausted.
Preliminary Accreditation	The organization demonstrates compliance with selected standards in the first of two surveys conducted under Early Survey Policy Option 1.

Weighted Decision Rules

Recently, the Joint Commission has reevaluated how a complex organization's overall accreditation decision should be impacted by a component's decision involving threats to patient safety, instances in which inaccurate information is provided to the Joint Commission, or a violation of other Accreditation Participation Requirements.

As such, the Joint Commission has revised the weighted decision rules so that, when a secondary component of a complex organization meets rules of Conditional Accreditation or Preliminary Denial of Accreditation as a consequence of invoking the Immediate Threat to Life Policy or not complying with the Information Accuracy and Truthfulness Policy or Accreditation Participation Requirement, that accreditation decision would apply equally to the component and the complex organization of which the component is a part. *See* Table 2 on page APP-35 for more information on the weighted decision rules.

Essential Laboratory Function

In a similar change, the Joint Commission has revised the impact of the accreditation decision of pathology and clinical laboratory services on a hospital's overall accreditation decision. The *2005 Hospital Accreditation Standards (HAS)* lists pathology and clinical laboratory services as an "essential" hospital service and requires that a hospital provide or provide for these services in order to be eligible for accreditation.

Because of the essential nature of pathology and clinical laboratory services, the Joint Commission has determined that a hospital's status should not be protected should the level of standards compliance for laboratory services be lower than that of the hospital since the performance of all other essential hospital services is considered in the hospital's status. Therefore, should a hospital laboratory receive an accreditation decision of Provisional Accreditation, Conditional Accreditation, or Preliminary Denial of Accreditation, the hospital would receive the same decision.

Table 2. Weighted Decision Rules

Primary Program	Secondary Programs
One program in a complex organization is to be identified as "primary" (this is not a change from the previous rule).	If one of the secondary programs meets a rule for Preliminary Denial of Accreditation, the overall decision for the organization will be Conditional Accreditation.
If the primary program meets a rule for Provisional Accreditation, Conditional Accreditation, or Preliminary Denial of Accreditation, the overall decision for the organization will be Provisional Accreditation, Conditional Accreditation, or Preliminary Denial of Accreditation, respectively.	If one of the secondary programs meets a rule for Conditional Accreditation, the overall decision for the organization will be Provisional Accreditation.
	If two or more of the secondary programs meet rules for Preliminary Denial of Accreditation, the overall decision for the organization will be Preliminary Denial of Accreditation.
	If two or more of the secondary programs meet rules for Conditional Accreditation, the overall decision for the organization will be Conditional Accreditation.
	If the primary or any secondary program meets a rule for Provisional Accreditation, the overall decision for the organization will be Provisional Accreditation.

Award Display and Use

The Joint Commission provides each accredited organization with one certificate of accreditation per site. There is no charge for the initial certificate(s). Additional certificates may be purchased. Such requests should be sent to the Certificate Coordinator, Division of Accreditation Operations at the Joint Commission.

The certificate and all copies remain the Joint Commission's property. They must be returned if the following situations occur:
- The organization is issued a new certificate reflecting a name change

or
- The organization's accreditation status is changed, withdrawn, or denied, for any reason

An organization accredited by the Joint Commission must be accurate in describing to the public the nature and meaning of its accreditation and its award.* When an organization receives an accreditation award, the Joint Commission sends the organization guidelines for characterizing the accreditation award.

---

* See APR 11 on page APR-7 in the "Accreditation Participation Requirements" chapter

Accreditation award certificates will include language about educating patients and their families on how to contact the Joint Commission.

An organization may not engage in any false or misleading advertising of the accreditation award. Any such advertising may be grounds to deny accreditation. For example, an organization may not represent its accreditation as being awarded by any of the Joint Commission's corporate members.

These include the American College of Physicians, the American College of Surgeons, the American Dental Association, the American Hospital Association, and the American Medical Association. The Joint Commission has permission to reprint the seals of its corporate members on the certificates of accreditation. However, these seals must not be reproduced or displayed separately from the certificate.

Any organization that materially misleads the public about any matter relating to its accreditation must undertake corrective advertising of a degree acceptable to the Joint Commission in the same medium in which the misrepresentation occurred. If an organization fails to undertake the required corrective advertising following the communication of false or misleading advertising about its accreditation status, the organization may be subject to loss of accreditation.

The Joint Commission's logo is a registered trademark. An accredited organization may use the logo if it follows the following guidelines:
- The logo must remain in the same proportional relationship as provided and should not be displayed any larger than an organization's own logo
- The logo's format cannot be changed, the name may not be separated from the symbol, and it must be printed in the original color
- Graphic devices such as seals, other words, or slogans cannot be added to the logo except for the words "Accredited by"

These guidelines apply to logo use on all print materials, Internet Web pages, and promotional items, such as coffee mugs, T-shirts, and notepads. Contact the Department of Communications at the Joint Commission at 630/792-5631 for questions about using the Joint Commission logo.

Before the Next Survey

This section provides information relevant to organizations between Joint Commission surveys. Material includes the duration of an accreditation award; the process for continuing accreditation; how to notify the Joint Commission in the event of organizational changes including the opening or closing of a unit or services, addition or deletion of components, leadership changes, mergers, consolidations, and acquisitions; and unscheduled and unannounced for-cause surveys.

Re-entering the Accreditation Process

In order for a previously accredited organization to be designated as "new" and be subject to only a four-month track record period for demonstrating standards compliance, it must not have participated in the accreditation process during the previous six months. If an organization is re-entering the accreditation process before six

Accreditation Policies and Procedures

months have passed, it must demonstrate a continuing 12-month track record of compliance with the standards.

Duration of Accreditation Award

An accreditation award is continuous until the organization has its next full survey, which is usually around three years unless revoked for cause or as otherwise outlined in this chapter. Accreditation is effective on the first day after the Joint Commission completes the organization's survey. An organization may request a full accreditation survey more frequently than once every three years. The Joint Commission will, at its discretion and in accordance with its mission, determine whether to honor the request. Such requests should be sent to the organization's account representative.

Continuous Compliance

The Joint Commission expects an accredited organization to be in continuous compliance with all applicable standards and EPs. It may ask an organization to supply, in writing, information about compliance with standards. It may also survey an organization at any time with or without notice in response to complaints, media coverage, or other information that raises questions about the adequacy of patient health and safety protections (*see* "Unscheduled and Unannounced 'For-Cause' Surveys" on page APP-39). The Joint Commission might also conduct a survey if an organization fails to respond to a request for more information.

An organization's failure to permit a survey can be viewed by the Joint Commission as the organization no longer wanting to participate in the accreditation process. Therefore, the Joint Commission will begin proceedings to deny accreditation to the organization.*

Continuing Accreditation

The Joint Commission does not automatically renew an organization's accreditation. An organization seeking to continue its accreditation must reapply for accreditation, undergo a full accreditation survey, and be found in compliance with the standards and intent statements.

Accreditation Renewal Process

The Joint Commission will notify an organization approximately six to nine months before the organization's triennial accreditation due date that it needs to complete an application for a resurvey and provide information about how the application can be accessed, completed, and transmitted to the Joint Commission electronically via the organization's extranet site. The organization should call 630/792-5800 if it has not received such a notification four months before its accreditation due date.

Note: *Effective January 1, 2006, all triennial surveys will be conducted on an unannounced basis. As such, the accreditation renewal process will change. Please consult future issues of* Perspectives *or the 2006 revision of this book for more information on the anticipated changes.*

---

* *See* APR 3 on page APR-2 in the "Accreditation Participation Requirements" chapter.

Generally, the Joint Commission conducts a triennial survey in the time period between 45 calendar days before the organization's three-year survey due date and 45 calendar days after the due date. The Joint Commission notifies the organization of the survey date at least four weeks before the survey. If there are any specific dates within the 45 calendar days before and after the due date range that would conflict with other organization activities, the organization should identify those dates in the application as dates to avoid.

Accreditation Decision During Triennial Survey

An organization's previous accreditation decision remains in effect until a decision is made either to accredit or to preliminarily deny accreditation to the organization.

Notification of Changes Made Between Surveys

Accreditation is neither automatically transferred nor continued if significant changes occur within the organization. When significant changes occur, the organization must notify the Joint Commission in writing not more than 30 calendar days after such change is made. The organization must also notify the Joint Commission in writing if it opens or closes any units or services.

When an organization offers at least 25% of its services at a new location or in a significantly altered physical plant, the organization must also fill out and submit to the Joint Commission Part 2: Basic Building Information of the Statement of Conditions™ (SOC) Compliance Document, Part 3E or 3F of the Statement of Fire Safety (SFS), and Part 4: Plan for Improvement, should *Life Safety Code®* deficiencies be present (for a copy of the SOC, visit the Joint Commission's Web site at http://www.jcaho.org, select Accredited Organizations, then your accreditation program, then Standards, and then Statement of Conditions™). Failure to provide timely notification to the Joint Commission of these changes may result in the loss of accreditation.

Mergers, Consolidations, and Acquisitions

In the case of a merger, consolidation, or acquisition, the Joint Commission may decide that the organization responsible for services must have a survey. Barring exceptional circumstances, the Joint Commission continues the accreditation of the organization undergoing the kind of changes described above until it determines whether an extension survey is necessary.

Note: *When an accredited organization acquires another organization and an extension survey is conducted, the survey findings resulting from the extension survey would be maintained separately from, and would not be reflected in, the accreditation decision acquiring organization for 12 months following the acquisition. After the 12-month period, any outstanding standards compliance problems in the acquired component(s) would be reflected in the accreditation decision of the acquiring organization.*

Extension Surveys

An extension survey is conducted at an accredited organization or at a site that is owned and operated by the organization if the accredited organization's current

Accreditation Policies and Procedures

accreditation is not due to expire for at least nine months and when at least one of the conditions above is met. The results of an extension survey may affect the organization's accreditation decision.

An extension survey of the organization may be necessary if the organization has the following:
- Instituted a new service or program for which the Joint Commission has standards
- Changed ownership and there are a significant number of changes in the management and clinical staff or operating policies and procedures
- Offered at least 25% of its services at a new location or in a significantly altered physical plant
- Expanded its capacity to provide services by 25% or more as measured by patient volume, pieces of equipment, or other relevant measures
- Provided a more intensive level of service
or
- Merged with, consolidated with, or acquired an unaccredited site, service, or program for which there are applicable Joint Commission standards and EPs

An extension survey may also occur with the following situations:
- The Joint Commission grants an organization's request to continue its current accreditation beyond the conclusion of the three-year cycle*
or
- An organization has merged, consolidated, or acquired an accredited organization whose accreditation expiration date is within three months of the merger, consolidation, or acquisition, while its own accreditation expiration date is at least nine months away.

Unscheduled and Unannounced "For-Cause" Surveys

The Joint Commission may perform either an unscheduled survey or an unannounced survey when it becomes aware of potentially serious standards compliance or patient care or safety issues, or it has other valid reasons for surveying in an accredited organization.[†]

Note: *The "for-cause" unscheduled or unannounced surveys should not be confused with "regular unannounced" surveys, as described on page APP-5.*

Either type of survey can take place at any point in an organization's three-year accreditation cycle. The Joint Commission usually provides the organization with 24 to 48 hours' advance notice of an unscheduled survey. No preliminary report is generated after an unscheduled survey whether announced or unannounced.

Note: *Organizations are charged for these surveys, regardless of the outcome. The cost of the survey can be obtained by calling the Pricing Unit at 630/792-5115. However, organizations are not charged for random unannounced surveys (for additional information on random unannounced surveys, see page APP-40).*

---

* Such requests are granted only for unusual or compelling reasons.

† *See* APR 3 on page APR-2 in the "Accreditation Participation Requirements" chapter.

No advance notice is provided for unannounced surveys. Reasons for unannounced surveys include occurrence of any event or series of events in an accredited organization that creates the following significant situations:
- Concern that a continuing threat may exist to the safety or care of patients at risk or
- Indication that the organization is not or has not been in compliance with the Joint Commission's Information Accuracy and Truthfulness Policy

Such a survey can either include all the organization's services or only those areas where a serious concern may exist.

Results of any unannounced or unscheduled surveys may generate follow-up activities and can affect an organization's current accreditation decision. The Joint Commission may deny accreditation if the organization does not allow the Joint Commission to conduct unscheduled or unannounced surveys.

Random Unannounced Surveys

The Joint Commission also conducts unannounced surveys on a 5% random sample of accredited organizations. The survey is generally conducted 9 to 30 months following the accreditation date (that is, the date after the last day of the full survey). An organization will receive no advance notice of the random unannounced survey. One surveyor conducts each such survey for one day. Organizations are not charged for random unannounced surveys.

Note: *As part of the move toward all accreditation surveys being conducted on an unannounced basis in 2006, the Joint Commission will no longer conduct random unannounced surveys after January 1, 2006.*

During the random unannounced survey, the surveyor assesses both fixed and variable components, or performance areas. Fixed components are identified each year for organizations based on the highest priority focus areas and selected National Patient Safety Goals. Fixed components are identified based on the degree of actual or perceived risk to the care of patients posed by noncompliance with standards related to these elements. Fixed components for each accreditation program are published in *Joint Commission Perspectives*® and are listed on the Joint Commission Web site. Variable components are identified through the PFP. Presurvey information run through PFP identifies prioritized organization-specific PFAs to be evaluated. (*See* the PFP section of this chapter for more on presurvey information.) The surveyor may also expand the scope of the random unannounced survey based on findings at the time of the survey.

No random unannounced surveys will be conducted at an organization undergoing an unannounced triennial survey.

Review and Appeal Procedures

After any Preliminary Denial of Accreditation decision, the organization has the right to make a detailed presentation before a Review Hearing Panel. The Accreditation Committee will then review the findings of the Review Hearing Panel and either deny accreditation to the organization or select an appropriate alternative

Accreditation Policies and Procedures

accreditation decision. The organization may appeal any decision of the Accreditation Committee to deny accreditation before the decision becomes the final decision of the Joint Commission.

The following outline details review and appeal procedures.

I. **Evaluation by the Joint Commission Staff**
   A. **Review and Determination by Joint Commission Staff.** Following a triennial or other survey activity, the Joint Commission staff shall review survey findings, survey documents, and any other relevant materials or information received from any source. Except as provided in paragraphs I.B, I.C, and I.D, Joint Commission staff shall, in accordance with decision rules approved by the Accreditation Committee of the Board of Commissioners, do the following:
   1. Determine or recommend to the Accreditation Committee that the organization be accredited, as described in paragraph VII of these procedures
   or
   2. Recommend to the Accreditation Committee that the organization be conditionally accredited
   or
   3. Determine that the organization be conditionally accredited, if the organization does not submit Evidence of Standards Compliance (ESC) in accordance with paragraph I.B.I.a or I.B.I.b
   or
   4. Recommend to the Accreditation Committee that the organization be preliminarily denied accreditation; or
   5. Defer consideration while additional information regarding the organization's compliance status is reviewed by the Joint Commission staff
   or
   6. Determine or recommend to the Accreditation Committee that the organization be preliminarily accredited in accordance with the Early Survey Policy set forth on pages APP-7–APP-10
   or
   7. Recommend to the Accreditation Committee that the organization be initially denied Preliminary Accreditation in accordance with the Early Survey Policy set forth on pages APP-7–APP-10

   B. **Determination to Recommend Conditional Accreditation Based on Full Triennial Surveys.**
   1. Notification to Organization of Areas of Noncompliance with Standards. In the case of full triennial surveys, if the Joint Commission staff, based on survey findings, survey documents, and any other relevant materials or information received from any source, determines to recommend that the organization be conditionally accredited, it will outline its findings and determination. The organization may do the following:

a. Accept the findings and determination of the staff through submission of the ESC

or

b. Submit to the Joint Commission, through ESC any clarification of its compliance with Joint Commission standards at the time of the survey that is not reflected in the Accreditation Report, along with an explanation of why such documentation was not available for review at the time of the survey

2. Consideration of the Organization's Response. Joint Commission staff shall review the organization's submission of any additional information and shall, in accordance with decision rules approved by the Accreditation Committee, do the following:

a. Recommend to the Accreditation Committee that the organization be conditionally accredited

or

b. Recommend to the Accreditation Committee that the organization be preliminarily denied accreditation

or

c. Recommend to the Accreditation Committee that the organization be accredited, as described in paragraph VII of these procedures

C. Determination to Recommend That Accreditation Be Preliminarily Denied Based on Full Triennial or Other Survey Activity.

1. Notification to Organization of Areas of Noncompliance with Standards. In the case of full triennial surveys, if the Joint Commission staff, based on survey findings, survey documents, and any other relevant materials or information received from any source, determines, in accordance with decision rules approved by the Accreditation Committee, to recommend to the Accreditation Committee that the organization be preliminarily denied accreditation, it will outline its findings and determination. The organization may do the following:

a. Accept the findings and determination of the staff through submission of the ESC

or

b. Submit to the Joint Commission through the ESC any clarification of its compliance with Joint Commission standards at the time of the survey that is not reflected in the Accreditation Report, along with an explanation of why such information was not available for review at the time of the survey

2. Consideration of the Organization's Response. Joint Commission staff members shall review the organization's submission of any additional information and shall, in accordance with decision rules approved by the Accreditation Committee, do the following:

a. Recommend to the Accreditation Committee that the organization be conditionally accredited

or

b. Recommend to the Accreditation Committee that the organization be preliminarily denied accreditation

or

c. Recommend to the Accreditation Committee that the organization be accredited, as described in paragraph VII of these procedures.

D. **Decisions by the President of the Joint Commission.** Notwithstanding anything outlined in paragraphs I.A–I.C.1 of these procedures to the contrary, if the findings of any survey identify any condition that poses a threat to public or resident safety, the president of the Joint Commission, or if the president is not available, a vice president of the Joint Commission designated by the president to do so, may promptly decide that the organization be immediately placed in Preliminary Denial of Accreditation. This action and the findings that led to this action shall be reported by telephone and in writing to the organization's chief executive officer and in writing to the authorities having jurisdiction. The president's or his or her designee's decision shall be promptly reviewed by the Accreditation Committee in accordance with paragraph II of these procedures.

II. Review by the Accreditation Committee

A. **Scope of Review.** The Accreditation Committee shall consider the Joint Commission president's, or the president's designee's, decision and the Joint Commission staff's report and recommendation and may review the survey findings, survey documents, any other relevant materials or information received from any source, including any additional information supplied by the organization in response to this information or, in the case of a Preliminary Denial of Accreditation decision by the president or his or her designee, information supplied by the organization regarding corrective actions taken in response to the identification of a serious threat to resident or public health or safety.

B. **Decision.** Following such consideration, the Accreditation Committee shall do the following:
1. Accredit the organization, as described in paragraph VII of these procedures
2. Or conditionally accredit the organization
3. Or preliminarily deny accreditation to the organization or confirm a decision by the president or his or her designee to preliminarily deny accreditation
4. Or defer consideration while additional information regarding the organization's compliance status is gathered and reviewed by Joint Commission staff

5. Or order a resurvey or partial resurvey of the organization and an evaluation of the results, to the extent appropriate, by the Joint Commission staff. Thereafter, Joint Commission staff shall transmit its report and recommendation to the Accreditation Committee for action, as provided in paragraph II.C of these procedures.
6. Or preliminarily accredit the organization
7. Or initially deny Preliminary Accreditation to those organizations that apply for Early Survey Policy Option 1

C. **Deferred Consideration.** When the Accreditation Committee defers consideration pursuant to paragraph II.B.4 or II.B.5 of these procedures, Joint Commission staff shall review and report to the Accreditation Committee concerning the organization's compliance decision. The Accreditation Committee may order any resurvey or partial resurvey necessary to determine such decision.

Following such consideration and review, the Accreditation Committee shall do the following:
1. Accredit the organization, as described in paragraph VII of these procedures
2. Or conditionally accredit the organization
3. Or preliminarily deny accreditation or confirm a decision of the president or his or her designee to preliminarily deny accreditation to the organization
4. Or defer consideration while additional information regarding the organization's compliance status is gathered and reviewed by the Joint Commission staff
5. Or order an additional resurvey or partial resurvey of the organization and an evaluation of the results, to the extent appropriate, by the Joint Commission staff. Thereafter, Joint Commission staff shall transmit its report and recommendations to the Accreditation Committee for action, as provided in paragraph II.C of these procedures.
6. Or preliminarily accredit the organization
7. Or preliminarily deny Preliminary Accreditation to those organizations applying under Early Survey Policy Option 1

III. Conditional Accreditation

A. **Survey to Determine Implementation of the Evidence of Standards Compliance (ESC).** Within approximately six months from the date the organization is notified of its Conditional Accreditation decision, the Joint Commission shall conduct a survey of the organization to determine the degree to which deficiencies have been corrected or improvements implemented, although the Joint Commission upon occasion may shorten that time period, as appropriate.

B. **Review and Determination by Joint Commission Staff.** Joint Commission staff shall review the survey findings, survey documents, and any other relevant materials or information received from any source. In accor-

dance with decision rules approved by the Accreditation Committee, the Joint Commission staff shall do the following:
1. Determine or recommend to the Accreditation Committee that the organization be accredited, as described in paragraph VII of these procedures
2. Or recommend to the Accreditation Committee that the organization be preliminarily denied accreditation
3. Or defer consideration while additional information regarding the organization's compliance status is gathered and reviewed by the Joint Commission staff. At the conclusion of this review, one of the recommendations outlined in paragraph III.D of these procedures shall be made to the Accreditation Committee.

C. **Action by the Accreditation Committee.** Following review of the recommendations of the Joint Commission staff, the Accreditation Committee shall do the following:
1. Accredit the organization, as described in paragraph VII of these procedures
2. Or preliminarily deny accreditation to the organization
3. Or defer consideration while additional information regarding the organization's compliance status is gathered and reviewed by the Joint Commission staff
4. Or order a resurvey or partial resurvey of the organization and an evaluation of the results, to the extent appropriate, by the Joint Commission staff. Thereafter, Joint Commission staff shall transmit its report and recommendation to the Accreditation Committee for action, as provided in paragraph III.C of these procedures.

D. **Charges to the Organization.** The full costs of the Conditional Accreditation process shall be paid by the organization that receives Conditional Accreditation.

IV. **Review Hearing Panels**
A. **Right to a Hearing Before a Review Hearing Panel.** An organization that has been preliminarily denied accreditation* or Preliminary Accreditation pursuant to paragraph II.B.3, II.B.7, II.C.3, II.C.7, or III.C.2 of these procedures is entitled to a hearing in which to make a detailed presentation before a Review Hearing Panel if the Joint Commission receives the organization's written request for the hearing within five business days after the organization receives the written notice of the Accreditation Committee's decision, including confirmation of a decision by the president, or his or her designee, to preliminarily deny accreditation, as provided in paragraph I.D of these procedures. A Review Hearing Panel shall be com-

---

* The Preliminary Denial of Accreditation decision, if subsequently changed to other than Denial of Accreditation, following review and action by the Accreditation Committee, is no longer disclosable as part of the organization's accreditation decision history.

posed of two health care professionals not on the Accreditation Committee and one member of the Accreditation Committee who is familiar with the organization's decision.

B. Notice of the Time and Place of the Presentation Before a Review Hearing Panel. The presentation before the Review Hearing Panel shall be held at the Joint Commission's headquarters except when the president of the Joint Commission, or his or her designee, determines otherwise for good cause shown. At least 30 calendar days before the presentation, the Joint Commission shall send the organization written notice of the time and place of the hearing and copies of any supplemental materials or information received from any source that the organization does not already have and that may affect any accreditation decision. The notice shall advise the organization of the agenda to be followed and, if feasible, of the identity and professional qualifications of the panel members. At least 10 calendar days before the scheduled hearing date, the organization must submit to the Joint Commission any materials it wishes to be considered by the Review Hearing Panel.

C. Procedure for the Conduct of a Hearing. A Review Hearing Panel may proceed with only two of the three panel members present, provided one of them is the member of the Accreditation Committee. Representatives of the organization may make oral and written presentations and may be accompanied by legal counsel. Presentations or information concerning actions taken by the organization subsequent to the survey upon which the Preliminary Denial of Accreditation decision was based are not considered relevant to the validity of the decision. A Joint Commission surveyor who participated in the survey will ordinarily appear at the hearing.

D. Report of Review Hearing Panel. After a hearing has been completed, the Review Hearing Panel shall review the facts regarding the original Preliminary Denial of Accreditation decision. The panel will submit a written report of its findings on factual matters for consideration by the Accreditation Committee.

E. Charges to the organization. The organization will be charged a nominal fee for the conduct of a Review Hearing Panel.

V. Second Consideration by the Accreditation Committee

A. Scope of Review. The report of the Review Hearing Panel shall be considered by the Accreditation Committee.

B. Decision. Following such consideration, the Accreditation Committee shall do the following:
1. Accredit or preliminarily accredit the organization, as described in paragraph VII of these procedures
   or
2. Conditionally accredit the organization
   or

Accreditation Policies and Procedures

3. Deny accreditation to the organization
   or
4. Defer consideration while additional information regarding the organization's compliance status is gathered and reviewed by Joint Commission staff
   or
5. Order a resurvey or partial resurvey of the organization and an evaluation of the results, to the extent appropriate, by the Joint Commission staff

VI. **Review by the Board Appeal Review Committee**
   A. **Review Request.** An organization that has been denied accreditation or Preliminary Accreditation pursuant to paragraph V.B.3 of these procedures is entitled to request a review of the decision by the Board Appeal Review Committee if the Joint Commission receives the organization's request for review within five business days after the organization receives the written notice of the Accreditation Committee's decision. The Board Appeal Review Committee is composed of four members of the Board of Commissioners who are not members of the Accreditation Committee.

   B. **Notice of Time and Procedure for Review.** The Joint Commission shall send the organization a copy of the report of the Review Hearing Panel at least 20 business days before the meeting of the Board Appeal Review Committee at which the organization's request for review will be considered. Two members of the Board Appeal Review Committee will constitute a quorum. This meeting will generally be held by telephone conference, except when it is held in conjunction with meetings of the Board of Commissioners or other committee(s) of the Board of Commissioners. The organization must submit any materials that it wishes the Board Appeal Review Committee to consider at least 10 calendar days before the scheduled meeting date. The Board Appeal Review Committee shall review the decision of the Accreditation Committee, which considered the report of the Review Hearing Panel, and any written materials submitted by the organization, and shall do one of the following:
   1. Deny accreditation or Preliminary Accreditation to the organization, after finding that there is substantial evidence to support the Accreditation Committee's decision
      or
   2. Make an independent evaluation of the Accreditation Committee's decision and then decide to conditionally accredit, preliminarily accredit, or accredit the organization, as described in paragraph VII of these procedures.

   The action taken by the Board Appeal Review Committee shall constitute the final accreditation decision of the Joint Commission.

C. Participation. No member of the Accreditation Committee or of the Review Hearing Panel who participated in an accreditation decision or review of findings on factual matters concerning an organization shall participate in any deliberations or vote of the Board Appeal Review Committee in its review of that accreditation decision or report of findings on factual matters. This provision shall not preclude any commissioner who participated in a review hearing as a member of the Review Hearing Panel from presenting and responding to questions about the report of that Review Hearing Panel to the Board Appeal Review Committee.

VII. Procedure Relating to Not Compliant Standards and Determination of Corrected Not Compliant Standards

A. A decision of the Joint Commission staff pursuant to paragraph I.A.1, I.B.2.c, or I.C.2.c of these procedures, of the Accreditation Committee pursuant to paragraph II.B.1, II.C.1, or III.C.1 of these procedures, or of a Board Appeal Review Committee, as provided in paragraph VI.B of these procedures, to accredit an organization may be made contingent upon satisfactory correction of not compliant standards or, when appropriate, upon compliance with interim life safety measures. The organization may be conditionally accredited or its accreditation may be withdrawn if it does not correct or document the correction of the specified not compliant standards within the time specified in the notice of the decision to the organization, or, when applicable, fails to demonstrate compliance with the interim life safety measures. Joint Commission staff, through the use of surveys or partial surveys or through other means, such as ESC and MOS, shall determine whether the organization has corrected the not compliant standards within the time provided or, when applicable, has demonstrated compliance with interim life safety measures, and shall report its findings to the organization. If the Joint Commission staff determines that the organization has not corrected the not compliant standards within the time provided or, when applicable, has not demonstrated compliance with interim life safety measures, the organization's status will change to Provisional Accreditation. Joint Commission shall report its findings to the organization, and, after reviewing any comments of the organization, as appropriate and in accordance with decision rules approved by the Accreditation Committee, do the following:
   1. Provide another opportunity to the organization to correct or document the correction of not compliant standards, as provided in any applicable decision rules approved by the Accreditation Committee
      or
   2. Determine or recommend that the organization be placed in Conditional Accreditation status with a conditional follow-up survey in approximately four months or other time as appropriate
      or

3. Recommend to the Accreditation Committee that the organization be preliminarily denied accreditation, if certain not compliant standards, specified in decision rules approved by the Accreditation Committee, have not been corrected or the correction of which has not been documented after the specified number of opportunities given to the organization to do so, and, when applicable and as specified in decision rules approved by the Accreditation Committee, the organization has failed to demonstrate compliance with interim life safety measures

B. If the Joint Commission staff determines to recommend to the Accreditation Committee that the organization be preliminarily denied accreditation in accordance with paragraph VII.A.3, or be conditionally accredited in accordance with VII.A.2, the staff shall submit its recommendation and any comments of the organization to the Accreditation Committee for action, as provided in paragraph II.B.1 through II.B.7.

VIII. Final Accreditation Decision

A. The action taken by the Joint Commission staff shall constitute the final decision of the Joint Commission to do the following:
 1. Accredit the organization, when taken pursuant to paragraph I.A.1, I.B.2.c, or I.C.2.c of these procedures
 or
 2. Conditionally accredit the organization, when taken pursuant to paragraph I.A.3 or VII.A.2 of these procedures
 or
 3. Preliminarily accredit the organization, when taken pursuant to paragraph I.A.6 of these procedures

B. The action taken by the Accreditation Committee shall constitute the final decision of the Joint Commission to do the following:
 1. Accredit the organization, when taken pursuant to paragraph II.B.1, II.C.1, or III.C.1 of these procedures
 or
 2. Conditionally accredit the organization, when taken pursuant to paragraph II.B.2 or II.C.2 of these procedures
 or
 3. Deny accreditation to the organization, when taken pursuant to paragraph II.B.3, II.C.3, III.C.2, or VII.B of these procedures, and the organization does not request the opportunity to make a presentation before a Review Hearing Panel pursuant to paragraph IV.A of these procedures
 or
 4. Preliminarily accredit the organization, when taken pursuant to paragraph II.B.6 of these procedures
 or
 5. Deny Preliminary Accreditation to the organization, when taken pursuant to paragraph II.B.7 of these procedures, and the organization applying for Early Survey Policy Option 1 or 2 does not request the opportunity to make a presentation before a Review Hearing Panel pursuant to paragraph IV.A of these procedures

C. The action taken by the Board Appeal Review Committee shall constitute the final decision of the Joint Commission to do the following:
1. Accredit the organization, conditionally accredit the organization, or deny accreditation, when taken pursuant to paragraph VI.B of these procedures

IX. Status of the Organization Pending a Final Decision and Effective Date of a Final Decision

A. The accreditation status of an accredited organization shall continue in effect pending any final accreditation decision.

B. A final decision to accredit, preliminarily accredit, or conditionally accredit an organization that follows an initial Accreditation Committee decision of Preliminary Denial of Accreditation pursuant to paragraph II.B shall be considered effective as of the first day after completion of the organization's survey from which the decision results.

C. A final decision to deny accreditation or Provisional Accreditation to an organization shall become effective as follows:
1. As of the date of the decision made by the Board Appeal Review Committee pursuant to paragraph VI.B of these procedures
or
2. At the expiration of the time during which an organization may, but does not, request a review by the Board Appeal Review Committee, pursuant to paragraph VI.A of these procedures
or
3. At the expiration of the time during which an organization may, but does not, request the opportunity to make a presentation before a Review Hearing Panel pursuant to paragraph IV.A of these procedures
or
4. On receipt by the Joint Commission, before a final decision, of notification from the organization that it withdraws its request for review of a Preliminary Denial of Accreditation decision before a Review Hearing Panel or its request for appeal of a Denial of Accreditation decision before the Board Appeal Review Committee

X. Notice

Any notice required by these accreditation procedures to be given to an organization shall be addressed to the organization at its post office address as shown in Joint Commission records and shall be sent to the organization by certified letter as forwarded by a recognized package delivery service. Any notice required to be given to the Joint Commission by the organization shall be sent by the organization in the same manner and shall be addressed to the Office of the Executive Vice President for Accreditation Operations, Joint Commission on Accreditation of Healthcare Organizations, One Renaissance Boulevard, Oakbrook Terrace, IL 60181.

Sentinel Events

I. Sentinel Events

In support of its mission to continuously improve the safety and quality of health care provided to the public, the Joint Commission reviews organizations' activities in response to sentinel events in its accreditation process, including all full accreditation surveys and random unannounced surveys.
- A sentinel event is an unexpected occurrence involving death or serious physical or psychological injury, or the risk thereof. Serious injury specifically includes loss of limb or function. The phrase "or the risk thereof" includes any process variation for which a recurrence would carry a significant chance of a serious adverse outcome.
- Such events are called "sentinel" because they signal the need for immediate investigation and response.
- The terms "sentinel event" and "medical error" are not synonymous; not all sentinel events occur because of an error and not all errors result in sentinel events.

II. Goals of the Sentinel Event Policy

The policy has four goals:
1. To have a positive impact in improving patient care, treatment, and services and preventing sentinel events
2. To focus the attention of an organization that has experienced a sentinel event on understanding the causes that underlie the event, and on changing the organization's systems and processes to reduce the probability of such an event in the future
3. To increase the general knowledge about sentinel events, their causes, and strategies for prevention
4. To maintain the confidence of the public and accredited organizations in the accreditation process

III. Standards Relating to Sentinel Events

Standards
Each Joint Commission accreditation manual contains standards in the "Improving Organization Performance" (PI) chapter that relate specifically to the management of sentinel events. These standards are PI.1.10, PI.2.20, PI.2.30, and PI.3.10.

Organization-Specific Definition of Sentinel Event
The Improving Organization Performance standard, PI.2.30, requires each accredited organization to define "sentinel event" for its own purposes in establishing mechanisms to identify, report, and manage these events. While this definition must be consistent with the general definition of sentinel event as published by the Joint

Commission, accredited organizations have some latitude in setting more specific parameters to define "unexpected," "serious," and "the risk thereof." At a minimum, an organization's definition must include those events that are subject to review under the Sentinel Event Policy as defined in Section IV of this chapter.

Expectations Under the Standards for an Organization's Response to a Sentinel Event

Accredited organizations are expected to identify and respond appropriately to all sentinel events (as defined by the organization in accordance with the preceding paragraph) occurring in the organization or associated with services that the organization provides, or provides for. Appropriate response includes conducting a timely, thorough, and credible root cause analysis; developing an action plan designed to implement improvements to reduce risk; implementing the improvements; and monitoring the effectiveness of those improvements.

Root Cause Analysis

Root cause analysis is a process for identifying the basic or causal factors that underlie variation in performance, including the occurrence or possible occurrence of a sentinel event. A root cause analysis focuses primarily on systems and processes, not on individual performance. It progresses from special causes* in clinical processes to common causes† in organizational processes and identifies potential improvements in processes or systems that would tend to decrease the likelihood of such events in the future or determines, after analysis, that no such improvement opportunities exist.

Action Plan

The product of the root cause analysis is an action plan that identifies the strategies that the organization intends to implement in order to reduce the risk of similar events occurring in the future. The plan should address responsibility for implementation, oversight, pilot testing as appropriate, time lines, and strategies for measuring the effectiveness of the actions.

Survey Process

When conducting an accreditation survey, the Joint Commission seeks to evaluate the organization's compliance with the applicable standards and to score those standards based on performance throughout the organization over time (for example, the preceding 12 months for a full accreditation survey). Surveyors are instructed not to seek out specific sentinel events beyond those already known to the Joint Commission.

If, in the course of conducting the usual survey activities, a sentinel event is identified, the surveyor will take the following steps:

---

* **Special cause** is a factor that intermittently and unpredictably induces variation over and above what is inherent in the system. It often appears as an extreme point (such as a point beyond the control limits on a control chart) or some specific, identifiable pattern in data.

† **Common cause** is a factor that results from variation inherent in the process or system. The risk of a common cause can be reduced by redesigning the process or system.

- Inform the CEO that the event has been identified
- Inform the CEO the event will be reported to the Joint Commission for further review and follow-up under the provisions of the Sentinel Event Policy

During the on-site survey, the surveyor(s) will assess the organization's compliance with sentinel event-related standards in the following ways:
- Review the organization's process for responding to a sentinel event
- Interview the organization's leaders and staff about their expectations and responsibilities for identifying, reporting, and responding to sentinel events
- Ask for an example of a root cause analysis that has been conducted in the past year to assess the adequacy of the organization's process for responding to a sentinel event. Additional examples may be reviewed if needed to more fully assess the organization's understanding of, and ability to conduct, root cause analyses. In selecting an example, the organization may choose a "closed case" or a "near miss"* to demonstrate its process for responding to a sentinel event.

IV. Reviewable Sentinel Events

Definition of Occurrences That Are Subject to Review by the Joint Commission Under the Sentinel Event Policy

The definition of a reviewable sentinel event takes into account a wide array of occurrences applicable to a wide variety of health care organizations. Any or all occurrences may apply to a particular type of health care organization. Thus, not all of the following occurrences may apply to your particular organization. The subset of sentinel events that is subject to review by the Joint Commission includes any occurrence that meets any of the following criteria:
- The event has resulted in an unanticipated death or major permanent loss of function, not related to the natural course of the patient's illness or underlying condition[†‡]
or

---

* **Near miss** Used to describe any process variation that did not affect an outcome but for which a recurrence carries a significant change of a serious adverse outcome. Such a "near miss" falls within the scope of the definition of a sentinel event but outside the scope of those sentinel events that are subject to review by the Joint Commission under its Sentinel Event Policy.

[†] A distinction is made between an adverse outcome that is primarily related to the natural course of the patient's illness or underlying condition (not reviewed under the Sentinel Event Policy) and a death or major permanent loss of function that is associated with the treatment (including "recognized complications") or lack of treatment of that condition, or otherwise not clearly and primarily related to the natural course of the patient's illness or underlying condition (reviewable). In indeterminate cases, the event will be presumed reviewable and the organization's response will be reviewed under the Sentinel Event Policy according to the prescribed procedures and time frames without delay for additional information such as autopsy results.

[‡] "Major permanent loss of function" means sensory, motor, physiologic, or intellectual impairment not present on admission requiring continued treatment or lifestyle change. When "major permanent loss of function" cannot be immediately determined, applicability of the policy is not established until either the patient is discharged with continued major loss of function, or two weeks have elapsed with persistent major loss of function, whichever occurs first.

- The event is one of the following (even if the outcome was not death or major permanent loss of function unrelated to the natural course of the patient's illness or underlying condition):
    - Suicide of a patient in a setting where the patient receives around-the-clock care, treatment, and services (for example, hospital, residential treatment center, crisis stabilization center)
    - Unanticipated death of a full-term infant
    - Infant abduction or discharge to the wrong family
    - Rape*
    - Hemolytic transfusion reaction involving administration of blood or blood products having major blood group incompatibilities
    - Surgery on the wrong patient or wrong body part[†]

Examples of reviewable sentinel events and nonreviewable events are provided in Table 1 (page SE-5).

How the Joint Commission Becomes Aware of a Sentinel Event

Each organization is encouraged, but not required, to report to the Joint Commission any sentinel event meeting the above criteria for reviewable sentinel events. Alternatively, the Joint Commission may become aware of a sentinel event by some other means such as communication from a patient, a family member, an employee of the organization, a surveyor, or through the media.

Reasons for Reporting a Sentinel Event to the Joint Commission

Although self-reporting a sentinel event is not required and there is no difference in the expected response, time frames, or review procedures, whether the organization voluntarily reports the event or the Joint Commission becomes aware of the event by some other means, there are several advantages to the organization that self-reports a sentinel event:
- Reporting the event enables the addition of the "lessons learned" from the event to be added to the Joint Commission's Sentinel Event Database, thereby contributing to the general knowledge about sentinel events and to the reduction of risk for such events in many other organizations
- Early reporting provides an opportunity for consultation with Joint Commission staff during the development of the root cause analysis and action plan

---

* *Rape*, as a reviewable sentinel event, is defined as unconsented sexual contact involving a patient and another patient, staff member, or other perpetrator while being treated or on the premises of the health care organization, including oral, vaginal, or anal penetration or fondling of the patient's sex organ(s) by another individual's hand, sex organ, or object. One or more of the following must be present to determine reviewability:
- Any staff-witnessed sexual contact as described above
- Sufficient clinical evidence obtained by the organization to support allegations of unconsented sexual contact
- Admission by the perpetrator that sexual contact, as described above, occurred on the premises

[†] All events of surgery on the wrong patient or wrong body part are reviewable under the policy, regardless of the magnitude of the procedure or the outcome.

Table 1. Examples of Reviewable and Nonreviewable Sentinel Events*

Examples of Sentinel Events That are Reviewable Under the Joint Commission's Sentinel Event Policy

Any patient death, paralysis, coma, or other major permanent loss of function associated with a medication error.

Any suicide of a patient in a setting where the patient is housed around-the-clock, including suicides following elopement from such a setting.

Any elopement, that is unauthorized departure, of a patient from an around-the-clock care setting resulting in a temporally related death (suicide or homicide) or major permanent loss of function.

Any procedure on the wrong patient, wrong side of the body, or wrong organ.

Any intrapartum (related to the birth process) maternal death.

Any perinatal death unrelated to a congenital condition in an infant having a birth weight greater than 2,500 grams.

Assault, homicide, or other crime resulting in patient death or major permanent loss of function.

A patient fall that results in death or major permanent loss of function as a direct result of the injuries sustained in the fall.

Hemolytic transfusion reaction involving major blood group incompatibilities.

> **Note:** An adverse outcome that is *directly related* to the natural course of the patient's illness or underlying condition, for example, terminal illness present at the time of presentation, is **not** reportable **except** for suicide in, or following elopement from, a 24-hour care setting (*see above*).

Examples of Sentinel Events That are Nonreviewable Under the Joint Commission's Sentinel Event Policy

Any "near miss."

Full return of limb or bodily function to the same level as prior to the adverse event by discharge or within two weeks of the initial loss of said function.

Any sentinel event that has not affected a recipient of care (patient, client, resident).

Medication errors that do not result in death or major permanent loss of function.

Suicide other than in an around-the-clock care setting or following elopement from such a setting.

* **Note:** *This list may not apply to all settings.*

continued on next page

Table 1. Examples of Reviewable and Nonreviewable Sentinel Events* (continued)

A death or loss of function following a discharge "against medical advice (AMA)."

Unsuccessful suicide attempts.

Unintentionally retained foreign body without major permanent loss of function.

Minor degrees of hemolysis with no clinical sequelae.

> **Note:** In the context of its performance improvement activities, an organization may choose to conduct intensive assessment, for example, root cause analysis, for some nonreportable events. Please refer to the "Improving Organization Performance" chapter of this Joint Commission publication.

- The organization's message to the public that it is doing everything possible to ensure that such an event will not happen again is strengthened by its acknowledged collaboration with the Joint Commission to understand how the event happened and what can be done to reduce the risk of such an event in the future

Required Response to a Reviewable Sentinel Event

If the Joint Commission becomes aware (either through voluntary self-reporting or otherwise) of a sentinel event that meets the above criteria (*see* page SE-4) and the event has occurred in an accredited organization, the organization is expected to do the following:
- Prepare a thorough and credible root cause analysis and action plan within 45 calendar days of the event or of becoming aware of the event
- Submit to the Joint Commission its root cause analysis and action plan, or otherwise provide for Joint Commission evaluation of its response to the sentinel event under an approved protocol (*see* Section VI), within 45 calendar days of the known occurrence of the event

The Joint Commission will then determine whether the root cause analysis and action plan are acceptable. If the determination that an event is reviewable under the Sentinel Event Policy occurs more than 45 calendar days following the known occurrence of the event, the organization will be allowed 15 calendar days for its response. If the organization fails to submit an acceptable root cause analysis within the 45 calendar days (or within 15 calendar days, if the 45 calendar days have already elapsed), it will be at risk for being placed on Accreditation Watch by the Accreditation Committee. An organization that experiences a sentinel event that does not meet the criteria for review under the Sentinel Event Policy is expected to complete a root cause analysis but does not need to submit it to the Joint Commission.

Review of Root Cause Analyses and Action Plans
A root cause analysis will be considered acceptable if it has the following characteristics:
- The analysis focuses primarily on systems and processes, not on individual performance
- The analysis progresses from special causes in clinical processes to common causes in organizational processes
- The analysis repeatedly digs deeper by asking "Why?"; then, when answered, "Why?" again, and so on
- The analysis identifies changes that could be made in systems and processes (either through redesign or development of new systems or processes) which would reduce the risk of such events occurring in the future
- The analysis is thorough and credible

To be thorough, the root cause analysis must include the following:
- A determination of the human and other factors most directly associated with the sentinel event and the process(es) and systems related to its occurrence
- An analysis of the underlying systems and processes through a series of "Why?" questions to determine where redesign might reduce risk
- An inquiry into all areas appropriate to the specific type of event as described in Table 2 (*see* page SE-8)
- An identification of risk points and their potential contributions to this type of event
- A determination of potential improvement in processes or systems that would tend to decrease the likelihood of such events in the future, or a determination, after analysis, that no such improvement opportunities exist

To be credible, the root cause analysis must do the following:
- Include participation by the leadership of the organization and by individuals most closely involved in the processes and systems under review
- Be internally consistent (that is, not contradict itself or leave obvious questions unanswered)
- Provide an explanation for all findings of "not applicable" or "no problem"
- Include consideration of any relevant literature

An action plan will be considered acceptable if it does the following:
- Identifies changes that can be implemented to reduce risk or formulates a rationale for not undertaking such changes
- Identifies, in situations where improvement actions are planned, who is responsible for implementation, when the action will be implemented (including any pilot testing), and how the effectiveness of the actions will be evaluated

All root cause analyses and action plans will be considered and treated as confidential by the Joint Commission. A detailed listing of the minimum scope of root cause analysis for specific types of sentinel events is included in Table 2.

Accreditation Watch Designation
An organization is placed on Accreditation Watch when a reviewable sentinel event has occurred and has come to the Joint Commission's attention, and a thorough

Table 2. Minimum Scope of Root Cause Analysis for Specific Types of Sentinel Events

Detailed inquiry into these areas is expected when conducting a root cause analysis for the specified type of sentinel event. Inquiry into areas not checked (or listed) should be conducted as appropriate to the specific event under review.

	Suicide (24-Hour Care)	Medication Error	Procedural Complication	Wrong Site Surgery	Treatment Delay	Restraint Death	Elopement Death	Assault/Rape/Homicide	Transfusion Death	Infant Abduction
Behavioral assessment process*	X					X	X	X		
Physical assessment process†	X		X	X	X	X	X			
Patient identification process		X		X					X	
Patient observation procedures	X					X	X	X	X	
Care planning process	X		X			X	X			
Continuum of care	X				X	X				
Staffing levels	X	X	X	X	X	X	X	X	X	X
Orientation and training of staff	X	X	X	X	X	X	X	X	X	X
Competency assessment/credentialing	X	X	X			X	X	X	X	X
Supervision of staff‡		X	X			X	X		X	
Communication with patient/family	X			X	X	X	X			X
Communication among staff members	X	X	X	X	X	X			X	X
Availability of information	X	X	X	X	X	X			X	
Adequacy of technological support		X	X							
Equipment maintenance/management		X	X			X				
Physical environment§	X	X	X				X	X	X	X
Security systems and processes	X						X	X		X
Control of medications: storage/access		X							X	
Labeling of medications		X							X	

* Includes the process for assessing patient's risk to self (and to others, in cases of assault, rape, or homicide where a patient is the assailant).
† Includes search for contraband.
‡ Includes supervision of physicians-in-training.
§ Includes furnishings; hardware (for example, bars, hooks, rods); lighting; distractions.

and credible root cause analysis of the sentinel event and action plan has not been completed in specified time frames. Although Accreditation Watch status is not an official accreditation category, it can be publicly disclosed by the Joint Commission.

Follow-up Activities

After the Joint Commission has determined that an organization has conducted an acceptable root cause analysis and developed an acceptable action plan, the Joint

Commission will notify it that the root cause analysis and action plan are acceptable and will assign an appropriate follow-up activity, typically a measure of success* (MOS) or follow-up survey within six months.

V. The Sentinel Event Database

To achieve the third goal of the Sentinel Event Policy, "to increase the general knowledge about sentinel events, their causes, and strategies for prevention," the Joint Commission collects and analyzes data from the review of sentinel events, root cause analyses, action plans, and follow-up activities. These data and information form the content of the Joint Commission's Sentinel Event Database.

The Joint Commission is committed to developing and maintaining this Sentinel Event Database in a fashion that will protect the confidentiality of the organization, the caregiver, and the patient. Included in this database are three major categories of data elements:
1. Sentinel event data
2. Root cause data
3. Risk reduction data

Aggregate data relating to root causes and risk-reduction strategies for sentinel events that occur with significant frequency will form the basis for future error-prevention advice to organizations through *Sentinel Event Alert* and other media. The Sentinel Event Database is also a major component of the evidence base for the National Patient Safety Goals.

VI. Procedures for Implementing the Sentinel Event Policy

Voluntary Reporting of Reviewable Sentinel Events to the Joint Commission

If an organization wishes to report an occurrence in the subset of sentinel events that are subject to review by the Joint Commission, the organization will be asked to complete a form to be sent to the Joint Commission's Office of Quality Monitoring by mail or by facsimile transmission (630/792-5636). Copies of the sentinel event reporting form may be obtained by calling the Sentinel Event Hotline at 630/792-3700 or the Office of Quality Monitoring at 630/792-5642. This form may also be accessed via the Joint Commission Web site at http://www.jcaho.org.

Reviewable Sentinel Events That Are Not Reported by the Organization

If the Joint Commission becomes aware of a sentinel event subject to review under the Sentinel Event Policy which was not reported to the Joint Commission by the organization, the CEO of the organization is contacted, and a preliminary assess-

---

* For more information about measures of success, see the "The New Joint Commission Accreditation Process" chapter in this book.

ment of the sentinel event is made. An event that occurred more than one year before the date the Joint Commission became aware of the event will not, in most cases, be reviewed under the Sentinel Event Policy. In such a case, a written response will be requested from the organization, including a summary of processes in place to prevent similar occurrences.

Determination That a Sentinel Event Is Reviewable Under the Sentinel Event Policy

Based on available factual information received about the event, Joint Commission staff will apply the above definition (page SE-3) to determine whether the event is reviewable under the Sentinel Event Policy. Challenges to a determination that an event is reviewable will be resolved through consultation with senior staff in the Division of Accreditation Operations.

Initial On-Site Review of a Sentinel Event

An initial on-site review of a sentinel event will usually not be conducted unless it is determined that there is a potential ongoing threat to patient health or safety or potentially significant noncompliance with Joint Commission standards. If an on-site ("for-cause") review is conducted, the organization will be billed an appropriate amount based on the established fee schedule to cover the costs of conducting such a survey.

Disclosable Information

If the Joint Commission receives an inquiry about the accreditation status of an organization that has experienced a reviewable sentinel event, the organization's accreditation status will be reported in the usual manner without making reference to the sentinel event. If the inquirer specifically references the specific sentinel event, the Joint Commission will acknowledge that it is aware of the event and currently is working or has worked with the organization through the sentinel event review process.

Initiation of Accreditation Watch

If the Joint Commission becomes aware that an organization has experienced a reviewable sentinel event, but the organization fails to submit or otherwise make available an acceptable root cause analysis and action plan, or otherwise provide for Joint Commission evaluation its response to the sentinel event under an approved protocol, within 45 calendar days of the event, or of its becoming aware of the event, or within 15 calendar days if the determination that the event is reviewable under the Sentinel Event Policy occurs more than 45 calendar days following the known occurrence of the event, unless Joint Commission staff for good reason has agreed to a short extension of time, a recommendation will be made to the Accreditation Committee to place the organization on Accreditation Watch. If the Accreditation Committee places the organization on Accreditation Watch, the organization will then be permitted an additional 15 calendar days to submit an acceptable root cause analysis and action plan, or otherwise provide for Joint Commission evaluation of its response to the sentinel event under an approved protocol.

The organization will be offered advisory assistance in performing a root cause analysis of the event.

Accreditation Watch status is considered publicly disclosable information.

In all cases of an organization refusing to permit review of information regarding a reviewable sentinel event in accordance with the Sentinel Event Policy and its approved protocols, the initial response by the Joint Commission is assignment of Accreditation Watch. Continued refusal may result in loss of accreditation.

Submission of Root Cause Analysis and Action Plan

The organization that experiences a sentinel event subject to the Sentinel Event Policy is asked to submit two documents (in addition to the sentinel event reporting form discussed on page SE-0): (1) the complete root cause analysis, including its findings; and (2) the resulting action plan that describes the organization's risk reduction strategies and a strategy for evaluating their effectiveness. The template, "A Framework for a Root Cause Analysis and Action Plan in Response to a Sentinel Event," is available to organizations as an aid in organizing the steps in a root cause analysis and developing an action plan. This three-page form can be obtained by calling the Sentinel Event Hotline at 630/792-3700 or by accessing it on the Joint Commission Web site at http://www.jcaho.org.

The root cause analysis and action plan are not to include the patient's name or the names of caregivers involved in the sentinel event.

Alternatively, if the organization has concerns about waivers of confidentiality protections as a result of sending the root cause analysis documents to the Joint Commission, the following alternative approaches to a review of the organization's response to the sentinel event are acceptable:
1. A review of the root cause analysis and action plan documents brought to Joint Commission headquarters by organization staff then taken back to the organization on the same day
2. An on-site visit by a specially trained surveyor to review the root cause analysis and action plan
3. An on-site visit by a specially trained surveyor to review the root cause analysis and findings without directly viewing the root cause analysis documents through a series of interviews and a review of relevant documentation. For purposes of this review activity, "relevant documentation" includes, at a minimum, any documentation relevant to the organization's process for responding to sentinel events, the patient's medical record, and the action plan resulting from the analysis of the subject sentinel event. The latter serves as the basis for appropriate follow-up activity.
4. When the organization affirms that it meets specified criteria respecting the risk of waiving confidentiality protections for root cause analysis information shared with the Joint Commission, an on-site visit by a specially trained surveyor to conduct the following:
    a. Interviews and review relevant documentation, including the patient's medical record, to obtain information about the following:

- The process the organization uses in responding to sentinel events
- The relevant policies and procedures preceding and following the organization's review of the specific event, and the implementation thereof, sufficient to permit inferences about the adequacy of the organization's response to the sentinel event

b. A standards-based survey of the patient care, treatment, and services and the organization management functions relevant to the sentinel event under review.

Any one of the four alternatives will result in a sufficient charge to the organization to cover the average direct costs of the visit. Inquiries about the fee should be directed to the Joint Commission's Pricing Unit at 630/792-5115.

The Joint Commission must receive a request for review of an organization's response to a sentinel event using any of these alternative approaches within at least five business days of the self-report of a reviewable event or of the initial communication by the Joint Commission to the organization that it has become aware of a reviewable sentinel event.

The Joint Commission's Response

Staff assesses the acceptability of the organization's response to the reviewable sentinel event, including the thoroughness and credibility of any root cause analysis information reviewed and the organization's action plan. If the root cause analysis and action plan are found to be thorough and credible, the response will be accepted and an appropriate follow-up activity will be assigned.

If the response is unacceptable, staff will provide consultation to the organization on the criteria that have not yet been met and will allow an additional 15 calendar days beyond the original submission period for the organization to resubmit its response. This additional time is provided only if the organization's initial submission of its root cause analysis and action plan was within the time frame as outlined above.

If the response continues to be unacceptable, staff will recommend to the Accreditation Committee that the organization be placed on Accreditation Watch and be required to address the inadequacies and to submit, or make available for review, a new root cause analysis and action plan within 15 calendar days of notification that the Accreditation Committee has found the response to be unacceptable and has placed the organization on Accreditation Watch, or staff will provide for further Joint Commission evaluation of the organization's response to the event.

Depending on the organization's initial response to the Accreditation Watch decision, the Joint Commission will determine whether an on-site visit should be made to help the organization conduct an appropriate root cause analysis and develop an action plan.

When the organization's response (initial or revised) is found to be acceptable, the Joint Commission issues a letter that does the following:
- Reflects the Joint Commission's determination to (1) continue or modify the organization's current accreditation status and (2) terminate the Accreditation Watch if previously assigned

- Assigns an appropriate follow-up activity, typically an MOS or a follow-up visit to be conducted within six months

If on review the organization's response is still not acceptable or the organization fails to respond, staff will recommend to the Accreditation Committee that the organization be placed in Preliminary Denial of Accreditation. If approved by the Accreditation Committee, this accreditation decision would be considered publicly disclosable information and the process for resolution of Preliminary Denial of Accreditation would be initiated.

Action Plan Follow-up Activity

The follow-up activity will assess (based on applicable standards) the following:
- The organization's response to additional relevant information obtained since completion of the root cause analysis
- The implementation of system and process improvements identified in the action plan
- The means by which the organization will continue to assess the effectiveness of those efforts
- The organization's response to data collected to measure the effectiveness of the actions
- The resolution of any outstanding requirements for improvement

A decision to maintain or change the organization's accreditation status as a result of the follow-up activity or to assign additional follow-up requirements will be based on existing decision rules unless otherwise determined by the Accreditation Committee.

Handling Sentinel Event–Related Documents

Handling of any submitted root cause analysis and action plan is restricted to specially trained staff in accordance with procedures designed to protect the confidentiality of the documents.

Upon completion of the Joint Commission review of any submitted root cause analysis and action plan and the abstraction of the required data elements for the Joint Commission's Sentinel Event Database, the original root cause analysis documents and any copies will be destroyed. Upon request, the original documents will be returned to the organization.

The action plan resulting from the analysis of the sentinel event will initially be retained to serve as the basis for the follow-up activity. Once the action plan has been implemented to the satisfaction of the Joint Commission as determined through follow-up activities, the Joint Commission will destroy the action plan.

Oversight of the Sentinel Event Policy

The Accreditation Committee of the Joint Commission's Board of Commissioners is responsible for overseeing the implementation of this policy and procedure. In addition to reviewing and deciding individual cases involving Accreditation Watch, the Accreditation Committee periodically audits root cause analyses and action plans reviewed by staff. For the purposes of these audits, the Joint Commission temporarily retains random samples of these documents. Upon completion of the audit, these documents are also destroyed.

For more information about the Joint Commission's Sentinel Event Policy and Procedures, visit the Joint Commission's Web site at http://www.jcaho.org or call the Sentinel Event Hotline at 630/792-3700.

National Patient Safety Goals

This chapter addresses the National Patient Safety Goals and requirements. Organizations providing care relevant to each of the goals will be responsible for implementing the applicable requirements or, with Joint Commission approval, effective alternatives.

As with Joint Commission standards, accredited organizations are evaluated for continuous compliance with the specific requirements associated with the National Patient Safety Goals. Compliance with these requirements is assessed by the Joint Commission through on-site surveys and Evidences of Standards Compliance (ESCs). In midcycle, the organization also assesses its own compliance in the Periodic Performance Review (PPR).* Organizations are judged to be either compliant or not compliant with each goal. If an organization does not fully comply with all the requirements associated with a goal, the organization will be assigned a requirement for improvement for the goal in the same way that noncompliance with an element of performance (EP) for a standard generates a requirement for improvement for that standard. All requirements for improvement generate follow-up requirements, and can impact the accreditation decision, as determined by established accreditation decision rules. Failure to resolve a requirement for improvement for a goal can ultimately lead to loss of accreditation.

Note: *Readers might notice that some goals appear to be misnumbered or "missing" from the numerical sequence. This is not a typographical error. Some goals do not apply to hospitals and therefore have not been included in this chapter.*

---

* For those programs required to complete a PPR.

The purpose of the Joint Commission's National Patient Safety Goals is to promote specific improvements in patient safety. The goals highlight problematic areas in health care and describe evidence and expert-based solutions to these problems. Recognizing that sound system design is intrinsic to the delivery of safe, high-quality health care, the goals focus on systemwide solutions, wherever possible.

Although the requirements associated with the National Patient Safety Goals are generally more prescriptive than Joint Commission standards requirements, organizations may request Joint Commission approval of specific alternative approaches to meeting National Patient Safety Goal requirements. The Joint Commission also provides guidance on how to achieve effective compliance with each goal's requirements. This guidance includes detailed answers to Frequently Asked Questions (FAQs).

Three of the requirements associated with the 2004 National Patient Safety Goals that related to preventing wrong site, wrong procedure, and wrong person surgery have been incorporated into the Universal Protocol for ambulatory care, critical access hospitals, hospitals, and office-based surgery, effective July 1, 2004. The 2004 goals and requirements are now replaced by the Universal Protocol for these programs, and their compliance with these three requirements are now scored at the Universal Protocol, which is also provided in this chapter on pages NPSG-5–NPSG-6.

The National Patient Safety Goals are derived primarily from informal recommendations made in the Joint Commission's safety newsletter, *Sentinel Event Alert*. The Sentinel Event database, which contains de-identified aggregate information on sentinel events reported to the Joint Commission, is the primary, but not the sole, source of information from which the *Alerts*, as well as the National Patient Safety Goals, are derived. A broadly representative Sentinel Event Advisory Group works with Joint Commission staff on a continuing basis to determine priorities for, and develop, goals and associated requirements. As part of this development process, candidate goals and requirements are sent to the field for review and comment. Selected existing and new goals and requirements are annually recommended by the Advisory Group to the Joint Commission's Board of Commissioners for final review and approval. The Advisory Group also assists the Joint Commission in evaluating potential alternatives to goal requirements that have been suggested by individual organizations.

Note: *New goals and requirements are indicated in* **bold**.

Goal 1
Improve the accuracy of patient identification.

Requirement 1A
Use at least two patient identifiers (neither to be the patient's room number) whenever administering medications or blood products; taking blood samples and other specimens for clinical testing, or providing any other treatments or procedures.

Note: *The preceding requirement is not scored here. It is scored at standard PC.5.10, EP 4.*

Goal 2
Improve the effectiveness of communication among caregivers.

Requirement 2A
For verbal or telephone orders or for telephonic reporting of critical test results, verify the complete order or test result by having the person receiving the order or test result "read-back" the complete order or test result.

Note: *The preceding requirement is not scored here. It is scored at standard IM.6.50, EP 4.*

Requirement 2B
Standardize a list of abbreviations, acronyms and symbols that are not to be used throughout the organization.

Note: *The preceding requirement is not scored here. It is scored at standard IM.3.10, EP 2.*

Requirement 2C
A Measure, assess and, if appropriate, take action to improve the timeliness of reporting, and the timeliness of receipt by the responsible licensed caregiver, of critical test results and values.

Goal 3
Improve the safety of using medications.

Requirement 3A
Remove concentrated electrolytes (including, but not limited to, potassium chloride, potassium phosphate, sodium chloride >0.9%) from patient care units.

Note: *The preceding requirement is not scored here. It is scored at standard MM.2.20, EP 9.*

Requirement 3B
Standardize and limit the number of drug concentrations available in the organization.

Note: *The preceding requirement is not scored here. It is scored at standard MM.2.20, EP 8.*

Requirement 3C
A Identify and, at a minimum, annually review a list of look-alike/sound-alike drugs used in the organization, and take action to prevent errors involving the interchange of these drugs.

Goal 5
Improve the safety of using infusion pumps.

Requirement 5A
A Ensure free-flow protection on all general-use and PCA (patient controlled analgesia) intravenous infusion pumps used in the organization.

Goal 7
Reduce the risk of health care–associated infections.

Requirement 7A
Comply with current Centers for Disease Control and Prevention (CDC) hand hygiene guidelines.*

Note: *The preceding requirement is not scored here. It is scored at standard IC.4.10, EP 2.*

Requirement 7B
A Manage as sentinel events all identified cases of unanticipated death or major permanent loss of function associated with a health care–associated infection.

Goal 8
Accurately and completely reconcile medications across the continuum of care.

Requirement 8A
A During 2005, for full implementation by January 2006, develop a process for obtaining and documenting a complete list of the patient's current medications upon the patient's admission to the organization and with the involvement of the patient. This process includes a comparison of the medications the organization provides to those on the list.

Requirement 8B
A A complete list of the patient's medications is communicated to the next provider of service when it refers or transfers a patient to another setting, service, practitioner or level of care within or outside the organization.

Goal 9
Reduce the risk of patient harm resulting from falls.

---

* Organizations are required to comply with all 1A, 1B, 1C CDC recommendations or requirements.

Requirement 9A
A Assess and periodically reassess each patient's risk for falling, including the potential risk associated with the patient's medication regimen, and take action to address any identified risks.

Universal Protocol
Wrong site, wrong procedure, and wrong person surgery can be prevented. This universal protocol is intended to achieve that goal. It is based on the consensus of experts from the relevant clinical specialties and professional disciplines and is endorsed by nearly 50 professional medical associations and organizations.

In developing this protocol, consensus was reached on the following principles:
- Wrong site, wrong procedure, wrong person surgery can and must be prevented.
- A robust approach—using multiple, complementary strategies—is necessary to achieve the goal of eliminating wrong site, wrong procedure, wrong person surgery.
- Active involvement and effective communication among all members of the surgical team is important for success.
- To the extent possible, the patient (or legally designated representative) should be involved in the process.
- Consistent implementation of a standardized approach using a universal, consensus-based protocol will be most effective.
- The protocol should be flexible enough to allow for implementation with appropriate adaptation when required to meet specific patient needs.
- A requirement for site marking should focus on cases involving right/left distinction, multiple structures (fingers, toes), or levels (spine).
- The universal protocol should be applicable or adaptable to all operative and other invasive procedures that expose patients to harm, including procedures done in settings other than the operating room.

In concert with these principles, the following steps, taken together, comprise the Universal Protocol for Eliminating Wrong Site, Wrong Procedure, Wrong Person Surgery™ (Universal Protocol):
- Pre-operative verification process
  - Purpose: To ensure that all of the relevant documents and studies are available prior to the start of the procedure and that they have been reviewed and are consistent with each other and with the patient's expectations and with the team's understanding of the intended patient, procedure, site and, as applicable, any implants. Missing information or discrepancies must be addressed before starting the procedure.
  - Process: An ongoing process of information gathering and verification, beginning with the determination to do the procedure, continuing through all settings and interventions involved in the preoperative preparation of the patient, up to and including the "time out" just before the start of the procedure.
- Marking the operative site
  - Purpose: To identify unambiguously the intended site of incision or insertion.

- ○ Process: For procedures involving right/left distinction, multiple structures (such as fingers and toes), or multiple levels (as in spinal procedures), the intended site must be marked such that the mark will be visible after the patient has been prepped and draped.
- "Time out" immediately before starting the procedure
  - ○ Purpose: To conduct a final verification of the correct patient, procedure, site and, as applicable, implants.
  - ○ Process: Active communication among all members of the surgical/procedure team, consistently initiated by a designated member of the team, conducted in a "fail-safe" mode, i.e., the procedure is not started until any questions or concerns are resolved.

UP 1

The organization fulfills the expectations set forth in the Universal Protocol and associated implementation guidelines.

Requirement 1A

A Conduct a preoperative verification process as described in the Universal Protocol.

Requirement 1B

A Mark the operative site as described in the Universal Protocol.

Requirement 1C

Conduct a "time out" immediately before starting the procedure as described in the Universal Protocol.

Note: *The preceding element of performance is not scored here. It is scored at standard PC.13.20, EP 9.*

Accreditation Participation Requirements

This chapter includes specific requirements for participation in the accreditation process and for maintaining an accreditation award. These differ from survey eligibility criteria in that the accreditation process may be initiated even when all accreditation participation requirements (APRs) have not yet been met.

For a hospital seeking accreditation for the first time, compliance with the APRs is assessed during the initial survey. For the accredited hospital, compliance with these requirements is assessed throughout the accreditation cycle through on-site surveys, the Periodic Performance Review (PPR), Evidence of Standards Compliance (ESCs), and periodic updates of hospital-specific data and information. Hospitals are either compliant or not compliant with APRs. When a hospital does not comply with an APR, the hospital will be assigned a requirement for improvement in the same context that noncompliance with a standard or element of performance (EP) generates a requirement for improvement. However, refusal to permit performance of an unscheduled or unannounced for-cause survey (APR 3) or falsification of information (APR 10), will immediately lead to Preliminary Denial of Accreditation. All requirements for improvement can impact the accreditation decision and follow-up requirements, as determined by established accreditation decision rules. Failure to resolve a requirement for improvement can ultimately lead to loss of accreditation.

Application for Accreditation

APR 1
When requested, the hospital provides the Joint Commission with all official records and reports of public or publicly recognized licensing (for example, a state license), examining, reviewing, or planning bodies.*

Element of Performance for APR 1
A 1. The hospital provides the Joint Commission with all official records and reports of licensing, examining, reviewing, or planning bodies.

APR 2
The hospital immediately reports any changes in the information provided in the application for accreditation and any changes made between surveys.†

Rationale for APR 2
A hospital that experiences a significant change in ownership or control, location, capacity, or the categories of services offered must notify the Joint Commission in writing not more than 30 days after such changes. The Joint Commission may decide that the hospital must be resurveyed when a significant merger or consolidation has taken place. The Joint Commission continues the hospital's accreditation until it determines whether a resurvey is necessary. Failure to provide timely notification to the Joint Commission of ownership, merger or consolidation, and service changes may result in interruption or loss of accreditation.

Element of Performance for APR 2
A 1. The hospital notifies the Joint Commission not more than 30 days before or after a significant change in ownership or control, location, capacity, or the categories of services offered.

Acceptance of Survey

APR 3
A hospital permits the performance of an unscheduled or unannounced for-cause survey‡ at the discretion of the Joint Commission.

---

* *See also* page APP-19 in the "Accreditation Policies and Procedures" chapter.

† *See also* page APP-20.

‡ *See also* page APP-39 for an explanation of the difference between an unscheduled and unannounced for-cause survey. In addition, *see* the last paragraph of "Continuous Compliance" on page APP-37.

Rationale for APR 3
The Joint Commission may perform either an unscheduled or unannounced for-cause survey when it becomes aware of potentially serious patient care or safety issues in a hospital. Either type of survey can take place at any point in a hospital's three-year accreditation cycle. An unscheduled or unannounced survey can either include all of the hospital's services or address only those areas where a serious concern may exist. In addition, the Joint Commission conducts unannounced surveys on a random sample of accredited hospitals at 9 to 30 months following the accreditation date. A hospital's failure to permit an unscheduled or unannounced survey is grounds for withdrawal of accreditation.

Elements of Performance for APR 3
A 1. The hospital permits the performance of an unscheduled for-cause survey.

A 2. The hospital permits the performance of an unannounced for-cause survey.

Performance Measurement*

APR 4
Not applicable

APR 5
The hospital selects and uses accepted core measure sets and/or non-core performance measures from at least one listed performance measurement system.

Rationale for APR 5
The hospital selects and uses core measures if appropriate to the population served, or other accepted performance measures from at least one listed performance measurement system (PMS) to meet current ORYX requirements.

If core measures are not applicable, the hospital identifies clinical measures based on current ORYX requirements. The hospital submits data for its measures to the performance measurement system(s) at least quarterly, and such submissions identify monthly data points. A hospital applying for initial survey must notify the Joint Commission of its measure selection(s) no later than the time of survey. Each hospital must also notify the Joint Commission of any subsequent additions or changes to its measure selections.

---

* Hospitals are also encouraged to keep up-to-date on any changes in ORYX requirements by reviewing recent issues of *Joint Commission Perspectives*® or going to the Performance Measurement area on the Joint Commission's Web site at http://www.jcaho.org/pms/index.htm.

Elements of Performance for APR 5

A 1. The hospital has selected a sufficient number of core measure sets and/or non-core performance measures to meet current ORYX requirements.

A 2. The hospital notifies the Joint Commission of its core measure sets and/or non-core performance measures selections by the date requested.

A 3. The hospital notifies the Joint Commission of any changes in its core measure sets and/or non-core performance measures selections.

A 4. Each individual core measure set and/or non-core performance measure is used for at least four consecutive quarters.

APR 6

The hospital ensures that aggregate data for the selected core measure set and/or non-core performance measures are submitted to the Joint Commission at least quarterly.

Rationale for APR 6

Hospital-specific aggregate data, reported as monthly data points, must be submitted four times per year by established deadlines from the performance measurement system to the Joint Commission for use in the accreditation process, as required by the Joint Commission. The Joint Commission has defined the type and format of performance measurement data to be submitted in a fashion consistent with nationally-recognized standards.

The submission of hospital-specific data will be performed by the selected performance measurement system(s) and will include comparative data for other hospitals in the same performance measurement system that have selected the same performance measures.

Element of Performance for APR 6

A 1. The hospital ensures that aggregate data for the selected core measure set and/or non-core performance measure are submitted four times a year in accordance with established time lines to the Joint Commission.

APR 7

Not applicable

Public Information Interviews

APR 8
The hospital provides notice of an upcoming full accreditation survey and of the opportunity for a public information interview.*

Rationale for APR 8
A hospital must provide an opportunity for the public to participate in a public information interview (PII) during a full survey. The public includes the following:
- Patients and their families
- Patient advocates and advocacy groups
- Members of the community for whom services are provided
- Hospital personnel and staff

The hospital is responsible for making the PII process widely known and effective as a source of compliance information in the accreditation process. The Joint Commission requires a hospital scheduled for a full survey to post announcements of the survey date, the opportunity for a PII, and how to request an interview. To maximize participation, postings must be made throughout the hospital in the form provided by the Joint Commission (*see* Public Notice Form on page APP-24). This example may be used by the hospital, or the hospital may design its own Public Notice form that conveys the same information as in this example. Hospitals should post notices in public eating areas, on bulletin boards near major entrances, and in treatment or residential areas. In addition, if all staff members are not likely to see such postings, the hospital must provide each staff member with a written announcement of the survey.

The hospital must also provide potential PII participants with sufficient advance notice. The Joint Commission requires hospitals to post public notices at least 30 days before the scheduled survey date. Notices must remain posted until the survey is completed.

The hospital should also promptly initiate community advertising or other communications as soon as it receives notice of the survey date. Appropriate steps to take in notifying the community of the opportunity for PIIs include the following:
- Informing all advocacy groups (such as organized patient groups and unions) that have substantively communicated with the hospital in the previous 12 months
- Reaching other members of the community, for example, through a public service announcement on radio or television, a classified advertisement in a local newspaper, or notice in a community newsletter or other publication

---
* *See also* pages APP-22–APP-25.

- Informing individuals who inquire about the survey of the survey date(s) and opportunity to participate

Element of Performance for APR 8
A 1. The hospital provides notice of an upcoming full survey and of the opportunity of a PII.

APR 9
The hospital notifies the Joint Commission of any requests for a public information interview.*

Rationale for APR 9
The hospital must promptly forward to the Joint Commission all written requests to participate in a PII. Hospitals receiving an oral request should instruct the individual(s) to make the request in writing and mail it to the Joint Commission. The hospital should provide the individual(s) needing assistance in doing this with the necessary support. The hospital is responsible for notifying the interviewee(s) of the exact date, time, and place of the PII.

Elements of Performance for APR 9
A 1. The hospital notifies the Joint Commission of any requests for a PII.

A 2. The hospital notifies any interviewee (s) of the exact date, time, and place of the PII.

Misrepresentation of Information

APR 10
The hospital does not misrepresent information in the accreditation process.†

Rationale for APR 10
Information provided by the hospital and used by the Joint Commission for the accreditation process must be accurate and truthful. Such information may be the following:
- Provided orally
- Obtained through direct observation by Joint Commission surveyors
- Derived from documents supplied by the hospital to the Joint Commission
- Involve data submitted electronically by the hospital through the performance measurement system to the Joint Commission

---

* *See also* pages APP-10 and APP-12.

† *See also* page APP-10.

Accreditation Participation Requirements

The Joint Commission requires each hospital seeking accreditation to engage in the accreditation process in good faith. Any hospital that fails to participate in good faith by falsifying information presented in the accreditation process may have its accreditation denied or removed by the Joint Commission.

For the purpose of this requirement, falsification is defined as the fabrication, in whole or in part, and through commission or omission, of any information provided by an applicant or accredited hospital to the Joint Commission. This includes any redrafting, reformatting, or content deletion of documents. However, the hospital may submit additional material that summarizes or otherwise explains the original information submitted to the Joint Commission. These additional materials must be properly identified, dated, and accompanied by the original documents.

Element of Performance for APR 10
A 1. The hospital provides accurate and truthful information throughout the accreditation process.

APR 11
The hospital does not publicly misrepresent its accreditation status or the scope of facilities and services to which the accreditation applies.*

Rationale for APR 11
Hospitals accredited by the Joint Commission must be accurate when describing to the public the nature and meaning of their accreditation. On request, the Joint Commission's Department of Communications will provide accredited hospitals with appropriate guidelines for characterizing the accreditation award. A hospital may not engage in any false or misleading advertising with respect to the accreditation award. Any such advertising may be grounds for denying or revoking accreditation.

Elements of Performance for APR 11
A 1. The hospital accurately represents its accreditation status as to the scope of facilities and services to which the accreditation applies.

A 2. The hospital does not engage in any false or misleading advertising with respect to the accreditation award.

APR 12
Accredited hospitals or hospitals seeking accreditation are not permitted to use Joint Commission full-time, part-time, or intermittent surveyors to provide any accreditation-related consulting services.

---

* *See also* pages APP-35 and APP-36.

Rationale for APR 12

Consulting services include, but are not limited to, the following:
- Helping a hospital to meet Joint Commission standards
- Helping a hospital to complete its PPR
- Assisting a hospital to remedy areas identified in its PPR as needing improvements
- Conducting mock surveys for a hospital
- Providing consultation to a hospital to address Priority Focus Process (PFP) information

Element of Performance for APR 12

A 1. The hospital does not use Joint Commission full-time, part-time, or intermittent surveyors to provide any accreditation-related consulting services.

Survey Observers

APR 13

A hospital that applies for survey is obligated to accept Joint Commission on Accreditation of Healthcare Organizations' surveyor management staff and/or a member of the Board of Commissioners to observe a survey under two specific circumstances:
- Observation and mentoring of surveyors as part of surveyor management and development
- Preceptorship of new surveyors

The observer will not participate in the on-site survey process in any fashion, including the scoring of standards compliance. The presence of an observer will not result in any additional charge to the hospital nor will it be accepted as "de facto" grounds for score revisions or decision appeal.

Element of Performance for APR 13

A 1. The hospital accepts Joint Commission on Accreditation of Healthcare Organizations' surveyor management staff and/or a member of the Board of Commissioners to observe a survey under either of the two specific circumstances.

Periodic Performance Review

APR 14

The hospital fulfills the Periodic Performance Review (PPR) requirement at the midpoint of its accreditation cycle.

Rationale for APR 14
Full Periodic Performance Review

The hospital must complete and transmit to the Joint Commission a PPR and plan of action and identify appropriate measures of success (MOS) at the 18-month point in the accreditation cycle. The hospital also participates in a conference call with Joint Commission staff to reach final agreement on the elements of the plan of action and MOS. The plan of action addresses all standards areas identified as being not in compliance. At the time of the hospital's triennial survey, the surveyors will validate whether the MOS data indicate that performance has been sustained.

The results of the PPR do not affect a hospital's accreditation decision at the 18-month point of the accreditation cycle. In the unlikely event that the Joint Commission or the hospital identifies a continuing situation that represents a potential threat to health or safety through the PPR, a special announced survey will be initiated to facilitate resolution of the situation.

The hospital, in concert with the medical staff, demonstrates that physicians were appropriately involved in the completion of the PPR and development of action plans.

Option 1

If the hospital selects option 1 as an alternative to the full PPR, the hospital must attest that after careful consideration with legal counsel, the hospital has decided not to participate in the full PPR and instead will complete a PPR and plan of action and identify appropriate MOS at the 18-month point in the accreditation cycle. The hospital may elect to participate in a conference call related to standards issues with Joint Commission staff at the 18-month in the accreditation cycle. The plan of action addresses all standards areas identified as being not in compliance. At the time of the hospital's triennial survey, the surveyors will validate whether the MOS data indicate that performance has been sustained.

The hospital, in concert with the medical staff, demonstrates that physicians were appropriately involved in the completion of the PPR and development of action plans.

Option 2

If the hospital selects option 2 as an alternative to the full PPR it must attest that after careful consideration with legal counsel, the hospital has decided not to participate in the full PPR and instead intends to undergo a limited survey at the midpoint in its accreditation cycle. Following the survey, the hospital must submit a plan of action with appropriate MOS for any recommendation cited at the survey. The hospital also participates in a conference call with Joint Commission staff to reach final agreement on the elements of the plan of action and MOS. At the time of thehospital's triennial survey, the surveyors will validate whether the MOS data indicate that performance has been sustained.

Option 3

If the hospital selects option 3 as an alternative to the full PPR, it must attest that, after careful consideration with legal counsel, it has decided not to participate in the full PPR and instead intends to undergo a limited survey at the midpoint in its accreditation cycle. Following the survey, the hospital may elect to participate in a conference call to discuss standards-related issues with Joint Commission staff. At the time of the hospital's triennial survey, the surveyors will receive no information relating to the hospital's option 3 survey findings.

Elements of Performance for APR 14

A 1. The hospital completes the full PPR and plan of action at the 18-month point in the accreditation cycle and, in concert with the medical staff, demonstrates that it has involved physicians in their completion.

or

The hospital attests that after careful consideration with legal counsel, it has decided not to participate in the full PPR and completes option 1, and, in concert with the medical staff, demonstrates that it has involved physicians in the PPR and plan of action.

or

The hospital attests that, after careful consideration with legal counsel, it has decided not to participate in the full PPR and completes option 2 at the midpoint in the accreditation cycle.

or

The hospital attests that, after careful consideration with legal counsel, it has decided not to participate in the full PPR and completes option 3 at the midpoint in the accreditation cycle.

A 2. For the full PPR and Option 2, the hospital participates in a conference call with the Joint Commission staff to reach final agreement on the elements of the plan of action.

Ethics, Rights, and Responsibilities

Overview

The **goal** of the ethics, rights, and responsibilities function is to improve care, treatment, services, and outcomes by recognizing and respecting the rights of each patient and by conducting business in an ethical manner. Care, treatment, and services are provided in a way that respects and fosters dignity, autonomy, positive self regard, civil rights, and involvement of patients. Care, treatment, and services consider the patient's abilities and resources; the relevant demands of his or her environment; and the requirements and expectations of the providers and those they serve. The family is involved in care, treatment, and service decisions with the patient's approval.

A hospital's adherence to ethical care and business practices significantly affects the patient's experience of and response to care, treatment, and services. The standards in this chapter address the following processes and activities related to ethical care and business practices:
- Managing the hospital's relationships with patients and the public in an ethical manner
- Considering the values and preferences of patients, including the decision to discontinue care, treatment, and services
- Helping patients understand and exercise their rights
- Informing patients of their responsibilities in care, treatment, and services
- Recognizing the hospital's responsibilities under law

Patients deserve care, treatment, and services that safeguard their personal dignity and respect their cultural, psychosocial, and spiritual values. These values often influence the patient's perceptions and needs. By understanding and respecting these values, providers can meet care, treatment, and service needs and preferences.

Standards

The following is a list of all standards for this function. They are presented here for your convenience without footnotes or other explanatory text. If you have a question about a term used here, please check the Glossary.

Note: *A revised standard numbering system is being used with the reformatted standards. This revised numbering system will allow for more flexibility to add standards while maintaining the current label for each standard.*

Organization Ethics

RI.1.10 The hospital follows ethical behavior in its care, treatment, and services and business practices.

RI.1.20 The hospital addresses conflicts of interest.

RI.1.30 The integrity of decisions is based on identified care, treatment, and service needs of the patients.

RI.1.40 When care, treatment, and services are subject to internal or external review that results in the denial of care, treatment, services, or payment, the hospital makes decisions regarding the provision of ongoing care, treatment, services, or discharge based on the assessed needs of the patients.

Individual Rights

RI.2.10 The hospital respects the rights of patients.

RI.2.20 Patients receive information about their rights.

RI.2.30 Patients are involved in decisions about care, treatment, and services provided.

RI.2.40 Informed consent is obtained.

RI.2.50 Consent is obtained for recording or filming made for purposes other than the identification, diagnosis, or treatment of the patients.

RI.2.60 Patients receive adequate information about the person(s) responsible for the delivery of their care, treatment, and services.

RI.2.70 Patients have the right to refuse care, treatment, and services in accordance with law and regulation.

RI.2.80	The hospital addresses the wishes of the patient relating to end-of-life decisions.
RI.2.90	Patients and, when appropriate, their families are informed about the outcomes of care, treatment, and services that have been provided, including unanticipated outcomes.
RI.2.100	The hospital respects the patient's right to and need for effective communication.
RI.2.110	Not applicable
RI.2.120	The hospital addresses the resolution of complaints from patients and their families.
RI.2.130	The hospital respects the needs of patients for confidentiality, privacy, and security.
RI.2.140	Patients have a right to an environment that preserves dignity and contributes to a positive self image.
RI.2.150	Patients have the right to be free from mental, physical, sexual, and verbal abuse, neglect, and exploitation.
RI.2.160	Patients have the right to pain management.
RI.2.170	Patients have a right to access protective and advocacy services.
RI.2.180	The hospital protects research subjects and respects their rights during research, investigation, and clinical trials involving human subjects.
RI.2.190	In hospitals that provide opportunities for work, a defined policy addresses situations in which patients work.

Individual Responsibilities

RI.3.10	Patients are given information about their responsibilities while receiving care, treatment, and services.

Understanding the Parts of This Chapter

To help you navigate this reformatted standards chapter, it may be helpful to think of its parts this way:
- The **standard** is the "goal."
- The **rationale** explains why it's important to achieve this goal.
- The **elements of performance** identify the step(s) needed to achieve this goal.

These parts are defined as follows.

Standard A statement that defines the performance expectations and/or structures or processes that must be in place in order for a hospital to provide safe, high-quality care, treatment, and services. A hospital is either "compliant" or "not compliant" with a standard.

Accreditation decisions are based on simple counts of the standards that are determined to be "not compliant."

Rationale A statement that provides background, justification, or additional information about a standard. A standard's rationale is not scored. In some instances, the rationale for a standard is self-evident. Therefore, not every standard has a written rationale.

Elements of performance (EPs) The specific performance expectations and/or structures or processes that must be in place in order for a hospital to provide safe, high-quality care, treatment, and services. The scoring of EP compliance determines a hospital's overall compliance with a standard. EPs are evaluated on the following scale:

        0   Insufficient compliance
        1   Partial compliance
        2   Satisfactory compliance
       NA Not applicable

You will find a **measure of success** icon—Ⓜ—next to some EPs. Measures of success (MOS) need to be developed for certain EPs when a standard is judged to be out of compliance through either the Periodic Performance Review (PPR) or the onsite survey. An MOS is defined as a quantifiable measure, usually related to an audit, that can be used to determine whether an action has been effective and is being sustained.*

Assessing Your Compliance

Once you are familiar with the parts of this chapter, you can begin to assess your compliance with its requirements. The scoring category for each EP is noted next to the EP. If you would like to assess your hospital's performance, mark your scores for the EPs and the standards by following the simple steps described below.

---

* For more information about measures of success, *see* the "The New Joint Commission Accreditation Process" chapter in this book.

Ethics, Rights, and Responsibilities

Two components are scored for each EP: (1) compliance with the requirement itself **and** (2) compliance with the track record* for that requirement. Scoring has been simplified, and track record achievements (which have always been part of the scoring) have been appropriately modified.

Note: *Some standards and EPs do not apply to a particular type of organization; these standards and EPs are marked "not applicable" and the related text is not included. Your hospital is not expected to comply with standards and EPs marked "not applicable."*

In addition, some standards and EPs that do apply to organizations may not apply to the specific care, treatment, and services that your individual hospital provides. Although these standards and EPs are included in the manual, you are not expected to comply with them. If you are unsure about the standards or EPs that apply to your hospital, please contact the Joint Commission's Standards Interpretation Group at 630/792-5900.

Step 1: Score Your Compliance with Each Element of Performance

Before you can determine your compliance with the standards, you must score your compliance with each EP. There are three scoring criterion categories: A, B, and C (described below). Please note that for each EP scoring criterion category, your hospital must meet the performance requirement itself and the track record achievements (*see* "Track Record Achievements").

Category A

These EPs relate to the presence or absence of the requirement(s) and are scored either yes (2) or no (0); however, score 1 for partial compliance is also possible based on track record achievements.

If an A EP has multiple components designated by bullets, your hospital must be compliant with all the bullets to receive a score of 2. If your hospital does not meet one or more requirements in the bullets, you will receive a score of 0.

Category B

Category B EPs are scored in two steps:
1. As with category A EPs, category B EPs relate to the presence or absence of the requirement(s). If your hospital *does not meet* the requirement(s), the EP is scored 0; there is no need to assess your compliance with the principles of good process design.
2. If your hospital *does meet* the requirement(s), but there is concern about the quality or comprehensiveness of the effort, then and only then should you assess the qualitative aspect of the EP. That is, review the applicable principles of good process design and ask how the principles were applied in the situation under discussion. Good process design has the following characteristics:

---

* **Track record** The amount of time that an organization has been in compliance with a standard, element of performance, or other requirement.

- Is consistent with your hospital's mission, values, and goals
- Meets the needs of patients
- Reflects the use of currently accepted practices (doing the right thing, using resources responsibly, using practice guidelines)
- Incorporates current safety information and knowledge such as sentinel event data and National Patient Safety Goals
- Incorporates relevant performance improvement results

This two-part evaluation applies to both simple and bulleted B EPs. First, the EPs are assessed to determine if the requirements are present. If the EP has multiple components designated by bullets, as with the category A EPs, your hospital must meet the requirements in *all* the bulleted items to get a score of 2. If your hospital meets *none* of the requirements in the bullets, it receives a score of 0. If your hospital meets *at least one, but not all*, of the bulleted requirements, it will receive a score of 1 for the EPs.

Use the following rules to determine your EP score:
- Your EP score is 0 if your hospital does not meet the requirement(s); you *do not* need to assess your compliance with the preceding applicable principles of good process design
- Your EP score is 1 if your hospital does meet the requirement(s), but considered only *some* of the preceding applicable principles of good process design
- Your EP score is 2 if your hospital does meet the requirement(s) *and* considered *all* the preceding principles of good process design

Category C

C EPs are scored 0, 1, or 2 based on the number of times your hospital does not meet the EP. These EPs are frequency based and require totaling the number of occurrences (that is, results of performance or nonperformance) related to a particular EP. Each situation discovered by a surveyor(s) will be counted as a separate occurrence.

Note: *Multiple events of the same type related to a single patient and single practitioner/staff member are counted as one occurrence only.*

Use the following rules to determine your EP score:
- Your EP score is 2 if you find one or fewer occurrences of noncompliance with the EP
- Your EP score is 1 if you find two occurrences of noncompliance with the EP
- Your EP score is 0 if you find three or more occurrences of noncompliance with the EP

If an EP in the C category has multiple requirements designated by bullets, the following scoring guidelines apply:
- If there are fewer than 2 findings in all bullets, the EP is scored 2
- If there are three or more findings in all bullets, the EP is scored 0
- In all other combinations of findings, the EP is scored 1

Track Record Achievements

In addition to meeting the requirement(s) in each EP, regardless of category, your hospital must also meet the following track record achievements:

Score	Initial Survey	Full Survey
2	4 months or more	12 months or more
1	2 to 3 months	6 to 11 months
0	Fewer than 2 months	Fewer than 6 months

Sample Sizes

If during an onsite survey, your hospital has been found to be not compliant with one or more standards, you must demonstrate Evidence of Standards Compliance (ESC) for each standard that is not compliant. The ESC must address compliance at the EP level; when an EP within a noncompliant standard requires an MOS, your hospital must demonstrate achievement with the MOS when completing the ESC.

Note: *Not every EP requires an MOS. EPs that do require an MOS are clearly marked in this chapter. Organizations are required to demonstrate achievement with an MOS only for EPs within a noncompliant standard that require an MOS. Organizations do not need to demonstrate achievement with an MOS for any EP within a compliant standard.*

When demonstrating achievement with the MOS during the ESC process, your hospital is **required** to use the following sample sizes, which were established because of their statistical significance, their relative simplicity in application, and their sensitivity to an organization's population size:
- For a population size of fewer than 30 cases, sample 100% of available cases
- For a population size of 30 to 100 cases, sample 30 cases
- For a population size of 101 to 500 cases, sample 50 cases
- For a population size greater than 500 cases, sample 70 cases

Note: *Hospitals are encouraged, but not required, to follow this sample size when demonstrating achievement with an MOS for an EP within a noncompliant standard after conducting a full, Option 1, or Option 2 Periodic Performance Review (PPR).*

When conducting PPR (optional use) or demonstrating an ESC (mandatory use), use the following percentages to determine your score: 90% through 100% of your sample size is in compliance = score 2; 80% through 89% (two instances of noncompliance) of your sample size is in compliance = score 1; less than 80% (three or more instances of noncompliance) of your sample size is in compliance = score 0.

In addition, the following information should govern your hospital's selection of samples:
- The appropriate sample size should be determined by the specific population related to the survey findings
- The sampling approach should involve either systematic random sampling (for example, your hospital selects every second or third case for review) or simple random sampling (for example, your hospital uses a series of random numbers generated by a computer to identify the cases to be reviewed)

- If your hospital chooses not to use these sample sizes while conducting PPR options 1 or 2, you should make sure that your sample size is sufficiently large enough to ensure statistical significance
- When submitting a clarifying ESC, if your hospital selects records as part of its sample, the records should be from a period of no more than three months before the last date of the survey
- Assessment of MOS compliance is conducted for a four-month period following the date of ESC approval. Your hospital should select records as a part of your sample following the date of ESC approval and use the required sample sizes. MOS percentage compliance rates are derived from the average of all four months.

Step 2: Use Your EP Scores to Gauge Your Compliance with the Standards

Now that you have evaluated and scored each EP for a particular standard, use these simple rules to determine your compliance with the standard itself:
- Your hospital is not in compliance (that is, "not compliant") with the standard if any EP is scored 0
- Otherwise, your hospital is in compliance with a standard if 65% or more of its EPs are scored 2

Ethics, Rights, and Responsibilities

Standards, Rationales, Elements of Performance, and Scoring

Organization Ethics

Introduction
A hospital has an ethical responsibility to the patients and community it serves. To fulfill this responsibility, ethical care, treatment, and service practices and ethical business practices must go hand in hand. Furthermore, the hospital provides care, treatment, and services within its scope, stated mission and philosophy, and applicable law and regulation.

The hospital's system of ethics supports honest and appropriate interactions with patients. The system of ethics also includes patients whenever possible in decisions about their care, treatment, and services, including ethical issues.

Standard RI.1.10
The hospital follows ethical behavior in its care, treatment, and services and business practices.

Elements of Performance for RI.1.10

B 1. The hospital identifies ethical issues and issues prone to conflict.

B 2. The hospital develops and implements a process to handle these issues when they arise.

B 3. The hospital's policies and procedures reflect ethical practices for marketing, admission, transfer, discharge, and billing.

B 4. Marketing materials accurately represent the hospital and address the care, treatment, and services that the hospital can provide, directly or by contractual arrangement.

C Ⓜ 5. Patients receive information about charges for which they will be responsible.

B 6. The effectiveness and safety of care, treatment, and services does not depend on the patient's ability to pay.

C Ⓜ 7. The leaders ensure that care, treatment, and services are not negatively affected when the hospital grants a staff member's request to be excused from participating in an aspect of the care, treatment, and services.

Standard RI.1.20
The hospital addresses conflicts of interest.

Rationale for RI.1.20
Potential conflicts of interest can arise in subtle and obvious circumstances. The hospital needs to be aware of potential conflicts of interest and review relationships with other entities carefully to ensure that its mission and responsibility to the patients and community it serves is not harmed by any professional, ownership, contractual, or other relationships.

Elements of Performance for RI.1.20
A   1.   The hospital defines what constitutes a conflict of interest.

C Ⓜ   2.   The hospital discloses existing or potential conflicts of interest for those who provide care, treatment, and services as well as governance.

B   3.   The hospital reviews its relationship and its staff's relationships with other care providers, educational institutions, and payers to ensure that those relationships are within law and regulation and determine if conflicts of interest exist.

B   4.   The hospital addresses conflicts of interest when they arise.

Standard RI.1.30
The integrity of decisions is based on identified care, treatment, and service needs of the patients.

Rationale for RI.1.30
Decisions are based on the patients' care, treatment, and service needs, regardless of how the hospital compensates or shares financial risk with its leaders, managers, staff, and licensed independent practitioners.

Elements of Performance for RI.1.30
B   1.   The hospital has policies and procedures that address the integrity of clinical decision making.

C Ⓜ   2.   To avoid compromising the quality of care, decisions are based on the patient's identified care, treatment, and service needs and in accordance with hospital policy.

B   3.   Policies and procedures and information about the relationship between the use of care, treatment, and services and financial incentives are available to all patients, staff, licensed independent practitioners, and contracted providers, when requested.

Standard RI.1.40
When care, treatment, and services are subject to internal or external review that results in the denial of care, treatment, services, or payment, the hospital makes decisions regarding the provision of ongoing care, treatment, and services, or discharge based on the assessed needs of the patients.

Ethics, Rights, and Responsibilities

Rationale for RI.1.40
When an individual requests or presents for care, treatment, and services, the hospital is professionally and ethically responsible for providing care, treatment, and services within its capability, mission, and applicable law and regulation. At times, indications for such care, treatment, and services can contradict the recommendations of an external entity performing a utilization review (for example, insurance companies, managed care reviewers, and federal or state payers). If such a conflict arises, care, treatment, service, and discharge decisions are made based on the patients' identified needs, regardless of the recommendations of the external agency.

Elements of Performance for RI.1.40
C Ⓜ 1. The hospital makes decisions regarding the provision of ongoing care, treatment, services, or discharge based on the care, treatment, and services required by the patient.

C Ⓜ 2. The patient and/or the family is involved in these decisions.

Individual Rights

Introduction
A mere list of rights cannot guarantee those rights. Rather, a hospital shows its support of rights by how its staff interacts with patients and involves them in decisions about their care, treatment, and services. These standards focus on how the hospital respects the culture and rights of patients during those interactions. This begins with respecting their right to treatment, care, and service.

Standard RI.2.10
The hospital respects the rights of patients.

Elements of Performance for RI.2.10
B 1. The hospital's policies and practices address the rights of patients to care, treatment, and services within its capability and mission and in compliance with law and regulation.

C Ⓜ 2. Each patient has a right to have his or her cultural, psychosocial, spiritual, and personal values, beliefs, and preferences respected.

C Ⓜ 3. The hospital supports the right of each patient to personal dignity.

C Ⓜ 4. The hospital accommodates the right to pastoral and other spiritual services for patients.

Standard RI.2.20

Patients receive information about their rights.

Elements of Performance for RI.2.20

C Ⓜ 1. Information on rights is provided to each patient.

2. Not applicable

3. Not applicable

4. Not applicable

C Ⓜ 5. Information on the extent to which the hospital is able, unable, or unwilling to honor advance directives is given upon admission if the patient has an advance directive.

C Ⓜ 6. The patient has the right to access, request amendment to, and receive an accounting of disclosures regarding his or her own health information as permitted under applicable law.

Standard RI.2.30

Patients are involved in decisions about care, treatment, and services provided.

Rationale for RI.2.30

Making decisions about care, treatment, and services sometimes presents questions, conflicts, or other dilemmas for the hospital and the patients, family, or other decision makers. These dilemmas may involve issues about admission; care, treatment, and services; or discharge. The hospital works with patients, and when appropriate, their families, to resolve such dilemmas.

Elements of Performance for RI.2.30

C Ⓜ 1. Patients are involved in decisions about their care, treatment, and services.

C Ⓜ 2. Patients are involved in resolving dilemmas about care, treatment, and services.

C Ⓜ 3. A surrogate decision maker, as allowed by law, is identified when a patient cannot make decisions about his or her care, treatment, and service.

C Ⓜ 4. The legally responsible representative approves care, treatment, and service decisions.*

C Ⓜ 5. The family, as appropriate and as allowed by law, with permission of the patient or surrogate decision maker, is involved in care, treatment, and service decisions.

---

* In some states, law dictates that urgent care, family planning, and/or behavioral health services can be provided to a minor without the approval or consent of a parent or guardian.

Ethics, Rights, and Responsibilities

Standard RI.2.40
Informed consent is obtained.

Rationale for RI.2.40
The goal of the informed consent process is to establish a mutual understanding between the patient and the physician or other licensed independent practitioner who provides the care, treatment, and services about the care, treatment, and services that the patient receives. This process allows each patient to fully participate in decisions about his or her care, treatment, and services.

Elements of Performance for RI.2.40

B 1. The hospital's policies describe the following:
- Which procedures or care, treatment, and services require informed consent
- The process used to obtain informed consent
- How informed consent is to be documented in the record
- When a surrogate decision maker, rather than the patient, may give informed consent
- When procedures or care, treatment, and services normally requiring informed consent may be given without informed consent

C Ⓜ 2. Informed consent is obtained and documented in accordance with the hospital's policy.

B 3. A complete informed consent process includes a discussion of the following elements:*
- The nature of the proposed care, treatment, services, medications, interventions, or procedures
- Potential benefits, risks, or side effects, including potential problems related to recuperation
- The likelihood of achieving care, treatment, and service goals
- Reasonable alternatives to the proposed care, treatment, and service
- The relevant risks, benefits, and side effects related to alternatives, including the possible results of not receiving care, treatment, and services
- When indicated, any limitations on the confidentiality of information learned from or about the patient

Standard RI.2.50
Consent is obtained for recording or filming[†] made for purposes other than the identification, diagnosis, or treatment of the patients.

---

* Documentation of the items listed in EP 3 may be in a form, progress notes, or elsewhere in the record.

[†] Recording or filming refers to photographic, video, electronic, or audio media.

Rationale for RI.2.50

Recording or filming of care, treatment, and services provided to patients can be useful for many purposes, but such recording or filming is likely to compromise the patient's privacy and confidentiality. Therefore, the hospital should obtain consent from the patient for recording or filming.

Elements of Performance for RI.2.50

C Ⓜ 1. When recording or filming are to be used only for internal organizational purposes (for example, performance improvement and education), there is documentation of consent, which may be obtained as part of general consent to treatment or another form, if a statement is included in the form regarding the use of recordings or filming for such internal purposes.

C Ⓜ 2. When recording or films are made for external purposes that will be heard or seen by the public (for example, commercial filming, television programs, marketing), there is documentation of a specific, separate consent that includes the circumstances of the use of the recording or film.

C Ⓜ 3. Except for the circumstances set forth in EP 4 (below), there is documentation of consent before recording or filming.

C Ⓜ 4. The following occurs in situations in which the patient is unable to give informed consent before recording or filming:
- The recording or filming may occur before consent, provided it is within the established policy of the hospital and the policy is established through an appropriate ethical mechanism (for example, an ethics committee) that includes community input
- The recording or film remains in the hospital's possession and is not used for any purpose until and unless consent is obtained
- If consent for use cannot subsequently be obtained, the recording or film is either destroyed or the nonconsenting patient must be removed from the recording or film

A 5. Patients have the right to request cessation of recording or filming.

A 6. Patients have the right to rescind consent for use up until a reasonable time before the recording or film is used.

C Ⓜ 7. Anyone who engages in recording or filming (who is not already bound by the hospital's confidentiality policy) signs a confidentiality statement to protect the patient's identity and confidential information.

Standard RI.2.60

Patients receive adequate information about the person(s) responsible for the delivery of their care, treatment, and services.

Ethics, Rights, and Responsibilities

Elements of Performance for RI.2.60

C Ⓜ 1. The information provided includes the following:
- The name of the physician or other practitioner primarily responsible for their care, treatment, and services
- The name of the physician or other practitioner who will provide the care, treatment, and services

C Ⓜ 2. The information is given to the patient on a timely basis as defined by the hospital.

Standard RI.2.70
Patients have the right to refuse care, treatment, and services in accordance with law and regulation.

Elements of Performance for RI.2.70

A 1. Patients have the right to refuse care, treatment, and services in accordance with law and regulation.

A 2. When the patient is not legally responsible, the surrogate decision maker, as allowed by law, has the right to refuse care, treatment, and services on the patient's behalf.

Standard RI.2.80
The hospital addresses the wishes of the patient relating to end-of-life decisions.

Elements of Performance for RI.2.80

B 1. Policies, in accordance with law and regulation, address advance directives and the framework for forgoing or withdrawing life-sustaining treatment and withholding resuscitative services.

C Ⓜ 2. Adults are given written information about their right to accept or refuse medical or surgical treatment, including forgoing or withdrawing life-sustaining treatment or withholding resuscitative services.

A 3. The existence or lack of an advance directive does not determine an individual's access to care, treatment, and services.

C Ⓜ 4. Documentation indicates whether or not the patient has signed an advance directive.

A 5. The patient has the option to review and revise advance directives.

C Ⓜ 6. Appropriate staff are aware of the advance directive if one exists.

C Ⓜ 7. The hospital helps or refers the patients for assistance in formulating advance directives upon request.

B   8. The hospital has a mechanism for health care professionals and designated representatives to honor advance directives within the limits of the law and the hospital's capabilities.

C Ⓜ   9. The hospital documents and honors the patient's wishes concerning organ donation within the limits of the law or hospital capacity.

B   10. *For Outpatient Hospital Settings:* The hospital's policies address advance directives and specify whether the hospital will honor the directives.

C Ⓜ   11. *For Outpatient Hospital Settings:* The policies are communicated to patients and families when asked about or as appropriate to the care, treatment, and services provided.

C Ⓜ   12. *For Outpatient Hospital Settings*: Upon request, the hospital helps patients formulate medical advance directives or refers them for assistance.

13. Through 20. Not applicable

C Ⓜ   21. The policies are consistently implemented.

Standard RI.2.90

Patients and, when appropriate, their families are informed about the outcomes of care, treatment, and services that have been provided, including unanticipated outcomes.

Elements of Performance for RI.2.90

At a minimum, the patient and when appropriate, his or her family, is informed about the following (EPs 1–2):

C Ⓜ   1. Outcomes of care, treatment, and services that have been provided that the patient (or family) must be knowledgeable about to participate in current and future decisions affecting the patient's care, treatment, and services.

C Ⓜ   2. Unanticipated outcomes of care, treatment, and services that relate to sentinel events considered reviewable* by the Joint Commission.

C Ⓜ   3. The responsible licensed independent practitioner or his or her designee informs the patient (and when appropriate, his or her family) about those unanticipated outcomes of care, treatment, and services (*see* EP 2 above).†

Standard RI.2.100

The hospital respects the patient's right to and need for effective communication.

---

* *See* the "Sentinel Events" chapter of this book for a definition of reviewable sentinel events.

† In settings where there is no licensed independent practitioner, the staff member responsible for the care of the patient is responsible for sharing information about such outcomes.

Ethics, Rights, and Responsibilities

Rationale for RI.2.100
The patient has the right to receive information in a manner that he or she understands. This includes communication between the hospital and the patient, as well as communication between the patient and others outside the hospital.

Elements of Performance for RI.2.100

B   1. The hospital respects the right and need of patients for effective communication.

B   2. Written information provided is appropriate to the age, understanding, and, as appropriate to the population served, the language of the patient.

C Ⓜ   3. The hospital facilitates provision of interpretation (including translation services) as necessary.

C Ⓜ   4. The hospital addresses the needs of those with vision, speech, hearing, language, and cognitive impairments.

B   5. The hospital offers telephone and mail service as appropriate to the setting and population.

Additional Elements of Performance for Hospital Settings That Provide Longer Term Care (More Than 30 Days)

Ⓜ   6. When a hospital restricts a patient's visitors, mail, telephone calls, or other forms of communication, the restrictions are determined with the patient's participation and, when appropriate, his or her family.

C Ⓜ   7. When a hospital restricts a patient's visitors, mail, telephone calls, or other forms of communication, the restrictions are documented along with justification in the clinical or case record.

C Ⓜ   8. When a hospital restricts a patient's visitors, mail, telephone calls, or other forms of communication, the restrictions are evaluated for therapeutic effectiveness.

Standard RI.2.110
Not applicable

Standard RI.2.120
The hospital addresses the resolution of complaints from patients and their families.

Elements of Performance for RI.2.120

C Ⓜ   1. The hospital informs patients, families, and staff about the complaint resolution process.

C Ⓜ   2. The hospital receives, reviews, and, when possible, resolves complaints from patients and their families.

C Ⓜ 3. The hospital responds to individuals making a significant (as defined by the hospital) or recurring complaint.

C Ⓜ 4. The hospital informs patients about their right to file a complaint with the state authority.

C Ⓜ 5. Patients can freely voice complaints and recommend changes without being subject to coercion, discrimination, reprisal, or unreasonable interruption of care, treatment, and services.

Standard RI.2.130
The hospital respects the needs of patients for confidentiality, privacy, and security.

Rationale for RI.2.130
This standard and its EPs allow flexibility in how a hospital can accomplish this requirement. Privacy, safety, and security can be demonstrated in various ways, for example, via policies and procedures, practices, or the design of the environment.

Elements of Performance for RI.2.130
C Ⓜ 1. The hospital protects confidentiality of information about patients.

C Ⓜ 2. The hospital respects the privacy of patients.

C Ⓜ 3. Patients who desire private telephone conversations have access to space and telephones appropriate to their needs and the care, treatment, and services provided.

C Ⓜ 4. The hospital provides for the safety and security of patients and their property.

5. Not applicable

6. Not applicable

Additional Element of Performance for Hospital Settings That Provide Longer Term Care (More Than 30 Days)
B 7. The number of patients in a room is appropriate to the hospital's goals and the patients' ages, developmental levels, clinical conditions, or diagnosis needs.

Standard RI.2.140
Patients have a right to an environment that preserves dignity and contributes to a positive self image.

Rationale for RI.2.140
The hospital creates a supportive environment for all patients. Because a program or unit at times becomes the patient's "home," the hospital provides an atmosphere

Ethics, Rights, and Responsibilities

that supports the patient's dignity. For example, in a long term care unit, patients have space to display greeting cards, calendars, and other personal items important to their well-being.

Elements of Performance for RI.2.140

B   1. The environment of care supports the positive self-image of patients and preserves their human dignity.

B   2. The hospital provides sufficient storage space to meet the personal needs of the patients.

B   3. The hospital allows patients to keep and use personal clothing and possessions, unless this infringes on others' rights or is medically or therapeutically contraindicated (as appropriate to the setting or service).

Standard RI.2.150

Patients have the right to be free from mental, physical, sexual, and verbal abuse, neglect, and exploitation.*

Note: See *standard PC.3.10, which addresses assessing and reporting of abuse, neglect, and exploitation.*

Elements of Performance for RI.2.150

B   1. The hospital addresses how it will, to the best of its ability, protect patients from real or perceived abuse, neglect, or exploitation from anyone, including staff, students, volunteers, other patients, visitors, or family members.

C Ⓜ   2. All allegations, observations, or suspected cases of abuse, neglect, or exploitation that occur in the hospital are investigated by the hospital.

Standard RI.2.160

Patients have the right to pain management.

Rationale for RI.2.160

Patients may experience pain. Unrelieved pain has adverse physical and psychological effects. The hospital respects and supports the right of patients to pain management. In accordance with the hospital's mission, this may occur through referral.

Element of Performance for RI.2.160

B   1. The hospital plans, supports, and coordinates activities and resources to ensure that pain is recognized and addressed appropriately and in accordance with the care, treatment, and services provided including the following:

---

* Taking advantage of another for one's own advantage or benefit.

- Assessing for pain
- Educating all relevant providers about assessing and managing pain
- Educating patients and families, when appropriate, about their roles in managing pain and the potential limitations and side effects of pain treatments

Standard RI.2.170
Patients have a right to access protective and advocacy services.

Elements of Performance for RI.2.170
C Ⓜ 1. When the hospital serves a population of patients who often need protective services (that is, guardianship and advocacy services, conservatorship, and child or adult protective services), it provides resources to help the family and the courts determine the patient's needs for such services.

B 2. When appropriate, the hospital maintains a list of names, addresses, and telephone numbers of pertinent state client advocacy groups such as the state authority and the protection and advocacy network.

C Ⓜ 3. The list is given to patients when requested.

B 4. The hospital develops and implements policies and procedures for the above requirements.

Standard RI.2.180
The hospital protects research subjects and respects their rights during research, investigation, and clinical trials involving human subjects.

Rationale for RI.2.180
A hospital that conducts research, investigations, or clinical trials involving human subjects knows that its first responsibility is to the health and well being of the research subjects. To protect and respect the research subjects' rights, the hospital reviews all research protocols. If another institution's Institutional Review Board (IRB) reviews the research protocols, the hospital does not need to perform this activity.

Elements of Performance for RI.2.180
C Ⓜ 1. The hospital reviews all research protocols in relation to its mission, values, and other guidelines and weighs the relative risks and benefits to the research subjects.

C Ⓜ 2. The hospital provides patients who are potential subjects in research, investigation, and clinical trials with adequate information* to participate or refuse to participate in research.

---

* **Adequate information** includes an explanation of the purpose of the research and expected duration of the subject's participation; a description of expected benefits, potential discomforts, and risks; alternative services that might prove advantageous to the individual; and a full explanation of the procedures to be followed.

Ethics, Rights, and Responsibilities

C Ⓜ 3. Patients are informed that refusing to participate or discontinuing participation at any time will not compromise their access to care, treatment, and services not related to the research.

C Ⓜ 4. Consent forms address the above elements of performance; indicate the name of the person who provided the information and the date the form was signed; and address the participant's right to privacy, confidentiality, and safety.

C Ⓜ 5. Subjects are told the extent to which their personally identifiable private information will be held in confidence.

C Ⓜ 6. All information given to subjects is in the medical record or research file along with the consent forms.

C Ⓜ 7. If a research-related injury (that is, physical, psychological, social, financial, or otherwise) occurs, the principal investigator attempts to address any harmful consequences the subject may have experienced as a result of research procedures.

Applicable Only to Hospital Settings That Provide Longer Term Care (More Than 30 Days)
Standard RI.2.190
In hospitals that provide opportunities for work, a defined policy addresses situations in which patients work.

Rationale for RI.2.190
Patients may be offered the opportunity to perform work for the hospital (for example, work therapy programs in grounds keeping or the library) that does not endanger them, other patients, or staff. If the hospital asks patients to perform such tasks (work), they have the right to refuse.

Elements of Performance for RI.2.190
B 1. Policies and procedures address situations in which patients work.

C Ⓜ 2. Policies and procedures are implemented.

C Ⓜ 3. Wages paid to patients are in accordance with applicable law and regulation.

C Ⓜ 4. Work is addressed in the care, treatment, and service plan.

C Ⓜ 5. Work is performed voluntarily.

Individual Responsibilities

Introduction
The safety of health care delivery is enhanced when patients, as appropriate to their condition, are partners in the health care process. Additionally, hospitals are entitled to reasonable and responsible behavior on the part of the patients, within their capabilities, and their families. The hospital identifies the responsibilities of the patients and their families and educates them about these responsibilities, particularly in regard to facilitating the safe delivery of care, treatment, and services.

The statement of responsibilities includes at least the following:
- **Providing information.** Patients and families, as appropriate, must provide, to the best of their knowledge, accurate and complete information about present complaints, past illnesses, hospitalization, medications, and other matters relating to their health. Patients and their families must report perceived risks in their care and unexpected changes in their condition. They can help the hospital understand their environment by providing feedback about service needs and expectations.
- **Asking questions.** Patients and families, as appropriate, must ask questions when they do not understand their care, treatment, and service or what they are expected to do.
- **Following instructions.** Patients and their families must follow the care, treatment, and service plan developed. They should express any concerns about their ability to follow the proposed care plan or course of care, treatment, and services. The hospital makes every effort to adapt the plan to the specific needs and limitations of the patients. When such adaptations to the care, treatment, and service plan are not recommended, patients and their families are informed of the consequences of the care, treatment, and service alternatives and not following the proposed course.
- **Accepting consequences.** Patients and their families are responsible for the outcomes if they do not follow the care, treatment, and service plan.
- **Following rules and regulations.** Patients and their families must follow the hospital's rules and regulations.
- **Showing respect and consideration.** Patients and their families must be considerate of the hospital's staff and property, as well as other patients and their property.
- **Meeting financial commitments.** Patients and their families should promptly meet any financial obligation agreed to with the hospital.

Standard RI.3.10
Patients are given information about their responsibilities while receiving care, treatment, and services.

Rationale for RI.3.10
The practice identifies patient and family responsibilities and educates them about these responsibilities as appropriate to the services provided. Patients are responsi-

ble for providing accurate and complete information about their symptoms or reason for visit, past illnesses, hospitalizations, medications (including prescribed and nonprescribed medications and herbals), and other matters of care. Patients are also responsible for acknowledging when they do not understand a contemplated treatment course or care decision.

Elements of Performance for RI.3.10

B 1. The hospital has a policy that defines the mechanism for communicating responsibilities of patients.

B 2. The policy includes the responsibilities for providing information, asking questions, following instructions, accepting consequences, following rules and regulations, showing respect and consideration, and meeting financial commitments.

C Ⓜ 3. Patients are informed about their responsibilities verbally, in writing, or both, based on hospital policy.

C Ⓜ 4. Patients are informed about their responsibilities initially and as needed thereafter.

Provision of Care, Treatment, and Services

Overview

Care, treatment, and services are provided through the successful coordination and completion of a series of processes that include appropriate initial assessment of needs; development of a plan for care, treatment, and services; the provision of care, treatment, and services; ongoing assessment of whether the care, treatment, and services provided are meeting the patient's needs, and either the successful discharge of the patient or referral or transfer of the patient for continuing care, treatment, and services.

The provision of care, treatment, and services to patients is composed of four core processes or elements:
1. Assessing patient needs
2. Planning care, treatment, and services
3. Providing the care, treatment, and services the patient needs
4. Coordinating care, treatment, and services

These core elements may also include the following activities:
- Providing access to the appropriate levels of care and/or disciplines for patients
- Providing interventions based on the plan for care, treatment, and services
- Teaching patients what they need to know about their care, treatment, and services
- Coordinating care, treatment, and services, if needed, when the patient is referred, transferred, or discharged

The elements that make up the provision of care, treatment, and services are related to each other through an integrated and cyclical process that may occur over minutes, hours, days, weeks, months, or years, depending on the setting and the needs of the patient. This cyclical process may occur among multiple organizations or within a single organization. The standards in this chapter address the processes in this cycle, including those provided for patient populations with unique needs or patients who are receiving interventions or services that are problem prone.

The core processes or elements of the provision of care, treatment, and services should not be seen as separate steps, rather as interrelated activities in an integrated and ongoing care process. The activities related to the provision of care, treatment, and services should be capable of moving easily between elements as required to meet patients' needs and maintain the continuity of care, treatment, and services.

Standards

The following is a list of all standards for this function. They are presented here for your convenience without footnotes or other explanatory text. If you have a question about a term used here, please check the Glossary.

Note: *A revised standard numbering system is being used with the reformatted standards. The revised numbering system will allow for more flexibility to add standards while maintaining the current number for each standard.*

Entry to Care, Treatment, and Services
PC.1.10 The hospital accepts for care, treatment, and services only those patients whose identified care, treatment, and service needs it can meet.

Assessment
PC.2.10 Not applicable

PC.2.20 The hospital defines in writing the data and information gathered during assessment and reassessment.

PC.2.30 Through PC.2.110 Not applicable

PC.2.120 The hospital defines in writing the time frame(s) for conducting the initial assessment(s).

PC.2.130 Initial assessments are performed as defined by the hospital.

PC.2.140 Not applicable

PC.2.150 Patients are reassessed as needed.

Additional Standard for Victims of Abuse
PC.3.10 Patients who may be victims of abuse or neglect are assessed. (*See standard RI.2.150.*)

PC.3.20 Through PC.3.50 Not applicable

Additional Standards for Patients Being Treated for Addictions
PC.3.60 Through PC.3.110 Not applicable

PC.3.120 The needs of patients receiving psychosocial services to treat alcoholism or other substance use disorders are assessed.

Provision of Care, Treatment, and Services

Additional Standard for Patients Being Treated for Emotional or Behavioral Disorders

PC.3.130   The needs of patients receiving treatment for emotional or behavioral disorders are assessed.

PC.3.140 Through PC.3.220   Not applicable

Diagnostic Services

PC.3.230   Diagnostic testing to determine the patient's health care needs is performed.

Planning Care, Treatment, and Services

PC.4.10   Development of a plan for care, treatment, and services is individualized and appropriate to the patient's needs, strengths, limitations, and goals.

Providing Care, Treatment, and Services

PC.5.10   The hospital provides care, treatment, and services for each patient according to the plan for care, treatment, and services.

PC.5.20   Not applicable

PC.5.30   Not applicable

PC.5.40   Not applicable

PC.5.50   Care, treatment, and services are provided in an interdisciplinary, collaborative manner.

PC.5.60   The hospital coordinates the care, treatment, and services provided to a patient as part of the plan for care, treatment, and services and consistent with the hospital's scope of care, treatment, and services.

Education

PC.6.10   The patient receives education and training specific to the patient's needs and as appropriate to the care, treatment, and services provided.

PC.6.20   Not applicable

PC.6.30   The patient receives education and training specific to the patient's abilities as appropriate to the care, treatment, and services provided by the hospital.

PC.6.40   Not applicable

PC.6.50 The hospital provides academic education to children and youth as needed.

Nutritional Care

PC.7.10 The hospital has a process for preparing and/or distributing food and nutrition products as appropriate to the care, treatment, and services provided.

Pain

PC.8.10 Pain is assessed in all patients.

PC.8.20 Not applicable

PC.8.30 Not applicable

PC.8.40 Not applicable

Access to the Outdoors

PC.8.50 Unless contraindicated, the hospital accommodates patients' needs to be outdoors when patients experience long lengths of stay.

Additional Standard For Hospitals with Behavioral Health Units

PC.8.60 In accordance with patients' needs, good standards of personal hygiene and grooming are taught and maintained, particularly bathing, brushing teeth, caring for hair and nails, and using the toilet, with due regard for privacy.

End-of-Life Care

PC.8.70 Comfort and dignity are optimized during end-of-life care.

Specific Procedures

PC.9.10 Not applicable

PC.9.20 Not applicable

Availability of Resuscitation Services

PC.9.30 Resuscitation services are available throughout the hospital.

Restraint and Seclusion

PC.10.10 Through PC.10.120 Not applicable

PC.11.10 The hospital's leaders determine the hospital's approach to the use of restraint for nonpsychiatric patients and limit its use to those situations where there is appropriate clinical justification.

Provision of Care, Treatment, and Services

PC.11.20 Performance improvement processes seek to identify opportunities to reduce the risks associated with restraint use through preventive strategies, innovative alternatives, and process improvements.

PC.11.30 Hospital policies and procedures guide appropriate and safe use of restraint.

PC.11.40 Any use of restraint (to which these standards apply) is initiated pursuant to either an individual order (standard PC.11.50) or an approved protocol (standard PC.11.60), the use of which is authorized by an individual order.

PC.11.50 Individual orders for initiating and renewing restraint are consistent with hospital policies and procedures and with the patient's needs and clinical condition.

PC.11.60 Protocols for restraint use contain criteria to ensure only clinically justified use.

PC.11.70 Patients in restraint are monitored.

PC.11.80 Not applicable

PC.11.90 Not applicable

PC.11.100 Each episode of restraint use is documented in the patient's medical record, consistent with hospital policies and procedures.

Behavioral Health Care Restraint and Seclusion

PC.12.10 The leaders establish and communicate the hospital's philosophy on restraint and seclusion to all staff with direct care responsibility.

PC.12.20 Staffing levels and assignments are set to minimize circumstances that give rise to restraint or seclusion use and to maximize safety when restraint and seclusion are used.

PC.12.30 Staff is trained and competent to minimize the use of restraint and seclusion and, when use is indicated, to use restraint or seclusion safely.

PC.12.40 The initial assessment of each patient at admission or intake assists in obtaining information about the patient that could help minimize the use of restraint or seclusion.

PC.12.50 Nonphysical techniques are the preferred intervention in behavior management.

PC.12.60 Restraint or seclusion is limited to emergencies in which there is an imminent risk of a patient physically harming himself or herself, staff, or others, and nonphysical interventions would not be effective.

PC.12.70 A licensed independent practitioner orders the use of restraint or seclusion.

PC.12.80 The patient's family is notified promptly of the initiation of restraint or seclusion.

PC.12.90 A licensed independent practitioner sees and evaluates the patient in person.

PC.12.100 Written or verbal orders for initial and continuing use of restraint and seclusion are time limited.

PC.12.110 Patients in restraint or seclusion are regularly reevaluated.

PC.12.120 Clinical leaders are told of instances in which patients experience extended or multiple episodes of restraint or seclusion.

PC.12.130 Patients in restraint or seclusion are assessed and assisted.

PC.12.140 Patients in restraint or seclusion are monitored.

PC.12.150 Restraint and seclusion are discontinued when the patient meets the behavior criteria for their discontinuation.

PC.12.160 The patient and staff participate in a debriefing about the restraint or seclusion episode.

PC.12.170 Medical records document that the use of restraint or seclusion is consistent with hospital policy.

PC.12.180 The hospital collects data on the use of restraint and seclusion.

PC.12.190 Hospital policies and procedures address prevention of restraint and seclusion and, when employed, guide their use.

Standards for Additional Special Procedures
Operative or Other High-Risk Procedures and/or the Administration of Moderate or Deep Sedation or Anesthesia

PC.13.10 Not applicable

PC.13.20 Operative or other procedures and/or the administration of moderate or deep sedation or anesthesia are planned.

PC.13.30 Patients are monitored during the procedure and/or administration of moderate or deep sedation or anesthesia.

PC.13.40 Patients are monitored immediately after the procedure and/or administration of moderate or deep sedation or anesthesia.

Additional Special Procedures
PC.13.50 Electroconvulsive therapy is used with adequate justification, documentation, and regard for patient safety.

PC.13.60 Psychosurgery or other surgical treatments for emotional, mental, or behavioral disorders are performed with adequate justification, documentation, and regard for patient safety.

PC.13.70 Use of behavior management procedures conforms to the patient's treatment plan and hospital policy.

PC.14.10 Through PC.14.30 Not applicable

Discharge or Transfer
PC.15.10 A process addresses the needs for continuing care, treatment, and services after discharge or transfer.

PC.15.20 The transfer or discharge of a patient to another level of care, treatment, and services, different professionals, or different settings is based on the patient's assessed needs and the hospital's capabilities.

PC.15.30 When patients are transferred or discharged, appropriate information related to the care, treatment, and services provided is exchanged with other service providers.

Waived Testing
PC.16.10 The hospital establishes policies and procedures that define the context in which waived test results are used in patient care, treatment, and services.

PC.16.20 The hospital identifies the staff responsible for performing and supervising waived testing.

PC.16.30 Staff performing tests have adequate, specific training and orientation to perform the tests and demonstrates satisfactory levels of competence.

PC.16.40 Approved policies and procedures governing specific testing-related processes are current and readily available.

PC.16.50 Quality control checks, as defined by the hospital, are conducted on each procedure.

PC.16.60 Appropriate quality control and test records are maintained.

Provision of Care, Treatment, and Services

Understanding the Parts of This Chapter

To help you navigate this reformatted standards chapter, it may be helpful to think of its parts this way:
- The **standard** is the "goal."
- The **rationale** explains why it's important to achieve this goal.
- The **elements of performance** identify the step(s) needed to achieve this goal.

These parts are defined as follows.

Standard A statement that defines the performance expectations and/or structures or processes that must be in place in order for a hospital to provide safe, high-quality care, treatment, and services. A hospital is either "compliant" or "not compliant" with a standard.

Accreditation decisions are based on simple counts of the standards that are determined to be "not compliant."

Rationale A statement that provides background, justification, or additional information about a standard. A standard's rationale is not scored. In some instances, the rationale for a standard is self-evident. Therefore, not every standard has a written rationale.

Elements of performance (EPs) The specific performance expectations and/or structures or processes that must be in place in order for a hospital to provide safe, high-quality care, treatment, and services. The scoring of EP compliance determines a hospital's overall compliance with a standard. EPs are evaluated on the following scale:

- **0** Insufficient compliance
- **1** Partial compliance
- **2** Satisfactory compliance
- **NA** Not applicable

You will find a **measure of success** icon—Ⓜ—next to some EPs. Measures of success (MOS) need to be developed for certain EPs when a standard is judged to be out of compliance through either the Periodic Performance Review (PPR) or the onsite survey. An MOS is defined as a quantifiable measure, usually related to an audit, that can be used to determine whether an action has been effective and is being sustained.*

Assessing Your Compliance

Once you are familiar with the parts of this chapter, you can begin to assess your compliance with its requirements. The scoring category for each EP is noted next to the EP. If you would like to assess your hospital's performance, mark your scores for the EPs and the standards by following the simple steps described below.

---

* For more information about measures of success, *see* the "The New Joint Commission Accreditation Process" chapter in this book.

Two components are scored for each EP: (1) compliance with the requirement itself **and** (2) compliance with the track record* for that requirement. Scoring has been simplified, and track record achievements (which have always been part of the scoring) have been appropriately modified.

Note: *Some standards and EPs do not apply to a particular type of organization; these standards and EPs are marked "not applicable" and the related text is not included. Your hospital is not expected to comply with standards and EPs marked "not applicable."*

In addition, some standards and EPs that do apply to organizations may not apply to the specific care, treatment, and services that your individual hospital provides. Although these standards and EPs are included in the manual, you are not expected to comply with them. If you are unsure about the standards or EPs that apply to your hospital, please contact the Joint Commission's Standards Interpretation Group at 630/792-5900.

Step 1: Score Your Compliance with Each Element of Performance

Before you can determine your compliance with the standards, you must score your compliance with each EP. There are three scoring criterion categories: A, B, and C (described below). Please note that for each EP scoring criterion category, your hospital must meet the performance requirement itself and the track record achievements (*see* "Track Record Achievements").

Category A
These EPs relate to the presence or absence of the requirement(s) and are scored either yes (2) or no (0); however, score 1 for partial compliance is also possible based on track record achievements.

If an A EP has multiple components designated by bullets, your hospital must be compliant with all the bullets to receive a score of 2. If your hospital does not meet one or more requirements in the bullets, you will receive a score of 0.

Category B
Category B EPs are scored in two steps:
1. As with category A EPs, category B EPs relate to the presence or absence of the requirement(s). If your hospital *does not meet* the requirement(s), the EP is scored 0; there is no need to assess your compliance with the principles of good process design.
2. If your hospital *does meet* the requirement(s), but there is concern about the quality or comprehensiveness of the effort, then and only then should you assess the qualitative aspect of the EP. That is, review the applicable principles of good process design and ask how the principles were applied in the situation under discussion. Good process design has the following characteristics:

---
* **Track record** The amount of time that an organization has been in compliance with a standard, element of performance, or other requirement.

- Is consistent with your hospital's mission, values, and goals
- Meets the needs of patients
- Reflects the use of currently accepted practices (doing the right thing, using resources responsibly, using practice guidelines)
- Incorporates current safety information and knowledge such as sentinel event data and National Patient Safety Goals
- Incorporates relevant performance improvement results

This two-part evaluation applies to both simple and bulleted B EPs. First, the EPs are assessed to determine if the requirements are present. If the EP has multiple components designated by bullets, as with the category A EPs, your hospital must meet the requirements in *all* the bulleted items to get a score of 2. If your hospital meets *none* of the requirements in the bullets, it receives a score of 0. If your hospital meets *at least one, but not all*, of the bulleted requirements, it will receive a score of 1 for the EPs.

Use the following rules to determine your EP score:
- Your EP score is 0 if your hospital does not meet the requirement(s); you *do not* need to assess your compliance with the preceding applicable principles of good process design
- Your EP score is 1 if your hospital does meet the requirement(s), but considered only *some* of the preceding applicable principles of good process design
- Your EP score is 2 if your hospital does meet the requirement(s) *and* considered *all* the preceding principles of good process design

Category C

C EPs are scored 0, 1, or 2 based on the number of times your hospital does not meet the EP. These EPs are frequency based and require totaling the number of occurrences (that is, results of performance or nonperformance) related to a particular EP. Each situation discovered by a surveyor(s) will be counted as a separate occurrence.

Note: *Multiple events of the same type related to a single patient and single practitioner/staff member are counted as* one occurrence only.

Use the following rules to determine your EP score:
- Your EP score is 2 if you find one or fewer occurrences of noncompliance with the EP
- Your EP score is 1 if you find two occurrences of noncompliance with the EP
- Your EP score is 0 if you find three or more occurrences of noncompliance with the EP

If an EP in the C category has multiple requirements designated by bullets, the following scoring guidelines apply:
- If there are fewer than 2 findings in all bullets, the EP is scored 2
- If there are three or more findings in all bullets, the EP is scored 0
- In all other combinations of findings, the EP is scored 1

Track Record Achievements

In addition to meeting the requirement(s) in each EP, regardless of category, your hospital must also meet the following track record achievements:

Score	Initial Survey	Full Survey
2	4 months or more	12 months or more
1	2 to 3 months	6 to 11 months
0	Fewer than 2 months	Fewer than 6 months

Sample Sizes

If during an onsite survey, your hospital has been found to be not compliant with one or more standards, you must demonstrate Evidence of Standards Compliance (ESC) for each standard that is not compliant. The ESC must address compliance at the EP level; when an EP within a noncompliant standard requires an MOS, your hospital must demonstrate achievement with the MOS when completing the ESC.

Note: *Not every EP requires an MOS. EPs that do require an MOS are clearly marked in this chapter. Organizations are required to demonstrate achievement with an MOS only for EPs within a noncompliant standard that require an MOS. Organizations do not need to demonstrate achievement with an MOS for any EP within a compliant standard.*

When demonstrating achievement with the MOS during the ESC process, your hospital is **required** to use the following sample sizes, which were established because of their statistical significance, their relative simplicity in application, and their sensitivity to an organization's population size:
- For a population size of fewer than 30 cases, sample 100% of available cases
- For a population size of 30 to 100 cases, sample 30 cases
- For a population size of 101 to 500 cases, sample 50 cases
- For a population size greater than 500 cases, sample 70 cases

Note: *Hospitals are encouraged, but not required, to follow this sample size when demonstrating achievement with an MOS for an EP within a noncompliant standard after conducting a full, Option 1, or Option 2 Periodic Performance Review (PPR).*

When conducting PPR (optional use) or demonstrating an ESC (mandatory use), use the following percentages to determine your score: 90% through 100% of your sample size is in compliance = score 2; 80% through 89% (two instances of noncompliance) of your sample size is in compliance = score 1; less than 80% (three or more instances of noncompliance) of your sample size is in compliance = score 0.

In addition, the following information should govern your hospital's selection of samples:
- The appropriate sample size should be determined by the specific population related to the survey findings
- The sampling approach should involve either systematic random sampling (for example, your hospital selects every second or third case for review) or simple random sampling (for example, your hospital uses a series of random numbers generated by a computer to identify the cases to be reviewed)

Provision of Care, Treatment, and Services

- If your hospital chooses not to use these sample sizes while conducting PPR options 1 or 2, you should make sure that your sample size is sufficiently large enough to ensure statistical significance
- When submitting a clarifying ESC, if your hospital selects records as part of its sample, the records should be from a period of no more than three months before the last date of the survey
- Assessment of MOS compliance is conducted for a four-month period following the date of ESC approval. Your hospital should select records as a part of your sample following the date of ESC approval and use the required sample sizes. MOS percentage compliance rates are derived from the average of all four months.

Step 2: Use Your EP Scores to Gauge Your Compliance with the Standards

Now that you have evaluated and scored each EP for a particular standard, use these simple rules to determine your compliance with the standard itself:

- Your hospital is not in compliance (that is, "not compliant") with the standard if any EP is scored 0
- Otherwise, your hospital is in compliance with a standard if 65% or more of its EPs are scored 2

Standards, Rationales, Elements of Performance, and Scoring

Entry to Care, Treatment, and Services

Agreeing to provide care, treatment, and services for a patient should be based both on the patient's needs and the scope of the services provided by the hospital. To do this, the hospital does the following:
- Establishes criteria to determine entry eligibility
- Defines the minimum information necessary to determine the patient's eligibility for entry to a program or service
- Defines the appropriate professionals and settings needed to provide the services offered consistent with the hospital's mission
- Makes entry decisions for appropriate care, treatment, and services offered by the hospital based on these criteria

Standard PC.1.10
The hospital accepts for care, treatment, and services only those patients whose identified care, treatment, and service needs it can meet.

Elements of Performance for PC.1.10

B 1. The hospital has a defined written process that includes the following:
- The information to be gathered to determine eligibility for entrance into the hospital
- The populations of patients accepted or not accepted by the hospital (for example, programs designed to treat adults that do not treat young children)
- The criteria to determine eligibility for entry into the system
- The procedures for accepting referrals

2. Through 8. Not applicable

C Ⓜ 9. The hospital accepts patients for care, treatment, and services according to established processes.

Assessment

The goal of assessment is to determine the appropriate care, treatment, and services to meet a patient's initial needs as well as his or her changing needs while in the setting.

Identifying and delivering appropriate care, treatment, and services depends on three processes:

1. *Collecting data* about each patient's health history; physical, functional, and psychosocial status; and needs as appropriate to the setting and circumstances
2. *Analyzing data* to produce information about patients' needs for care, treatment, and services and to identify the need for additional data
3. *Making care, treatment, and service decisions* based on information developed about each patient's needs and his or her response to care, treatment, and services

Qualified staff assesses each patient's care needs throughout the patient's contact with the hospital through assessments or screenings. These activities may also identify the need for additional assessments or planning. These assessments are as follows:
- Defined by the hospital
- Individualized to meet each patient's needs
- Address the needs of special populations

The process defined by the hospital identifies the patient's physical, cognitive, behavioral, emotional, and psychosocial status. This assessment identifies facilitating factors and possible barriers to the patient reaching his or her goals including the presenting problems and needs, such as the following:
- Symptoms that might be associated with a disease, condition, or treatment (such as pain, nausea, or dyspnea)
- Social barriers including cultural and language barriers
- Social and environmental factors
- Physical disabilities
- Vision and hearing impairments and disabilities
- Developmental disabilities
- Communicative disorders
- Cognitive disorders
- Emotional, behavioral, and mental disorders
- Substance abuse, dependence, and other addictive behaviors

The depth and frequency of the assessment or screening depend on a number of factors, including the patient's needs, program goals, and the care, treatment, and services provided. Assessment or screening activities may vary between settings, as defined by the clinical and other leaders of the hospital. Patient screenings, assessments and reassessments need to be done and documented within a reasonable time frame to identify the patient's needs and determine if these needs are being met.

Information gathered at the first contact can indicate the need for more data or a more intensive assessment of the patient's physical, psychological, cognitive and communicative skills or development, or social functioning. At a minimum, the need for further assessment is determined by the care, treatment, and services sought; the patient's presenting condition(s); and whether the patient agrees to care, treatment, and services.

Standard PC.2.10
Not applicable

Standard PC.2.20
The hospital defines in writing the data and information gathered during assessment and reassessment.

Elements of Performance for PC.2.20

B   1. The hospital's written definition of the data and information gathered during assessment and reassessment includes the following:
- The scope of assessment and reassessment activities by each discipline
- The content of the assessment and reassessment
- The criteria for when an additional or more in-depth assessment is done*

B   2. The screening, assessment, and reassessment activities described are within the scope of practice, state licensure laws, applicable regulations, or certification of the discipline doing the assessment.

A   3. If applicable, separate specialized assessment and reassessment information is identified for the various populations served.

B   4. The information defined by the hospital to be gathered during the initial assessment includes the following, as relevant to the care, treatment, and services:
- Physical assessment, as appropriate
- Psychological assessment, as appropriate
- Social assessment, as appropriate
- Each patient's nutrition and hydration status, as appropriate
- Each patient's functional status, as appropriate
- For patients receiving end-of-life care, the social, spiritual, and cultural variables that influence the perceptions and expressions of grief by the patient, family members, or significant others

B   5. The hospital has defined criteria for when nutritional plans must be developed.

Standards PC.2.30 Through PC.2.110
Not applicable

---

* For example, nutritional or functional risk assessments may be defined for at-risk patients. In such cases, nutritional risk criteria should be developed by dieticians or other qualified individuals, and functional risk criteria should be developed by rehabilitation specialists or other qualified individuals.

Provision of Care, Treatment, and Services

Standard PC.2.120
The hospital defines in writing the time frame(s) for conducting the initial assessment(s).

Elements of Performance for PC.2.120
A   1.   The hospital defines the time frame(s) for conducting the initial assessment(s).

The hospital specifies the following time frames for these assessments (EPs 2–5):

A   2.   A medical history and physical examination is completed within no more than 24 hours of inpatient admission

A   3.   A registered nurse completes a nursing assessment within 24 hours of inpatient admission

A   4.   A nutritional screening, when warranted by the patients' needs or condition, is completed within no more than 24 hours of inpatient admission

A   5.   A functional status screening, when warranted by the patient's needs or condition, is completed within no more than 24 hours of inpatient admission

Some of these elements may have been completed ahead of time, but must meet the following criteria:

A   6.   The history and physical must have been completed within 30 days before the patient was admitted or readmitted

A   7.   Updates to the patient's condition since the assessment(s) are recorded at the time of admission

Standard PC.2.130
Initial assessments are performed as defined by the hospital.

Elements of Performance for PC.2.130
C Ⓜ   1.   Each patient is assessed per hospital policy.

C Ⓜ   2.   Each patient's initial assessment is conducted within the time frame specified by the needs of the patient, hospital policy, and law and regulation.

A   3.   A registered nurse assesses the patient's need for nursing care in all settings, as required by law, regulation, or hospital policy.

Standard PC.2.140
Not applicable

Standard PC.2.150
Patients are reassessed* as needed.

Rationale for PC.2.150
Each patient may be reassessed for many reasons including the following:
- To evaluate his or her response to care, treatment, and services
- To respond to a significant change in status and/or diagnosis or condition
- To satisfy legal or regulatory requirements
- To meet time intervals specified by the hospital
- To meet time intervals determined by the course of the care, treatment, and services for the patient

Element of Performance for PC.2.150
C Ⓜ 1. Each patient is reassessed as needed.

Additional Standard for Victims of Abuse
Standard PC.3.10
Patients who may be victims of abuse or neglect are assessed. (*See* standard RI.2.150.)

Rationale for PC.3.10
Victims of abuse or neglect may come to a hospital in a variety of ways. The patient may be unable or may be reluctant to speak of the abuse, and it may not be obvious to the casual observer. Staff needs to be able to identify abuse or neglect as well as the extent and circumstances of the abuse or neglect to give the patient appropriate care.

Criteria for identifying and assessing victims of abuse, neglect, or exploitation should be used throughout the hospital. The assessment of the patient must be conducted within the context of the requirements of the law to preserve evidentiary materials and support future legal actions.

Elements of Performance for PC.3.10
A 1. The hospital develops or adopts criteria† for identifying victims in each of the following situations:
- Physical assault
- Rape
- Sexual molestation
- Domestic abuse
- Elder neglect or abuse
- Child neglect or abuse

---

* The scope and intensity of any further assessments are based on the patient's diagnosis; the setting; the patient's desire for care, treatment, and services; and the patient's response to any previous care, treatment, and services.

† The Family Violence Prevention Fund is one resource that can be contacted for further information at http://www.fvpf.org.

Provision of Care, Treatment, and Services

B   2. Appropriate staff* is educated about abuse or neglect and how to refer as appropriate.

A   3. A list of private and public community agencies that provide or arrange for assessment and care of abuse victims is maintained to facilitate appropriate referrals.

B   4. Victims of abuse or neglect are identified using the criteria developed or adopted by the hospital at entry into the system and on an ongoing basis.

B   5. The hospital's staff refers appropriately or conducts the assessment of victims of abuse or neglect.

A   6. All cases of possible abuse or neglect are reported to appropriate agencies according to hospital policy and law and regulation.

A   7. All cases of possible abuse or neglect are immediately reported in the hospital.

Standards PC.3.20 Through PC.3.110
Not applicable

Additional Standard for Patients Being Treated for Addictions
Obtaining and interpreting information about substance abuse, dependence, or other addictive behaviors is necessary to develop treatment plans. By gathering the data and information on the items listed in the standards, the clinician can assess the relationship of the physical state of each patient to the dependence; assess the nature of the patient's compulsion to use alcohol, drugs, or other addictive behaviors; assess the intensity of the patient's mental preoccupation with alcohol, drugs, or other addictive behaviors such as gambling; and distinguish between alcohol-related symptoms, drug-related symptoms, and symptoms of other addictive behaviors and other preexisting physical problems or pathologic behaviors.

Standard PC.3.120
The needs of patients receiving psychosocial services to treat alcoholism or other substance use disorders are assessed.

Elements of Performance for PC.3.120

A   1. The content of the assessment and reassessment of patients receiving psychosocial services to treat alcoholism includes at least the following:
- The patient's history of alcohol, nicotine, and other drug use, including age of onset, duration, intensity, patterns of use (for example, loss of control over amounts or frequencies of consumption, inability to consistently abstain from use, relapse), and consequences of use

---

* Staff should be able to screen for abuse and neglect as indicated by the patient's needs or conditions. The organization may define who conducts the full assessment for alleged or suspected abuse or neglect or refer to another organization.

- Types of previous treatment and responses to that treatment
- A history of mental, emotional, and behavioral problems; their co-occurrence with substance use problems; and their treatment
- A history of biomedical complications associated with alcohol, nicotine, or other drug use and the patient's level of awareness of the relationships between these behavioral conditions and his or her pattern of substance use
- A psychosocial assessment

B 2. As appropriate to the patient's age and specific clinical needs, the psychosocial assessment includes information about the following:
- Treatment acceptance or motivation for change
- Recovery environment features that serve as resources or obstacles to recovery, including the use of alcohol and other drugs by family members
- The patient's religion and spiritual orientation
- Any history of physical or sexual abuse, as either the abuser or the abused
- The patient's sexual history and orientation
- Environment and home
- Leisure and recreation
- Childhood history
- Military service history
- Financial status
- The patient's social, peer-group, and living situation
- The patient's family circumstances, including the constellation of the family group
- The patient's current living situation
- Social, ethnic, cultural, emotional, and health factors

B 3. Those responsible for the patient's care determine the need for family members to participate in the patient's care.

B 4. As appropriate, the following additional assessments are conducted:
- Vocational or education assessment
- Legal assessment
- Other functional evaluation of communication, self-care, and visual-motor functioning

Additional Standard for Patients Being Treated for Emotional or Behavioral Disorders
Standard PC.3.130

The needs of patients receiving treatment for emotional or behavioral disorders are assessed.

Elements of Performance for PC.3.130

A 1. The content of the assessment and reassessment of patients being treated for emotional and behavioral disorders includes at least the following:

- A history of mental, emotional, behavioral, and substance use problems; their co-occurrence; and treatment
- Current mental, emotional, and behavioral functioning, including a mental status examination
- Maladaptive or problem behaviors
- A psychosocial assessment

B 2. As appropriate to the patient's age and specific clinical needs, the psychosocial assessment includes information about the following:
- Environment and home
- Leisure and recreation
- Religion
- Childhood history
- Military service history
- Financial status
- The social, peer-group, and environmental setting from which the patient comes
- Sexual history, including abuse (either as the abuser or the abused)
- Physical abuse (either as the abuser or the abused)
- The patient's family circumstances, including the constellation of the family group
- The current living situation
- Social, ethnic, cultural, emotional, and health factors

B 3. Those responsible for the patient's care determine the need for family members to participate in the patient's care.

B 4. As appropriate, the following additional assessments are conducted:
- Vocational or educational assessment
- Legal assessment

C Ⓜ 5. The community resources currently used by the patient (especially for those with severe and persistent mental illness) are identified.

B 6. When indicated by the patient's age and specific clinical needs, the following are performed:
- A psychiatric evaluation
- Psychological assessments, including intellectual, projective, neuropsychological, and personality testing
- Other functional evaluations of communication, self-care, and visual-motor functioning

Standards PC.3.140 Through PC.3.220

Not applicable

Diagnostic Services

Standard PC.3.230
Diagnostic testing* necessary for determining the patient's health care needs is performed.

Elements of Performance for PC.3.230
C Ⓜ 1. Diagnostic testing and procedures are performed as ordered.

C Ⓜ 2. Diagnostic testing and procedures are performed in a timely manner as defined by the hospital.

C Ⓜ 3. When a test report requires clinical interpretation, relevant information is provided with the request.

Planning Care, Treatment, and Services
Planning includes creating an initial plan for care, treatment, and services appropriate to the patient's specific assessed needs, and then revising or maintaining the plan based on the patient's response. Planning for care, treatment, and services is individualized to meet the patient's unique needs and circumstances. Performed by qualified individuals, planning for care, treatment, and services involves using an interdisciplinary approach when warranted and involving the patient to the extent possible.

The plan may be modified or terminated based on reassessment; the patient's need for further care, treatment, and services; or the achievement of plan of care goals. This modification may result in planning for the patient's transfer to another setting or service or discharge from the hospital.

Standard PC.4.10
Development of a plan for care, treatment, and services is individualized and appropriate to the patient's needs, strengths, limitations, and goals.

Rationale for PC.4.10
Planning care, treatment, and services is not limited to developing a written plan. Rather, planning is a dynamic process that addresses the execution of care, treatment, and services. The plan for care, treatment, and services must be consistently re-evaluated to ensure that the patient's needs are met. Planning for care, treatment, and services includes the following:
- Integrating assessment findings in the care-planning process

---

* Diagnostic testing includes laboratory, radiologic, electrodiagnostic, and other functional tests and imaging technologies.

Provision of Care, Treatment, and Services

- Developing a plan for care, treatment, and services that includes patient care goals that are reasonable and measurable
- Regularly reviewing and revising the plan for care, treatment, and services
- Determining how the planned care, treatment, and services will be provided
- Documenting the plan for care, treatment, and services
- Monitoring the effectiveness of care planning and the provision of care, treatment, and services
- Involving patients and/or families in care planning

Elements of Performance for PC.4.10

B   1. Care, treatment, and services are planned to ensure that they are appropriate to the patient's needs.

B   2. Development of a plan for care, treatment, and services is based on the data from assessments.

       3. Not applicable

       4. Not applicable

       5. Not applicable

B   6. Patient needs, goals, time frames, settings, and services required to meet the patient needs and/or goals determine the plan for care, treatment, and services.

       7. Through 11. Not applicable

C Ⓜ 12. Evaluation of the patient is based on the patient care goals and the patient's plan for care, treatment, and services.

C Ⓜ 13. The goals of care, treatment, and services are revised when necessary.

B   14. Plans for care, treatment, and services are revised when necessary.

      15. Not applicable

      16. Not applicable

B   17. The plan for care, treatment, and services considers strategies to limit the use of restraints or seclusion as appropriate.

Providing Care, Treatment, and Services

Caring for patients involves providing individualized, planned, and appropriate interventions in settings responsive to specific individual needs. "Care" includes care, treatment, services, rehabilitation, habilitation, or another intervention provided to the patient by the hospital.

The goal of providing effective care, treatment, and services is met when the following are performed well:

- Intervening in a collaborative manner (in light of assessed patient needs)
- Educating the patient
- Promoting health and providing appropriate preventive care
- Providing supportive care, treating a disease or condition, and/or treating symptoms (such as pain, nausea, or dyspnea) using accepted professional standards of practice
- Meeting the patient's nourishment needs, if appropriate to the setting
- Helping patients with appropriate restorative services, including assistance with activities of daily living, such as eating, dressing, grooming, bathing, oral hygiene, ambulation, and toilet activities
- Rehabilitating physical, communicative, or psychosocial impairment or maintaining the patient's level of functioning
- Coordinating the care, treatment, and services provided to a patient
- Optimizing comfort and dignity during end-of-life care
- Involving families as indicated and acceptable to the patient

All interventions should respect and encourage the patient's ability to make choices, to develop and maintain a sense of achievement about attaining their personal health goals, and to choose to continue or modify participation in the care process.

The activities comprising care, treatment, and services may be performed by a variety of staff whose roles and responsibilities are determined by the component of care, treatment, and service being provided; relevant licensure; law and regulation; registration; certification; scope of practice; job description; or privileges.

Standard PC.5.10

The hospital provides care, treatment, and services for each patient according to the plan for care, treatment, and services.

Elements of Performance for PC.5.10

C Ⓜ 1. The hospital provides care, treatment, and services for each patient according to the plan for care, treatment, and services.

2. Not applicable

3. Not applicable

A 4. The hospital uses at least two patient identifiers (neither to be the patient's room number) whenever taking blood samples or administering medications or blood or blood products.

Standard PC.5.20

Not applicable

Provision of Care, Treatment, and Services

Standard PC.5.30
Not applicable

Standard PC.5.40
Not applicable

Standard PC.5.50
Care, treatment, and services are provided in an interdisciplinary, collaborative manner.

Rationale for PC.5.50
A collaborative, interdisciplinary approach to meeting the patient's needs and goals helps to coordinate care, treatment, and services and achieve optimal outcomes. The mix of disciplines involved and the intensity of the collaboration will vary as appropriate to each patient and the scope of services provided by the hospital. (*See* standards MS.2.10 and MS.2.20.) An interdisciplinary approach should not be interpreted as a requirement for an interdisciplinary care plan or the signing of other individual's notes. While an interdisciplinary care plan may be one method of accomplishing this goal, it is not required.

Element of Performance for PC.5.50
B 1. Care, treatment, and services are provided in an interdisciplinary, collaborative manner as appropriate to the needs of the patient and the hospital's scope of services.

Standard PC.5.60
The hospital coordinates the care, treatment, and services provided to a patient as part of the plan for care, treatment, and services and consistent with the hospital's scope of care, treatment, and services.

Rationale for PC.5.60
Throughout the provision of care, treatment, and services, patients should be matched with appropriate internal and external resources to meet their ongoing needs in a timely manner. Care, treatment, and services should be coordinated between providers and between settings, independent of whether they are provided directly or through written agreement.

Elements of Performance for PC.5.60
B 1. The hospital coordinates the care, treatment, and services provided through internal resources to a patient.

B 2. When external resources are needed, the hospital participates in coordinating care, treatment, and services with these resources.

B   3. The hospital has a process to receive or share relevant patient information to facilitate appropriate coordination and continuity when patients are referred to other care, treatment, and service providers.

B   4. There is a process to resolve duplication or conflict with either internal or external resources.

B   5. The plan of care, treatment, and services is designed to occur in a time frame that meets the patient's health needs.

Education

Standard PC.6.10
The patient receives education and training specific to the patient's needs and as appropriate to the care, treatment, and services provided.

Rationale for PC.6.10
Patients must be given sufficient information to make decisions and to take responsibility for self-management activities related to their needs. Patients and, as appropriate, their families are educated to improve individual outcomes by promoting healthy behavior and appropriately involving patients in their care, treatment, and service decisions.

Elements of Performance for PC.6.10

B   1. Education provided is appropriate to the patient's needs.

C Ⓜ 2. The assessment of learning needs addresses cultural and religious beliefs, emotional barriers, desire and motivation to learn, physical or cognitive limitations, and barriers to communication as appropriate.

B   3. As appropriate to the patient's condition and assessed needs and the hospital's scope of services, the patient is educated about the following:
- The plan for care, treatment, and services
- Basic health practices and safety
- The safe and effective use of medications
- Nutrition interventions, modified diets, or oral health
- Safe and effective use of medical equipment or supplies when provided by the hospital
- Understanding pain, the risk for pain, the importance of effective pain management, the pain assessment process, and methods for pain management
- Habilitation or rehabilitation techniques to help them reach the maximum independence possible

Standard PC.6.20
Not applicable

Standard PC.6.30
The patient receives education and training specific to the patient's abilities as appropriate to the care, treatment, and services provided by the hospital.

Rationale for PC.6.30
Learning styles vary, and the ability to learn can be affected by many factors including individual learning preferences and readiness to learn. Educational activities must be tailored to meet the patient's needs and abilities.

Elements of Performance for PC.6.30
B   1. Education provided is appropriate to the patient's abilities.

B   2. Education is coordinated among the disciplines providing care, treatment, and services.

B   3. The content is presented in an understandable manner.

B   4. Teaching methods accommodate various learning styles.

C Ⓜ   5. Comprehension is evaluated.

Standard PC.6.40
Not applicable

Standard PC.6.50
The hospital provides academic education to children and youth as needed.

Rationale for PC.6.50
Providing academic education helps maintain the educational and intellectual development of children and youth and helps to keep them from falling behind. When school-age children or youth are in the hospital for long periods, state or local laws may specify the requirements for meeting their schooling needs.

Elements of Performance for PC.6.50
A   1. The hospital defines the length of stay and absence from school that would require providing educational services in accordance with applicable law and regulation.

B   2. The hospital addresses the specific academic educational needs of children and youth.

Nutritional Care

This standard focuses on providing appropriate nutritional care, including food and nutrition therapy, in a timely and efficient manner using appropriate resources. Elements of nutritional care, such as screening or assessment and education, are addressed in other standards in this manual.

Standard PC.7.10
The hospital has a process for preparing and/or distributing food and nutrition products as appropriate to the care, treatment, and services provided.

Elements of Performance for PC.7.10

B 1. Food and nutrition products are provided for the patient as appropriate to care, treatment, and services.

C Ⓜ 2. Food and nutrition products are stored and prepared under proper conditions of sanitation, temperature, light, moisture, ventilation, and security.

C Ⓜ 3. Patients' cultural, religious, and ethnic food preferences are honored, when possible, unless contraindicated.

C Ⓜ 4. Substitutes of equal nutritional value are offered when patients refuse the food served.

5. Not applicable

A 6. Responsibilities are assigned for all activities involved in safely and accurately providing food and nutrition products.

C Ⓜ 7. Foods brought in by patients are stored appropriately.

8. Not applicable

9. Not applicable

10. Not applicable

C Ⓜ 11. Special diets and altered diet schedules are accommodated.

Pain

Standard PC.8.10
Pain is assessed in all patients.*

---

* Effective July 1, 2004.

Provision of Care, Treatment, and Services

Rationale for PC.8.10*

The identification and treatment of pain is an important component of the plan of care. Individuals are assessed based upon their clinical presentation, services sought, and in accordance with the care, treatment, and services provided.

Elements of Performance for PC.8.10

C Ⓜ 1. A comprehensive pain assessment is conducted as appropriate to the patient's condition and the scope of care, treatment, and services provided.

2. Not applicable

C Ⓜ 3. Regular reassessment and follow-up occur according to criteria developed by the hospital.

4. Not applicable

5. Not applicable

C Ⓜ 6. The assessment methods are appropriate to the patient's age and/or abilities.

C Ⓜ 7. When pain is identified, the patient is treated by the hospital or referred for treatment.

Standard PC.8.20
Not applicable

Standard PC.8.30
Not applicable

Standard PC.8.40
Not applicable

Access to the Outdoors

Standard PC.8.50
Unless contraindicated, the hospital accommodates patients' needs to be outdoors when patients experience long lengths of stay.[†]

---

* Effective July 1, 2004.

[†] For behavioral health care, this applies only to 24-hour settings.

Rationale for PC.8.50
Patient access to the outdoors can be therapeutic. The hospital can provide access on its own grounds, or it can use community resources.

Element of Performance for PC.8.50
B   1. The hospital arranges for safe access to the outdoors as appropriate to the population.

Additional Standard for Hospitals with Behavioral Health Units

Standard PC.8.60
In accordance with patients' needs, good standards of personal hygiene and grooming are taught and maintained, particularly bathing, brushing teeth, caring for hair and nails, and using the toilet, with due regard for privacy.

Elements of Performance for PC.8.60
C Ⓜ   1. Articles for grooming and personal hygiene appropriate to the patient's age, developmental level, and needs are readily available and accessible.

C Ⓜ   2. Patients are encouraged to take responsibility for maintaining their own living quarters and for day-to-day housekeeping activities of the program, as appropriate.

C Ⓜ   3. An oral care program is implemented as indicated by the patient's needs.

C Ⓜ   4. The hospital offers education on grooming activities based on each patient's needs.

C Ⓜ   5. As appropriate to the setting and length of stay, patients have access to the services of a barber or beautician, either in the hospital or community.

C Ⓜ   6. Patients get the help needed to perform these activities and, when indicated, assume responsibility for self care.

B   7. Incontinent patients are cleaned or bathed immediately after voiding or soiling, with due regard for privacy.

Provision of Care, Treatment, and Services

End-of-Life Care

Standard PC.8.70
Comfort and dignity are optimized during end-of-life care.*

Rationale for PC.8.70
The patient at or near the end of his or her life has the right to physical and psychological comfort. The hospital provides care that optimizes the dying patient's comfort and dignity and addresses the patient's and his or her family's psychosocial and spiritual needs.

Elements of Performance for PC.8.70
B   1. To the extent possible, as appropriate to the patient's and family's needs and the hospital's services, interventions address patient and family comfort, dignity, and psychosocial, emotional, and spiritual needs, as appropriate, about death and grief.

C Ⓜ   2. Staff is educated about the unique needs of dying patients and their families and caregivers.

Specific Procedures

Standard PC.9.10
Not applicable

Standard PC.9.20
Not applicable

Availability of Resuscitation Services

Standard PC.9.30
Resuscitation services are available throughout the hospital.

Elements of Performance for PC.9.30
B   1. Policies, procedures, processes, or protocols govern the provision of resuscitation services.

---

* Applies to all dying patients, not just hospice patients, for whom an organization may provide care, treatment, and services.

A   2.   Equipment is appropriate to the patient population (for example, adult, pediatric).

A   3.   Appropriate equipment is placed strategically throughout the hospital.

A   4.   Appropriate staff is trained and competent to recognize the need for and use of designated equipment in resuscitation efforts.

Standards PC.10.10 Through PC.10.120
Not applicable

Restraint and Seclusion

Applicability of these Restraint Standards in Acute Medical and Surgical (Nonpsychiatric) Care

Standards PC.11.10 through PC.11.100 apply to the use of restraint in medical and surgical care, which includes patients receiving pediatric, obstetrical, or rehabilitation care. This includes patients of any age who are as follows:
- Hospitalized in an acute care hospital to receive medical or surgical services
- In the emergency department for assessment, stabilization, or treatment for other than behavioral health care reasons
- In medical observation beds
- Undergoing same-day surgical or other ambulatory health care procedures
- Undergoing rehabilitation as an outpatient or inpatient

The specific device used to restrain a patient does not in itself determine whether these standards apply. Rather, it is the device's intended use (such as physical restriction), its involuntary application, and/or the identified patient need that determines whether use of the device triggers the application of these standards. Therefore, these standards do not apply to the following:
- Standard practices that include limitation of mobility or temporary immobilization related to medical, dental, diagnostic, or surgical procedures and the related post-procedure care processes (for example, surgical positioning, intravenous arm boards, radiotherapy procedures, protection of surgical and treatment sites in pediatric patients)
- Adaptive support in response to assessed patient need (for example, postural support, orthopedic appliances, tabletop chairs)
- Helmets
- Restraint use for behavioral health care reasons (to which the restraint standards in this manual for behavioral health care apply)
- Forensic and correction restrictions used for security

Introduction to the Restraint Standards in Acute Medical and Surgical (Nonpsychiatric) Care

In its broadest context, *restraint* is the direct application of physical force to a patient, with or without the patient's permission, to restrict his or her freedom of movement. The physical force may be human, mechanical devices, or a combination thereof. Restraint may be used in response to emergent, dangerous behavior; as an adjunct to planned care; as a component of an approved protocol; or, in some cases, as part of standard practice. Because restraint may be necessary for certain patients, health care organizations and providers need to be able to use restraint when essential to protect patients from harming themselves, other patients, or staff. They also need to be aware of the associated risks of both its use and nonuse.

Restraint has the potential to produce serious consequences, such as physical or psychological harm, loss of dignity, violation of a patient's rights, and even death. Because of the associated risks and consequences of use, hospitals are increasingly exploring ways to decrease restraint use through effective preventive strategies or the use of alternatives. For some hospitals, a restraint-free environment is appropriate to their patient populations and clinical services and is achievable now or in the future. But for many hospitals, restraint use may continue to be necessary in clinically justified situations and in the foreseeable future, given the hospital's populations and clinical services, the current state of knowledge, and availability of effective alternatives.

A physical, social, and organizational environment that limits restraint use to clinically appropriate and adequately justified situations and that seeks to identify opportunities to reduce the risks associated with restraint use through preventive strategies, innovative alternatives, and process improvements is an environment that helps hospital staff focus on the patient's well-being. The leaders' role is to help create such an environment. This requires planning and frequently new or reallocated resources, thoughtful education, and performance improvement. The result is an organization approach to restraint that protects the patient's health and safety and preserves his or her dignity, rights, and well-being.

Standard PC.11.10
The hospital's leaders determine the hospital's approach to the use of restraint for nonpsychiatric patients and limit its use to those situations where there is appropriate clinical justification.

Rationale for PC.11.10
Limiting restraint to clinically justified situations requires clear policies and procedures, well-trained staff, and the support of the hospital's leaders. Limiting restraint to those situations with appropriate clinical justification requires the following:
- The hospital's leaders determine the hospital's approach to the use of restraint in the care of nonpsychiatric patients
- Supportive plans, policies, and priorities
- Understanding the staffing needs associated with alternatives to restraint

- Ongoing staff orientation and education
- Patient and, as appropriate, family education

In particular, attention is directed toward the following:
- Refining medical, dental, surgical, and diagnostic patient assessment processes to identify earlier the potential risk of dangerous patient behavior and the prevention, as appropriate, of those behaviors
- Reviewing and, when necessary, redesigning patient care processes associated with restraint use
- Developing policy(ies), procedure(s) and protocols for properly using restraints
- Identifying, developing, and promoting preventive strategies to prevent restraint use and using safe and effective alternatives to restraint

Elements of Performance for PC.11.10

B 1. The hospital's leaders have determined the hospital's approach to the use of restraint in the care of nonpsychiatric patients.

B 2. Clinical justification is guided by clear criteria present in practice guidelines, practice parameters, pathways of care, or other standardized care processes developed by relevant professional organizations.

B 3. When criteria are not available, the qualified staff of a hospital establishes criteria or otherwise guides justification for the hospital's patient population and clinical services.

Standard PC.11.20

Performance improvement processes seek to identify opportunities to reduce the risks associated with restraint use through preventive strategies, innovative alternatives, and process improvements.

Rationale for PC.11.20

The measurement and assessment process related to restraint seeks to understand why restraint is used and incorporates this understanding into the hospital's plans and priorities to evaluate and, if appropriate, reduce its use. This understanding can be advanced by an initial baseline assessment of aggregate data on restraint episodes, followed by targeted monitoring.

Element of Performance for PC.11.20

B 1. The hospital measures and assesses its restraint use to identify opportunities to introduce preventive strategies, alternatives to use, and process improvements that reduce the risks associated with restraint use.

Standard PC.11.30

Hospital policies and procedures guide appropriate and safe use of restraint.

Provision of Care, Treatment, and Services

Rationale for PC.11.30
Several essential elements govern how a hospital uses restraint in a way that is appropriate to the population and patients. These essential elements ensure that any use of restraint, whether initiated by an individual order or through the use of a protocol, protects the patient and preserves his or her rights, dignity, and well-being.

Elements of Performance for PC.11.30
B   1. Policies and procedures include appropriate details as to how the hospital does the following:
- Protects the patient and preserves his or her rights, dignity, and well-being during use
- Bases use on the patient's assessed needs
- Makes decisions about least-restrictive methods
- Ensures safe application and removal by qualified staff
- Monitors and reassesses the patient during use, using qualified staff
- Meets patient needs during use
- Addresses risk associated with vulnerable patient populations, such as emergency, pediatric, and cognitively or physically limited patients
- Makes efforts to discuss the issue of restraint, when practical, with the patient and family around the time of its use
- When orders are needed, limits individual orders to licensed independent practitioners
- Requires renewal of orders in accordance with applicable law and regulation
- Documents restraint episodes in the medical record (*see* standard PC.11.100)

B   2. The policies and procedures are developed by appropriate staff and approved by the medical staff, nursing leadership, and, as appropriate, others.

Standard PC.11.40
Any use of restraint (to which these standards apply) is initiated pursuant to either an individual order (standard PC.11.50) or an approved protocol (standard PC.11.60), the use of which is authorized by an individual order.

Rationale for PC.11.40
Individual orders provide the framework for ensuring clinical justification of restraint use and for protecting patient rights, dignity, and well-being.

Elements of Performance for PC.11.40

A Ⓜ 1. Restraint (except for restraint initiated under a protocol as described in standard PC.11.60) is used upon the order of a licensed independent practitioner.*

A 2. If a licensed independent practitioner is not available to issue such an order, a registered nurse initiates restraint use based on an appropriate assessment of the patient.

A 3. In that case, a licensed independent practitioner is notified within 12 hours of the initiation of restraint, and a verbal or written order is obtained from that practitioner and entered into the patient's medical record.

A 4. If the initiation of restraint is based on a significant change in the patient's condition, the registered nurse immediately notifies a licensed independent practitioner.

A 5. A written order, based on an examination of the patient by a licensed independent practitioner, is entered into the patient's medical record within 24 hours of the initiation of restraint.

A 6. Continued use of restraint beyond the first 24 hours is authorized by a licensed independent practitioner renewing the original order or issuing a new order if restraint continues to be clinically justified.

A 7. Such renewal or new order is issued no less often than once each calendar day and is based on the licensed independent practitioner's examination of the patient.

Standard PC.11.50

Individual orders for initiating and renewing restraint are consistent with hospital policies and procedures and with the patient's needs and clinical condition.

Elements of Performance for PC.11.50

A 1. The individual order is consistent with hospital policies and procedures.

A 2. The individual order identifies a rationale for any variation from hospital policies and procedures for monitoring of the patient and for release from restraint before the order expires.

---

* This standard is not to be construed to limit the authority of a licensed independent practitioner to delegate tasks to other qualified health care staff (that is, physician assistants and nurse practitioners) to the extent recognized under state law or a state's regulatory mechanism. In the states that allow this delegation, hospitals that permit these individuals to order restraint for medical or surgical reasons are considered to be in compliance with this standard.

Provision of Care, Treatment, and Services

Standard PC.11.60
Protocols for restraint use contain criteria to ensure only clinically justified use.

Rationale for PC.11.60
During the treatment of certain specific conditions (for example, post-traumatic brain injury) or certain specific clinical procedures (for example, intubation), restraint may often be necessary to prevent significant harm to the patient. For specified conditions or procedures, protocols for restraint use may be established based on the frequent presentation in those conditions or procedures of behavior by patients that seriously endangers the patient or seriously compromises the effectiveness of the procedure.

Elements of Performance for PC.11.60

B 1. Restraint protocols include the following for assessing the patient:
- Criteria for applying restraint
- Criteria for monitoring the patient and reassessing the need for restraint
- Criteria for terminating restraint

A 2. A licensed independent practitioner issues a patient-specific order authorizing the use of restraint protocols.

A 3. Authorized staff maintains and terminates restraint in accordance with established criteria based on the individual patient needs and appropriate clinical justification.

B 4. Criteria for the use of restraint that are incorporated into such a protocol are as follows:
- Reflect the hospital policies and procedures on the appropriate and safe use of restraint
- Are approved by the medical staff, nursing leadership, and, as appropriate, others

Standard PC.11.70
Patients in restraint are monitored.

Rationale for PC.11.70
Monitoring determines the following:
- The patient's physical and emotional well-being
- That the patient's rights, dignity, and safety are maintained
- Whether less restrictive methods are possible
- Changes in the patient's behavior or clinical condition needed to initiate the removal of restraints
- Whether the restraint has been appropriately applied, removed, or reapplied

Elements of Performance for PC.11.70

B 1. Hospital policies and procedures, applicable state law, protocols, individual orders, the setting, and individual patient needs are used to establish the frequency, nature, and extent of monitoring of a patient in restraints.

A 2. A patient in restraints is monitored at least every two hours or sooner according to patient need and hospital policy.

C Ⓜ 3. Monitoring is accomplished by observation, interaction with the patient, or related direct examination of the patient by qualified staff.*

Standard PC.11.80
Not applicable

Standard PC.11.90
Not applicable

Standard PC.11.100
Each episode of restraint use is documented in the patient's medical record, consistent with hospital policies and procedures.

Elements of Performance for PC.11.100

B 1. Hospital policies and procedures establish the frequency, format (if appropriate), and content of entries in the patient's record relative to each episode of restraint use.

C Ⓜ 2. Documentation includes the following:
- Relevant orders for use
- Results of patient monitoring
- Reassessment
- Significant changes in the patient's condition

C Ⓜ 3. When restraint is used as part of a protocol, the patient's record contains the protocol or references the protocol.

Applicability of Behavioral Health Care Restraint and Seclusion Standards

The behavioral health care standards for restraint and seclusion apply to any use of restraint and seclusion for behavioral health care reasons.† All the standards in this

---

* Documentation of monitoring is in accordance with organization policies and procedures (*see* standard PC.11.30). Documentation is scored at standard PC.11.100.

† Behavioral health care reasons for the use of restraint or seclusion are primarily to protect the patient against injury to self or others because of an emotional or behavioral disorder. The restraint standards for medical or surgical purposes apply when the primary reason for use directly supports medical healing.

section—standards PC.12.10 through PC.12.190—apply to all *behavioral health care settings* in which restraint or seclusion is used, such as freestanding psychiatric hospitals, psychiatric units in general hospitals, and residential treatment centers. Selected standards—PC.12.60, PC.12.70, PC.12.90, PC.12.100, PC.12.110, PC.12.130, PC.12.140—apply to *nonbehavioral health care settings* in which restraint or seclusion is used for behavioral health reasons, with the exception of the cross-references to standard PC.12.30. The requirements that relate to staff qualification for this subset of standards appear in standard PC.11.30—restraint standards in acute medical and surgical care. Restraint or seclusion associated with a behavioral health care disorder is different from restraint used to promote medical/surgical healing. For example, standards PC.12.60, PC.12.70, PC.12.90, PC.12.100, PC.12.110, PC.12.130, and PC.12.140 apply to patients who are as follows:

- Hospitalized in an acute care hospital that does not have a psychiatric unit
- Hospitalized in an acute care hospital in other than a psychiatric unit to receive medical or surgical services
- In the emergency department for assessment, stabilization, or treatment, even if awaiting transfer to a psychiatric hospital or psychiatric unit
or
- Awaiting transfer from a nonpsychiatric bed to a psychiatric bed or psychiatric unit after receiving medical or surgical care

When the patient is awaiting transfer to a psychiatric unit, the transfer is accomplished as rapidly as possible. If the patient is in restraint or seclusion, emergency department staff or medical or surgical services staff collaborates with psychiatric staff to ensure appropriate evaluation of the patient, until the transfer occurs.

Exceptions to the Applicability of the Behavioral Health Care Restraint and Seclusion Standards

The standards for restraint and seclusion do not apply to the following:

- The use of restraint associated with acute medical or surgical care, which is covered under standards PC.11.10 through PC.11.100
- When a staff member(s) physically redirects or holds a child, without the child's permission, for 30 minutes or less; however, standard PC.12.30, which addresses staff competence and training, is applicable under these circumstances
- A time-out when the patient is restricted for 30 minutes or less from leaving an unlocked room and when its use is consistent with the patient's treatment plan
- Instances in which a patient is restricted to an unlocked room or area, consistent with a unit's rules or regulations and hospital policy(ies) and procedure(s)
- The use of restraint with patients who receive treatment through formal behavior management programs (to which the behavior management standard in this manual applies—standard PC.13.70). Such patients exhibit intractable behavior which is severely self-injurious or injurious to others, have not responded to traditional interventions, and are unable to contract with staff for safety (for example, understand the concept of and act on criteria for discontinuing restraint or seclusion).
- Forensic restrictions and restrictions imposed by correction and law enforcement authorities for security purposes. However, restraint or seclusion use related to the clinical care of a patient under forensic or correction restrictions is surveyed under these standards.

- Protective equipment such as helmets
- Adaptive support in response to the patient's assessed physical needs (for example, postural support, orthopedic appliances)
- Standard practices that include limitation of mobility or temporary immobilization related to medical, dental, diagnostic, or surgical procedures and the related postprocedure care processes (for example, surgical positioning, intravenous arm boards, radiotherapy procedures, protection of surgical and treatment sites in pediatric patients)

Introduction to the Behavioral Health Care Restraint and Seclusion Standards

Use of restraint and seclusion. The use of restraint and seclusion poses an inherent risk to the physical safety and psychological well-being of the patient and staff. Therefore, restraint and seclusion are used only in an emergency, when there is an imminent risk of a patient physically harming himself or herself or others, including staff. Nonphysical interventions are the first choice as an intervention, unless safety demands an immediate physical response.

Reducing the use of restraint and seclusion. Because restraint and seclusion have the potential to produce serious consequences, such as physical and psychological harm, loss of dignity, violation of a patient's rights, and even death, hospitals continually explore ways to prevent, reduce, and strive to eliminate restraint and seclusion use through effective performance improvement initiatives.

The leaders' role. The leaders' role is to create an environment that minimizes circumstances that give rise to restraint and seclusion use and that maximizes safety when restraint or seclusion is used. This requires allocating sufficient resources, providing initial and ongoing education, and integrating restraint and seclusion into performance improvement activities. The result is an organizational approach to restraint and seclusion that strives to prevent, reduce, and eliminate their use. When restraint and seclusion are used, there are procedures that protect the patient's health and safety while preserving his or her dignity, rights, and well-being.

The family's role. Throughout the standards, there are references to the involvement of the patient's family in the decisions and activities that relate to the use of restraint or seclusion. While this is intended to promote communication with providers and support and advocacy for the patient, there are instances in which family participation may be inappropriate because it could have a deleterious effect on the patient and his or her rights. In these instances, the standards related to family involvement would not apply.

Standard PC.12.10

The leaders establish and communicate the hospital's philosophy on restraint and seclusion to all staff with direct care responsibility.

Provision of Care, Treatment, and Services

Elements of Performance for PC.12.10

A   1. At a minimum, the hospital's philosophy addresses the following:
- Its commitment to prevent, reduce, and strive to eliminate restraint and seclusion
- Prevention of emergencies that have the potential to lead to use of restraint or seclusion
- Nonphysical interventions as preferred interventions
- Limitation of the use of restraint and seclusion to emergencies in which there is an imminent risk of a patient physically harming himself or herself or others, including staff
- Its responsibility to facilitate the discontinuation of restraint or seclusion as soon as possible
- Raising awareness among staff about how restraint or seclusion may be experienced by the patient
- Preserving the patient's safety and dignity when restraint or seclusion is used

A Ⓜ   2. This philosophy is communicated to all members of the hospital who have direct care responsibility.

Standard PC.12.20

Staffing levels and assignments are set to minimize circumstances that give rise to restraint or seclusion use and to maximize safety when restraint and seclusion are used.

Elements of Performance for PC.12.20

The hospital bases its staffing levels and assignments on a variety of factors, including the following:

A   1. Staff qualifications

B   2. The physical design of the environment

B   3. Diagnoses

B   4. Co-occurring conditions

B   5. Acuity levels

B   6. Age and developmental functioning of patients

Standard PC.12.30

Staff is trained and competent to minimize the use of restraint and seclusion and, when use is indicated, to use restraint or seclusion safely.

Elements of Performance for PC.12.30

A Ⓜ 1. The hospital educates staff about minimizing the use of restraint and seclusion and, *before* they participate in any use of restraint or seclusion, assesses the competence of staff to use them safely.

C Ⓜ 2. To minimize the use of restraint and seclusion, **all** direct care staff and any other staff involved in the use of restraint and seclusion receive ongoing training in and demonstrate an understanding of the following:
- The underlying causes of threatening behaviors exhibited by the patients
- That sometimes a patient may exhibit an aggressive behavior that is related to a patient's medical condition and not related to his or her emotional condition (for example, threatening behavior that may result from delirium in fevers or other medical conditions)
- How staff behaviors can affect the behaviors of the patients
- De-escalation, mediation, self-protection, and other techniques such as time-out
- How to recognize signs of physical distress in patients who are being held, restrained, or secluded

A 3. Staff members who are authorized to apply restraint or seclusion receive the training and demonstrate the competence cited in EP 2.

A 4. These direct care staff members also receive ongoing training in and demonstrate competence in the safe use of restraint, including physical holding techniques, take-down procedures, and the application and removal of mechanical restraints.

A 5. Staff members who are authorized to perform 15-minute assessments of patients in restraint or seclusion receive the training and demonstrate the competence cited in EP 2.

A 6. These staff members authorized to perform 15-minute assessments receive ongoing training and demonstrate competence in the following:
- Taking vital signs and interpreting their relevance to the physical safety of the patient in restraint or seclusion
- Recognizing nutritional and hydration needs
- Checking circulation and range of motion in the extremities
- Addressing hygiene and elimination
- Addressing physical and psychological status and comfort
- Helping patients meet behavior criteria for discontinuing restraint or seclusion
- Recognizing readiness for discontinuing restraint or seclusion
- Recognizing signs of any incorrect application of restraints
- Recognizing when to contact a medically trained licensed independent practitioner or emergency medical services to evaluate and/or treat the patient's physical status

Provision of Care, Treatment, and Services

A   7. Staff members who, in the absence of a licensed independent practitioner, are authorized to initiate restraint or seclusion, and/or perform evaluations/reevaluations of patients in restraint or seclusion to assess their readiness for discontinuation or establish the need to secure a new order, receive the training and demonstrate the competence cited above.

C Ⓜ   8. These staff members are also educated and demonstrate competence in the following:
- How age, developmental considerations, gender issues, ethnicity, and history of sexual or physical abuse may affect the way in which a patient reacts to physical contact
- Using behavior criteria for discontinuing restraint or seclusion and how to help patients in meeting these criteria

C Ⓜ   9. A sufficient number of staff with direct care responsibility receives additional training to ensure that an appropriate number of staff members are available at all times who are competent to initiate first aid and cardiopulmonary resuscitation.

A   10. The hospital has a plan for providing emergency medical services.

B   11. The viewpoints of patients who have experienced restraint or seclusion are incorporated into staff training and education to help staff better understand all aspects of restraint and seclusion.

B   12. Whenever possible, such patients contribute to the training and education curricula and/or participate in staff training and education.

Note: *Requirements related to ongoing education and the continuous assessment of staff competence are addressed in the "Management of Human Resources" chapter.*

Standard PC.12.40
The initial assessment of each patient at admission or intake assists in obtaining information about the patient that could help minimize the use of restraint or seclusion.

Elements of Performance for PC.12.40
The initial assessment of a patient who is at risk of harming himself or herself or others, including staff, identifies the following (EPs 1–5):

C Ⓜ   1. Techniques, methods, or tools that would help the patient control his or her behavior

       2. Not applicable

       3. Not applicable

C Ⓜ   4. Pre-existing medical conditions or any physical disabilities and limitations that would place the patient at greater risk during restraint or seclusion

2005 Hospital Accreditation Standards

C Ⓜ 5. Any history of sexual or physical abuse that would place the patient at greater psychological risk during restraint or seclusion.

C Ⓜ 6. As appropriate, the patient and/or family helps in identifying such techniques.

C Ⓜ 7. The patient and/or family are educated about the hospital's philosophy on restraint and seclusion to the extent that such information is not clinically contraindicated.

C Ⓜ 8. The family's role, including their notification of a restraint or seclusion episode, is discussed with the patient and, as appropriate, the patient's family.

A 9. This is done in conjunction with the patient's right to confidentiality.

A 10. The hospital determines whether the patient has an advance directive with respect to behavioral health care and ensures that direct care staff is aware of the behavioral health advance directive.

Standard PC.12.50
Nonphysical techniques are the preferred intervention in behavior management.

Element of Performance for PC.12.50
A 1. Nonphysical techniques are always the preferred intervention.*

Standard PC.12.60
Restraint or seclusion is limited to emergencies in which there is an imminent risk of a patient physically harming himself or herself, staff, or others, and nonphysical interventions would not be effective.

Elements of Performance for PC.12.60
C Ⓜ 1. Restraint or seclusion is used only when nonphysical interventions are ineffective or not viable and when there is an imminent risk of a patient physically harming himself or herself, staff, or others.

C Ⓜ 2. The type of physical intervention selected considers information learned from the patient's initial assessment.

A 3. The hospital does not permit restraint or seclusion for any other purpose, such as coercion, discipline, convenience, or retaliation by staff.

C Ⓜ 4. The use of restraint or seclusion is not based on a patient's restraint or seclusion history or solely on a history of dangerous behavior.

---

* Such interventions may include redirecting the patient's focus or employing verbal de-escalation.

Provision of Care, Treatment, and Services

Standard PC.12.70
A licensed independent practitioner* orders the use of restraint or seclusion.

Elements of Performance for PC.12.70

A 1. All restraint and seclusion are applied and continued pursuant to an order by the licensed independent practitioner who is primarily responsible for the patient's ongoing care, or his or her licensed independent practitioner designee, or other licensed independent practitioner.†

A 2. As soon as possible, but no longer than one hour after the initiation of restraint or seclusion, qualified staff does the following:
- Notifies and obtains an order (verbal or written) from the licensed independent practitioner
- Consults with the licensed independent practitioner about the patient's physical and psychological condition

A 3. The licensed independent practitioner does the following:
- Reviews with staff the physical and psychological status of the patient
- Determines whether restraint or seclusion should be continued
- Supplies staff with guidance in identifying ways to help the patient regain control so that restraint or seclusion can be discontinued
- Supplies an order

Standard PC.12.80
The patient's family is notified promptly of the initiation of restraint or seclusion.

Element of Performance for PC.12.80

C 🅜 1. In cases in which the patient has consented to have the family kept informed about his or her care, treatment, and services and the family has agreed to be notified, staff attempts to contact the family promptly to notify them of the restraint or seclusion episode.

Standard PC.12.90
A licensed independent practitioner sees and evaluates the patient in person.

---

* This standard is not to be construed to limit the authority of a doctor of medicine or osteopathy to delegate tasks to physician assistants and advanced practice nurses to the extent recognized under state law or a state's regulatory mechanism and allowed by the organization.

† Because restraint and seclusion use is limited to emergencies (in which a licensed independent practitioner may not be immediately available), the organization may authorize qualified, trained staff members who are not licensed independent practitioners to initiate restraint or seclusion before an order is obtained from the licensed independent practitioner. In addition, restraints and seclusion may be ordered by licensed practitioners (for example, registered nurses, licensed social workers) if permitted by state law and by the organization.

Elements of Performance for PC.12.90

A 1. The licensed independent practitioner primarily responsible for the patient's ongoing care, treatment, and services, or his or her licensed independent practitioner designee, or other licensed independent practitioner, evaluates the patient in person within 4 hours of the initiation of restraint or seclusion for patients ages 18 or older and within 2 hours of initiation for children and youth ages 17 and under.

A 2. At the time of the in-person evaluation, the licensed independent practitioner does the following:
- Works with the patient and staff to identify ways to help the patient regain control
- Revises the patient's plan for care, treatment, and services as needed
- If necessary, provides a new written order

A 3. The licensed independent practitioner evaluates the patient in person within 24 hours of the initiation of restraint or seclusion, if the patient is no longer in restraint or seclusion when an original verbal order expires.

A 4. For hospitals that use accreditation for Medicare deemed status purposes, a physician or other licensed independent practitioner must evaluate the patient within one hour of the initiation of restraint or seclusion, as required by the Centers for Medicare & Medicaid Services' (CMS') Interim Final Rule for Patient Rights, effective August 1, 1999.

Standard PC.12.100
Written or verbal orders for initial and continuing use of restraint and seclusion are time limited.

Rationale for PC.12.100
Time-limited orders do not mean that restraint or seclusion must be applied for the entire length of time for which the order is written. The standard for periodic assessment, the standard for monitoring and assisting, and the standard for reevaluation are intended to encourage the discontinuation of restraint or seclusion as soon as the patient meets the behavior criteria for its discontinuation.

When restraint or seclusion is terminated before the time-limited order expires, the original order can be used to reapply the restraint or seclusion if the patient is at imminent risk of physically harming himself or herself or others, and nonphysical interventions are not effective. However, when the original order expires, a new order for restraint or seclusion is obtained from the licensed independent practitioner primarily responsible for the patient's ongoing care, treatment, and services, or his or her licensed independent practitioner designee, or other licensed independent practitioner.

Provision of Care, Treatment, and Services

Elements of Performance for PC.12.100

A 1. Verbal and written orders for restraint and seclusion are limited to the following:
- 4 hours for patients ages 18 and older
- 2 hours for children and youth ages 9 to 17
- 1 hour for children under age 9

A 2. Orders for restraint or seclusion are not written as a standing order or on an as needed basis (that is, PRN).

C Ⓜ 3. If restraint or seclusion use needs to continue beyond the expiration of the time-limited order, a new order for restraint or seclusion is obtained from the licensed independent practitioner primarily responsible for the patient's ongoing care, treatment, and services, or his or her licensed independent practitioner designee, or other licensed independent practitioner.

Standard PC.12.110

Patients in restraint or seclusion are regularly reevaluated.

Elements of Performance for PC.12.110

B 1. By the time the order for restraint or seclusion expires, the patient is evaluated in person by one of the following:
- The licensed independent practitioner primarily responsible for the patient's ongoing care, treatment, and services
- His or her licensed independent practitioner designee
- Another licensed independent practitioner
  or
- A qualified, trained individual authorized by the hospital to perform this function

C Ⓜ 2. In conjunction with the patient's reevaluation, a new written or verbal order is given by the licensed independent practitioner primarily responsible for the patient's ongoing care, treatment, and services, or his or her licensed independent practitioner designee, or other licensed independent practitioner if the restraint or seclusion is to be continued.

C Ⓜ 3. The licensed independent practitioner or other qualified, authorized staff member reevaluates the efficacy of the patient's treatment plan and works with the patient to identify ways to help him or her regain control.

C Ⓜ 4. If the patient's licensed independent practitioner, or his or her licensed independent practitioner designee, is not the licensed independent practitioner who gives the order, the patient's licensed independent practitioner is notified of the patient's status if the restraint or seclusion is continued.

A   5.   The patient is reevaluated as follows:
- Every 4 hours for adults ages 18 and older
- Every 2 hours for children and youth ages 9 to 17
- Every hour for children under age 9

A   6.   The licensed independent practitioner conducts an in-person reevaluation at least every 8 hours for patients ages 18 years and older and every 4 hours for patients ages 17 and younger.

Standard PC.12.120
Clinical leaders are told of instances in which patients experience extended or multiple episodes of restraint or seclusion.

Rationale for PC.12.120
Information is communicated to the leadership to do the following:
- Assess whether additional resources are needed to facilitate discontinuation of restraint or seclusion

or
- Minimize recurrent instances of restraint and seclusion

Elements of Performance for PC.12.120
A   1.   The clinical leaders are immediately notified of any instance in which a patient remains in restraint or seclusion for more than 12 hours or experiences two or more separate episodes of restraint and/or seclusion of any duration within 12 hours.

A   2.   Thereafter, the clinical leaders are notified every 24 hours if either of the above conditions continues.

Standard PC.12.130
Patients in restraint or seclusion are assessed and assisted.

Elements of Performance for PC.12.130
C Ⓜ   1.   A staff member who is trained and competent in accordance with standard PC.12.30 assesses the patient at the initiation of restraint or seclusion and every 15 minutes thereafter.

B   2.   This assessment includes, as appropriate to the type of restraint or seclusion, the following:
- Signs of any injury associated with applying restraint or seclusion
- Nutrition and hydration
- Circulation and range of motion in the extremities
- Vital signs
- Hygiene and elimination

Provision of Care, Treatment, and Services

- Physical and psychological status and comfort
- Readiness for discontinuation of restraint or seclusion

C Ⓜ 3. Staff helps patients meet behavior criteria for discontinuing restraint or seclusion.

Standard PC.12.140
Patients in restraint or seclusion are monitored.

Elements of Performance for PC.12.140
A 1. Monitoring is done through continuous in-person observation by an assigned staff member who is competent and trained in accordance with standard PC.12.30.

C Ⓜ 2. After the first hour, a patient in seclusion without restraints may be continuously monitored using simultaneous video and audio equipment, if consistent with the patient's condition or wishes.

A 3. If the patient is in a physical hold, a second staff person is assigned to observe the patient.

Standard PC.12.150
Restraint and seclusion use are discontinued when the patient meets the behavior criteria for their discontinuation.

Elements of Performance for PC.12.150
C Ⓜ 1. As early as feasible in the restraint or seclusion process, the patient is made aware of the rationale for restraint or seclusion and the behavior criteria for its discontinuation.*

C Ⓜ 2. Restraint or seclusion is discontinued as soon as the patient meets his or her behavior criteria.

Standard PC.12.160
The patient and staff participate in a debriefing about the restraint or seclusion episode.

Rationale for PC.12.160
Debriefing is important in reducing the recurrent use of restraint and seclusion.

---

* Examples of behavior criteria include the ability of a patient to contract for safety, whether a patient is oriented to the environment, and/or cessation of verbal threats.

Elements of Performance for PC.12.160

B   1. The patient and, if appropriate, the patient's family participate with staff members who were involved in the episode and who are available in a debriefing about each episode of restraint or seclusion.

C Ⓜ   2. The debriefing occurs as soon as possible and appropriate, but no longer than 24 hours after the episode.

B   3. The debriefing is used to do the following:
- Identify what led to the incident and what could have been handled differently
- Ascertain that the patient's physical well-being, psychological comfort, and right to privacy were addressed
- Counsel the patient for any trauma that may have resulted from the incident
- When indicated, modify the patient's plan for care, treatment, and services

B   4. Information obtained and documented from debriefings is used in performance improvement activities.

Standard PC.12.170

Medical records document that the use of restraint or seclusion is consistent with hospital policy.

Elements of Performance for PC.12.170

C Ⓜ   1. The use of restraint or seclusion is recorded in the patient's medical record.

C Ⓜ   2. The focus of the entry(ies) is on the patient.

C Ⓜ   3. The medical record contains the following documentation:
- That the patient and/or family was told of the hospital's policy on restraint
- Any pre-existing medical conditions or any physical disabilities that would place the patient at greater risk during restraint and seclusion
- Any history of sexual or physical abuse that would place the patient at greater psychological risk during restraint or seclusion
- Each episode of use
- The circumstances that led to restraint or seclusion
- Consideration or failure of nonphysical interventions
- The rationale for the type of physical intervention selected
- Notification of the patient's family, as appropriate
- Written orders for use
- Behavior criteria for discontinuing restraint or seclusion
- Informing the patient of behavior criteria for discontinuing restraint or seclusion
- Each verbal order received from a licensed independent practitioner

Provision of Care, Treatment, and Services

- Each in-person evaluation and reevaluation of the patient
- 15-minute assessments of the patient's status
- Assistance provided to the patient to help him or her meet the behavior criteria for discontinuing restraint or seclusion
- Continuous monitoring
- Debriefing of the patient with staff
- Any injuries and treatment for these injuries
- Any deaths

B   4. Documentation is done in a manner that allows for data to be collected and analyzed for performance improvement activities (such as a restraint and seclusion log).

Standard PC.12.180
The hospital collects data on the use of restraint and seclusion.

Rationale for PC.12.180
The hospital collects restraint and seclusion data to monitor and improve its performance of processes that involve risks or may result in sentinel events. It uses the data to do the following:
- Ascertain that restraint and seclusion are used only as emergency intervention
- Identify opportunities for incrementally reducing the rate and increasing the safety of restraint and seclusion use
- Identify any need to redesign care processes

Elements of Performance for PC.12.180

B   1. The leaders determine the frequency with which data are aggregated.

A   2. Individual identifiers are used.

C Ⓜ   3. Data on all restraint and seclusion episodes are collected from and classified for all settings/units/locations by the following:
- Shift
- Staff who initiated the process
- The length of each episode
- Date and time each episode was initiated
- Day of the week each episode was initiated
- The type of restraint used
- Whether injuries were sustained by the patient or staff
- Age of the patient
- Gender of the patient

Particular attention is paid to the following (EPs 4–7):

B   4. Multiple instances of restraint or seclusion experienced by a patient within a 12-hour time frame

B   5. The number of episodes per patient

	6.	Instances of restraint or seclusion that extend beyond 12 consecutive hours
B		
B	7.	Use of psychoactive medications as an alternative for or to enable discontinuation of restraint or seclusion
B	8.	Licensed independent practitioners participate in measuring and assessing use of restraint and seclusion for all patients in the hospital.

Standard PC.12.190

Hospital policies and procedures address prevention of restraint and seclusion and, when employed, guide their use.

Elements of Performance for PC.12.190

Hospital policies and procedures include appropriate detail that addresses the following:

B	1.	Staffing levels
B	2.	Staff competence and training
B	3.	The initial assessment of the patient
B	4.	The role of nonphysical techniques in behavior management
B	5.	Time-out
B	6.	Limiting restraint or seclusion to emergencies
B	7.	Notification of the patient's family when restraint or seclusion is initiated
B	8.	Ordering of restraint and seclusion by a licensed independent practitioner
B	9.	In-person evaluations of the patient in restraint or seclusion
B	10.	Initiation of restraint and seclusion by staff other than a licensed independent practitioner
B	11.	Time-limited orders
B	12.	Reassessment of a patient in restraint or seclusion
B	13.	Monitoring the patient in restraint or seclusion
B	14.	Discontinuation of restraint or seclusion
B	15.	Post-restraint and seclusion practices
B	16.	Reporting injuries and deaths to the hospital's leadership and appropriate external agencies consistent with applicable law and regulation
B	17.	Documentation
B	18.	Data collection and the integration of restraint and seclusion into performance improvement activities

Standards for Additional Special Procedures

Operative or Other High-Risk Procedures and/or the Administration of Moderate or Deep Sedation or Anesthesia

Operative or other procedures and the administration of sedation or anesthesia often occur simultaneously. However, procedures do occur without sedation, and sedation or anesthesia is administered for noninvasive procedures (hyperbaric treatment, CT scan, MRI). Therefore, the following standards address both operative or other procedures and/or the administration of moderate or deep sedation or anesthesia.

Whenever an operative or other procedure is conducted, whether or not sedation or anesthesia is administered, appropriate staff must be involved in planning for and providing care to the patient. All procedures carry risk, but that risk is increased when sedation or anesthesia is administered.

The standards for sedation and anesthesia care apply when patients in any setting receive, for any purpose, by any route, the following:
- General, spinal, or other major regional anesthesia
or
- Moderate or deep sedation (with or without analgesia) that, in the manner used, may be reasonably expected to result in the loss of protective reflexes

Because sedation is a continuum, it is not always possible to predict how an individual patient receiving sedation will respond. Therefore, each hospital develops specific, appropriate protocols for the care of patients receiving sedation. These protocols are consistent with professional standards and address at least the following:
- Sufficient qualified individuals present to perform the procedure and to monitor the patient throughout administration and recovery. The individuals providing moderate or deep sedation and anesthesia have at a minimum had competency-based education, training, and experience in the following:
  1. Evaluating patients before performing moderate or deep sedation and anesthesia.
  2. Performing the moderate or deep sedation and anesthesia, including rescuing patients who slip into a deeper-than-desired level of sedation or analgesia. These include the following:
     a. Moderate sedation—are qualified to rescue patients from deep sedation and are competent to manage a compromised airway and to provide adequate oxygenation and ventilation
     b. Deep sedation—are qualified to rescue patients from general anesthesia and are competent to manage an unstable cardiovascular system as well as a compromised airway and inadequate oxygenation and ventilation
- Appropriate equipment for care and resuscitation
- Appropriate monitoring of vital signs, including, but not limited to, heart rates and oxygenation using pulse oximetry equipment, respiratory frequency and adequacy of pulmonary ventilation, the monitoring of blood pressure at regular intervals, and cardiac monitoring (by EKG or use of continuous cardiac monitoring device) in patients with significant cardiovascular disease or when dysrhythmias are anticipated or detected

- Documentation of care
- Monitoring of outcomes

Definitions of four levels of sedation and anesthesia include the following:

- **Minimal sedation (anxiolysis)**
  A drug-induced state during which patients respond normally to verbal commands. Although cognitive function and coordination may be impaired, ventilatory and cardiovascular functions are unaffected.
- **Moderate sedation/analgesia ("conscious sedation")**
  A drug-induced depression of consciousness during which patients respond purposefully to verbal commands (note, reflex withdrawal from a painful stimulus is not considered a purposeful response)—either alone or accompanied by light tactile stimulation. No interventions are required to maintain a patent airway, and spontaneous ventilation is adequate. Cardiovascular function is usually maintained.
- **Deep sedation/analgesia**
  A drug-induced depression of consciousness during which patients cannot be easily aroused but respond purposefully after repeated or painful stimulation. The ability to independently maintain ventilatory function may be impaired. Patients may require assistance in maintaining a patent airway and spontaneous ventilation may be inadequate. Cardiovascular function is usually maintained.
- **Anesthesia**
  Consists of general anesthesia and spinal or major regional anesthesia. It does not include local anesthesia. General anesthesia is a drug-induced loss of consciousness during which patients are not arousable, even by painful stimulation. The ability to independently maintain ventilatory function is often impaired. Patients often require assistance in maintaining a patent airway, and positive pressure ventilation may be required because of depressed spontaneous ventilation or drug-induced depression of neuromuscular function. Cardiovascular function may be impaired.

Standard PC.13.10
Not applicable

Standard PC.13.20
Operative or other procedures and/or the administration of moderate or deep sedation or anesthesia are planned.

Rationale for PC.13.20
Because the response to procedures is not always predictable and sedation-to-anesthesia is a continuum, it is not always possible to predict how an individual patient will respond. Therefore, qualified individuals are trained in professional standards and techniques to manage patients in the case of a potentially harmful event.

Provision of Care, Treatment, and Services

Elements of Performance for PC.13.20

B 1. Sufficient numbers of qualified staff (in addition to the licensed independent practitioner performing the procedure) are present* to evaluate the patient, help with the procedure, provide the sedation and/or anesthesia, monitor, and recover the patient.

A 2. Individuals administering moderate or deep sedation and anesthesia are qualified and have the appropriate credentials to manage patients at whatever level of sedation or anesthesia is achieved, either intentionally or unintentionally.

A 3. A registered nurse supervises perioperative nursing care.

B 4. Appropriate equipment to monitor the patient's physiologic status is available.

B 5. Appropriate equipment to administer intravenous fluids and drugs, including blood and blood components, is available as needed.

B 6. Resuscitation capabilities are available.

The following must occur before the operative and other procedures or the administration of moderate or deep sedation or anesthesia (EPs 7–10):

C Ⓜ 7. The anticipated needs of the patient are assessed to plan for the appropriate level of postprocedure care.

C Ⓜ 8. Preprocedural education, treatments, and services are provided according to the plan for care, treatment, and services.

A 9. The site, procedure, and patient are accurately identified and clearly communicated, using active communication techniques, during a final verification process such as a time-out before the start of any surgical or invasive procedure.

A 10. A presedation or preanesthesia assessment is conducted.

A 11. Before sedating or anesthetizing a patient, a licensed independent practitioner with appropriate clinical privileges plans or concurs with the planned anesthesia.

A 12. The patient is reevaluated immediately before moderate or deep sedation and before anesthesia induction.

Standard PC.13.30

Patients are monitored during the procedure and/or administration of moderate or deep sedation or anesthesia.

---

* For organizations providing obstetric or emergency operative services, this means they can provide anesthesia services as required by law and regulation.

Elements of Performance for PC.13.30

A   1.   Appropriate methods are used to continuously monitor oxygenation, ventilation, and circulation during procedures that may affect the patient's physiological status.

C Ⓜ   2.   The procedure and/or the administration of moderate or deep sedation or anesthesia for each patient is documented in the medical record.

Standard PC.13.40

Patients are monitored immediately after the procedure and/or administration of moderate or deep sedation or anesthesia.

Elements of Performance for PC.13.40

A   1.   The patient's status is assessed immediately after the procedure and/or administration of moderate or deep sedation or anesthesia.

C Ⓜ   2.   Each patient's physiological status, mental status, and pain level are monitored.

B   3.   Monitoring is at a level consistent with the potential effect of the procedure and/or sedation or anesthesia.

B   4.   Patients are discharged from the recovery area and the hospital by a qualified licensed independent practitioner or according to rigorously applied criteria approved by the clinical leaders.

C Ⓜ   5.   Patients who have received sedation or anesthesia in the outpatient setting are discharged in the company of a responsible, designated adult.

Additional Special Procedures

Standard PC.13.50

Electroconvulsive therapy is used with adequate justification, documentation, and regard for patient safety.

Elements of Performance for PC.13.50

B   1.   Written policies regulate electroconvulsive therapy.

C Ⓜ   2.   Whenever electroconvulsive therapy is used, the procedure is adequately justified and documented in the patient's medical record.

A   3.   Before initiating electroconvulsive therapy for a child or youth, two qualified, experienced child psychiatrists who are not directly involved in treating the child or youth do the following:
- Examine the child or youth
- Consult with the psychiatrist responsible for the child or youth
- Document their concurrence with the treatment in the child's or youth's medical record

Provision of Care, Treatment, and Services

A   4. Written consent for any electroconvulsive therapy is obtained from the patient and documented in the clinical/case record.

Standard PC.13.60
Psychosurgery or other surgical treatments for emotional, mental, or behavioral disorders are performed with adequate justification, documentation, and regard for patient safety.

Elements of Performance for PC.13.60
B   1. Written policies and procedures regulate psychosurgery or other surgical treatments for mental, emotional, or behavioral disorders.

B   2. Whenever these procedures are used, they are adequately justified and documented in the patient's medical record.

Standard PC.13.70
Use of behavior management procedures conforms to the patient's treatment plan and hospital policy.

Rationale for PC.13.70
Behavior management and treatment interventions should be therapeutic interventions that foster adaptive behaviors and not used exclusively for behavior control. Policies and procedures should require that the selection of interventions considers both appropriateness and minimizing restrictiveness of interventions.

Elements of Performance for PC.13.70
C Ⓜ   1. When behavior management procedures are used, they are included in the patient's plan for care, treatment, and services.

B   2. Written policies describe the following:
- The conditions under which specific behavior management procedures can be used and when they should not be used
- That any behavior management and plan for care, treatment, and services that includes the use of aversive procedures is reviewed and approved by both appropriate clinical leaders and a person(s) external to the hospital, such as an outside expert, an advocate, or a human rights committee
- That no procedure that physically hurts or is a psychological risk to the patient is allowed
- Time-outs are limited to no more than 30 minutes
- Time-outs occur in an unlocked room
- Time-outs educate the patient about the conditions under which time-outs are used
- Time-outs prohibit the use of intimidation, force, or threat

A   3. At a minimum, the following are prohibited:
- Procedures that deny any basic needs, such as nutritional diet, water, shelter, and essential, safe, and appropriate clothing
- Corporal punishment
- Fear-eliciting procedures
- Any behavior management and treatment intervention implemented by another patient
- Mechanical restraint and seclusion*

B   4. The hospital uses educational and positive reinforcement techniques (for example, alternative adaptive behaviors) wherever possible.

B   5. When more restrictive techniques are clinically necessary, the least restrictive alternative is used to avoid harm to the patient.

A   6. The hospital protects the patient's physical safety.

C Ⓜ   7. Patients and, as appropriate, their families participate in selecting behavior management and treatment interventions.

B   8. Other individuals may help implement a patient's behavior management program only as follows:
- If it is conducted as part of a structured treatment plan
- If it is conducted under the supervision of qualified staff
- If it is limited to empowering individuals to provide positive reinforcement
- If it does not become abusive

B   9. Group contingencies are based on collective group outcomes and not based on a single patient's behavior.

C Ⓜ   10. Qualified staff reviews, evaluates, and approves all behavior management procedures.

C Ⓜ   11. Time-out and procedures using restraining devices or aversive techniques are used only consistently with the patient's plan for care, treatment, and services, policies and procedures, and state and federal laws.

A   12. At a minimum, the following are included in the plan for care, treatment, and services and documented in the record:
- Target behavior
- Adaptive/replacement behavior
- Method of implementation—strategy, support, teaching methods, motivation and reward, if used, frequency, and circumstances under which the plan will be implemented

---

* The use of mechanical restraint and seclusion as treatment interventions under these standards is prohibited other than for patients who exhibit intractable behavior that is severely self-injurious or injurious to others, have not responded to traditional interventions, and are unable to contract with staff for safety (that is, understand the concept of, and act on, criteria for the discontinuation of restraint or seclusion). When restraint or seclusion is used in an emergency situation, its use needs to be in compliance with standards PC.12.10 through PC.12.190.

Provision of Care, Treatment, and Services

- Condition for discontinuation
- All interventions attempted

Standard PC.14.10
Not applicable

Standard PC.14.20
Not applicable

Standard PC.14.30
Not applicable

Discharge or Transfer
Patients may be discharged from the hospital entirely or discharged or transferred to another level of care, treatment, and services, to different health professionals, or to settings for continued services. The hospital's processes for transfer or discharge are based on the patients' assessed needs. To facilitate discharge or transfer, the hospital assesses the patient's needs, plans for discharge or transfer, facilitates the discharge or transfer process, and helps to ensure that continuity of care, treatment, and services is maintained.

Standard PC.15.10
A process addresses the needs for continuing care, treatment, and services after discharge or transfer.

Element of Performance for PC.15.10
B 1. The process addresses the following:
- The reason(s) for transfer or discharge
- The conditions under which transfer or discharge can occur
- Shifting responsibility for a patient's care from one clinician, organization, organizational program, or service to another (which could include transferring complete responsibility for the patient and his or her care, treatment, and services to others or referring the patient to others, such as one or more agencies or professionals, to provide one or more specific services)
- Mechanisms for internal and external transfer
- The accountability and responsibility for the patient's safety during transfer of both the hospital initiating the transfer and the organization receiving the patient

Standard PC.15.20

The transfer or discharge of a patient to another level of care, treatment, and services, different professionals, or different settings is based on the patient's assessed needs and the hospital's capabilities.

Rationale for PC.15.20

For some patients, effective planning addresses how needs will be met as they move to the next level of care, treatment, and services. For other patients, planning will consist of a clear understanding of how to access services in the future should the need arise.

Elements of Performance for PC.15.20

C Ⓜ 1. The patient's needs for continuing care to meet physical and psychosocial needs are identified.

C Ⓜ 2. Patients are told in a timely manner of the need to plan for discharge or transfer to another organization or level of care.

C Ⓜ 3. Planning for transfer or discharge involves the patient and all appropriate licensed independent practitioners, staff, and family members involved in the patient's care, treatment, and services.

C Ⓜ 4. When the patient is transferred, information provided to the patient includes the following:
- The reason they are being transferred
- Alternatives to transfer, if any

C Ⓜ 5. The discharge planning process is initiated early in the care, treatment, and services process.

C Ⓜ 6. When the patient is discharged, information provided to patients includes the following:
- The reason they are being discharged
- The anticipated need for continued care, treatment, and services* after discharge

C Ⓜ 7. When indicated, the patient is educated about how to obtain further care, treatment, and services to meet his or her identified needs.

C Ⓜ 8. When indicated and before discharge, the hospital arranges for or helps the family arrange for services needed to meet the patient's needs after discharge.

C Ⓜ 9. Written discharge instructions in a form the patient can understand are given to the patient and/or those responsible for providing continuing care.

---

* Available services include, as appropriate, special education, adult day care, case management, home health services, hospice, long term care facilities, ambulatory care, support groups, rehabilitation services, and community mental health services.

Standard PC.15.30
When patients are transferred or discharged, appropriate information related to the care, treatment, and services provided is exchanged with other service providers.

Rationale for PC.15.30
A patient may receive care, treatment, and services in many settings and may move from one hospital or provider to another. To facilitate the continuity of care, treatment, and services, information is provided to any organization or provider to which the patient is accepted, transferred, or discharged.

Elements of Performance for PC.15.30
C Ⓜ 1. The hospital communicates appropriate information to any organization or provider to which the patient is transferred or discharged.

C Ⓜ 2. The information shared includes the following, as appropriate to the care, treatment, and services provided:
- The reason for transfer or discharge
- The patient's physical and psychosocial status
- A summary of care, treatment, and services provided and progress toward goals
- Community resources or referrals provided to the patient

Waived Testing
The federal regulation governing laboratory testing, known as the Clinical Laboratory Improvement Amendments of 1988 (CLIA '88), classifies testing into four complexity levels: high complexity, moderate complexity, PPM (Provider Performed Microscopy, a sub-set of moderate complexity), and waived testing. The high, moderate, and PPM levels, otherwise called non-waived testing, have specific and detailed requirements regarding personnel qualifications, quality assurance, quality control, and other systems. Joint Commission requirements for the tests and laboratories or sites that perform them are located in the *Comprehensive Accreditation Manual for Laboratory and Point-of-Care Testing* (*CAMLAB*).

Waived testing is the most common complexity level performed by caregivers at the patient's bedside or point of care. The same laboratory test may be available by more than one method within a hospital, and those methods may be of different complexity levels. The list of methods that are approved as waived is under constant revision, so it is advisable to check the Food and Drug Administration (FDA), Centers for Disease Control and Prevention (CDC), or CMS' Web sites for the most up-to-date information regarding test categorization and complete CLIA requirements:
- http://www.fda.gov/cdrh/clia/index.html
- http://www.phppo.cdc.gov/clia
- http://www.cms.hhs.gov/clia

CLIA '88 identifies laboratory testing as an activity that occurs, not defined as "occurring" at a specific location. Any activity that evaluates any substance removed from a human body and translates that evaluation to a result becomes a laboratory test. The results may be stated as a number, presence or absence of a cell or reaction, or an interpretation, such as what occurs when recording a urine color. Test results that are used to assess a patient's condition or make a clinical decision about a patient are governed by CLIA '88.

Tests that produce a result measured as a number are called "quantitative" and are usually performed with the assistance of some type of instrument. Tests that produce a negative or positive result, such as occult bloods and urine pregnancy screens, are termed "qualitative" and are usually known as manual tests. Any test with analysis steps that rely on the use of an instrument to produce a result is an instrument-based test.

When a patient performs a test on himself or herself (for example, whole blood glucose testing by a patient on his or her own meter cleared by the FDA for home use), the action is not regulated. Testing performed by one individual on another individual while carrying out professional responsibilities is an activity regulated by CLIA '88. This distinction is important when caring for patients who monitor their own glucose or prothrombin times with home devices.

Standard PC.16.10*
The hospital establishes policies and procedures that define the context in which waived test results are used in patient care, treatment, and services.

Elements of Performance for PC.16.10*
B   1. Quantitative test result reports in the clinical record are accompanied by reference intervals specific to the test method used and are appropriate to the population served.

B   2. Criteria for confirmatory testing for each test, qualitative or quantitative, is specified in the written procedure as dictated by clinical usage and methodology limitations.

B   3. Actual usage is consistent with the hospital's policies and the manufacturer's recommendations for each waived test.

Standard PC.16.20
The hospital identifies the staff responsible for performing and supervising waived testing.

---

* Effective January 1, 2005.

Provision of Care, Treatment, and Services

Elements of Performance for PC.16.20

B   1. Staff members who perform testing are identified.

B   2. Staff members who direct or supervise testing are identified.

> **Note:** *These individuals may be employees of the hospital, contracted staff, or employees of a contracted service.*

Standard PC.16.30
Staff performing tests have adequate, specific training and orientation to perform the tests and demonstrate satisfactory levels of competence.

Rationale for PC.16.30
For waived tests to be performed properly, the staff performing them must be qualified to do so. Staff members who perform waived testing have specific training in each test performed. This training may be acquired through hospital or other training programs, such as those provided by other health care organizations or manufacturers.

Elements of Performance for PC.16.30*

C Ⓜ   1. Current competence of testing staff is demonstrated.

C Ⓜ   2. Each staff member who performs testing has been trained specifically to each test he or she is authorized to perform.

C Ⓜ   3. Each staff member who performs testing has been oriented according to the hospital's specific needs.

B   4. Testing that requires the use of an instrument is performed by staff with adequate and specific training on the use and care of that instrument.

C Ⓜ   5. Competence is assessed according to hospital policy at defined intervals, but at least at the time of orientation and annually thereafter.

B   6. These assessments have considered the following:
- The frequency by which staff members perform tests
- The technical backgrounds of the staff
- The complexity of the test methodology and the consequences of an inaccurate result

B   7. Methods to assess current competency include at least two of the following:
- Performing a test on an unknown specimen
- Having the supervisor or qualified delegate periodically observe routine work
- Monitoring each user's quality control performance
- Having written testing that is specific to the method assessed

B   8. The hospital evaluates and documents the information listed above.

> **Note:** *All staff who perform instrument-based testing, including but not limited to physicians, licensed independent practitioners, contracted staff, and RNs, must participate in training and competence demonstrations.*

Standard PC.16.40
Approved policies and procedures governing specific testing-related processes are current and readily available.

Rationale for PC.16.40
Current and up-to-date policies and procedures are an important reference tool in managing laboratory testing activities, particularly when individual staff members perform them infrequently. Testing policies and procedures include requirements that are in compliance with the manufacturer's recommendations regarding all of the following, as applicable:
- Specimen type (for example, a method for whole blood is not used for spinal fluid)
- Storage considerations for test components (for example, compliance with directions such as store away from direct light, temperature requirements, open container expiration dates, and so forth)
- Instrument maintenance and function checks such as calibration
- Quality control frequency and type
- Result follow-up recommendations (for example, out-of-range results' recommendation for retesting)
- Tests approved by the FDA for home use only are not used for professional purposes (for example, glucose meters cleared for home use only are not used in a hospital setting by nursing staff except as patient education)

Elements of Performance for PC.16.40

B   1. Written policies and procedures address all the following items:
- Collection, identification, and required labeling, as appropriate
- Specimen preservation, as appropriate
- Instrument calibration
- Quality control and remedial action
- Equipment performance evaluation
- Test performance

B   2. The policies and procedures for each item are applicable to the specific hospital.

> **Note:** *Reference to a manufacturer's manual is acceptable if appropriate modifications have been made to customize the manual's content for the hospital.*

C Ⓜ   3. Current and complete policies and procedures are readily available to the person performing the test.

Provision of Care, Treatment, and Services

A   4.   The director named on the waived testing certificate or a designee approves policies and procedures at defined intervals.

Standard PC.16.50
Quality control checks, as defined by the hospital, are conducted on each procedure.

Elements of Performance for PC.16.50

B   1.   The hospital has a written quality control plan that specifies how procedures will be controlled for quality, establishes timetables, and explains the rationale for choice of procedures and timetables.

B   2.   Quality control procedures are performed at least as frequently as recommended by the manufacturer, according to the hospital's policies.

C Ⓜ   3.   For instrument-based waived testing, quality control requirements include two levels of control, if commercially available.*

C Ⓜ   4.   Quality control procedures are performed at least once each day on each instrument used for patient testing.*

B   5.   The documented quality control rationale is based on the following:*
- How the test is used
- Reagent stability
- Manufacturers' recommendations
- The hospital's experience with the test
- Currently accepted guidelines

B   6.   At a minimum, manufacturers' instructions are followed.

Standard PC.16.60
Appropriate quality control and test records are maintained.

Elements of Performance for PC.16.60

C Ⓜ   1.   All quality control test results are documented, including internal, external, liquid, and electronic.

C Ⓜ   2.   Test results are documented.

              Note: *Test results may be located in the clinical record.*

B   3.   Quality control records, instrument problems, and individual results are correlated.

B   4.   A formal log is not required, but a functional audit trail is maintained that allows retrieval of results and associated quality control values for a minimum of two years.

---
* Effective January 1, 2005.

Medication* Management

Overview

Medication management is often an important component in the palliative, symptomatic, and curative treatment of many diseases and conditions. A safe medication management system addresses a hospital's medication processes, including the following (as applicable):
- Selection and procurement
- Storage
- Ordering and transcribing
- Preparing and dispensing
- Administration
- Monitoring

Effective and safe medication management involves multiple services and disciplines working closely together. These standards address activities involving various individuals within a hospital's medication management system, including, as appropriate to the setting, licensed independent practitioners, health care professionals, and staff involved in medication management processes.

A well-planned and implemented medication management system supports patient safety and improves the quality of care by doing the following:
- Reducing practice variation, errors, and misuse
- Monitoring medication management processes in regard to efficiency, quality, and safety
- Standardizing equipment and processes across the hospital to improve the medication management system
- Using evidence-based good practices to develop medication management processes
- Managing critical processes associated with medication management to promote safe medication management throughout the hospital
- Handling all medications in the same manner, including sample medications

An effective medication management system includes mechanisms for reporting potential and actual errors and a process to improve medication management processes and patient safety based on this information. The most effective feedback and improvement systems usually operate in hospitals with a nonpunitive culture.

---

* For the purpose of these standards, *medication* includes prescription medications, sample medications, herbal remedies, vitamins, nutraceuticals, over-the-counter drugs, vaccines, diagnostic and contrast agents used on or administered to persons to diagnose, treat, or prevent disease or other abnormal conditions; radioactive medications; respiratory therapy treatments; parenteral nutrition; blood derivatives; intravenous solutions (plain, with electrolytes and/or drugs); and any product designated by the Food and Drug Administration (FDA) as a drug. The definition of *medication* does not include enteral nutrition solutions (which are considered food products), oxygen, and other medical gases.

The "Medication Management" chapter (standards MM.1.10 through MM.8.10) addresses critical medication management processes, including those undertaken by the hospital and those provided through contracted pharmacy services. When pharmacy services are provided through a contract, the contract should address responsibility for these standards and performance expectations. A hospital receiving pharmacy services should monitor the performance of contracted services.

Medication Management

Standards

The following is a list of all standards for this chapter. They are presented here for your convenience without footnotes or other explanatory text. If you have a question about a term used here, please check the Glossary.

Note: *A revised standard numbering system is being used with the reformatted standards. This revised numbering system will allow for more flexibility to add standards while maintaining the current label for each standard.*

Patient-Specific Information

MM.1.10 Patient-specific information is readily accessible to those involved in the medication management system.

Selection and Procurement

MM.2.10 Medications available for dispensing or administration are selected, listed, and procured based on criteria.

Storage

MM.2.20 Medications are properly and safely stored throughout the hospital.

MM.2.30 Emergency medications and/or supplies, if any, are consistently available, controlled, and secure in the hospital's patient care areas.

MM.2.40 A process is established to safely manage medications brought into the hospital by patients or their families.

Ordering and Transcribing

MM.3.10 Only medications needed to treat the patient's condition are ordered.

MM.3.20 Medication orders are written clearly and transcribed accurately.

Preparing and Dispensing

MM.4.10 All prescriptions or medication orders are reviewed for appropriateness.

MM.4.20 Medications are prepared safely.

MM.4.30 Medications are appropriately labeled.

MM.4.40 Medications are dispensed safely.

MM.4.50 The hospital has a system for safely providing medications to meet patient needs when the pharmacy is closed.

MM.4.60 Not applicable

MM.4.70 Medications dispensed by the hospital are retrieved when recalled or discontinued by the manufacturer or the Food and Drug Administration for safety reasons.

MM.4.80 Medications returned to the pharmacy are appropriately managed.

Administering

MM.5.10 Medications are safely and accurately administered.

MM.5.20 Self-administered medications are safely and accurately administered.

Monitoring

MM.6.10 The effects of medication(s) on patients are monitored.

MM.6.20 The hospital responds appropriately to actual or potential adverse drug events and medication errors.

High-Risk Medications

MM.7.10 The hospital develops processes for managing high-risk or high-alert medications.

MM.7.20 Not applicable

MM.7.30 Not applicable

MM.7.40 Investigational medications are safely controlled and administered.

Evaluation

MM.8.10 The hospital evaluates its medication management system.

Understanding the Parts of This Chapter

To help you navigate this reformatted standards chapter, it may be helpful to think of its parts this way:
- The **standard** is the "goal."
- The **rationale** explains why it's important to achieve this goal.
- The **elements of performance** identify the step(s) needed to achieve this goal.

These parts are defined as follows.

Standard A statement that defines the performance expectations and/or structures or processes that must be in place in order for a hospital to provide safe, high-quality care, treatment, and services. A hospital is either "compliant" or "not compliant" with a standard.

Accreditation decisions are based on simple counts of the standards that are determined to be "not compliant."

Rationale A statement that provides background, justification, or additional information about a standard. A standard's rationale is not scored. In some instances, the rationale for a standard is self-evident. Therefore, not every standard has a written rationale.

Elements of performance (EPs) The specific performance expectations and/or structures or processes that must be in place in order for a hospital to provide safe, high-quality care, treatment, and services. The scoring of EP compliance determines a hospital's overall compliance with a standard. EPs are evaluated on the following scale:

> 0 Insufficient compliance
> 1 Partial compliance
> 2 Satisfactory compliance
> NA Not applicable

You will find a **measure of success** icon—Ⓜ—next to some EPs. Measures of success (MOS) need to be developed for certain EPs when a standard is judged to be out of compliance through either the Periodic Performance Review (PPR) or the onsite survey. An MOS is defined as a quantifiable measure, usually related to an audit, that can be used to determine whether an action has been effective and is being sustained.*

Assessing Your Compliance

Once you are familiar with the parts of this chapter, you can begin to assess your compliance with its requirements. The scoring category for each EP is noted next to the EP. If you would like to assess your hospital's performance, mark your scores for the EPs and the standards by following the simple steps described below.

---

* For more information about measures of success, *see* the "The New Joint Commission Accreditation Process" chapter in this book.

Two components are scored for each EP: (1) compliance with the requirement itself **and** (2) compliance with the track record* for that requirement. Scoring has been simplified, and track record achievements (which have always been part of the scoring) have been appropriately modified.

Note: *Some standards and EPs do not apply to a particular type of organization; these standards and EPs are marked "not applicable" and the related text is not included. Your hospital is not expected to comply with standards and EPs marked "not applicable."*

In addition, some standards and EPs that do apply to organizations may not apply to the specific care, treatment, and services that your individual hospital provides. Although these standards and EPs are included in the manual, you are not expected to comply with them. If you are unsure about the standards or EPs that apply to your hospital, please contact the Joint Commission's Standards Interpretation Group at 630/792-5900.

Step 1: Score Your Compliance with Each Element of Performance

Before you can determine your compliance with the standards, you must score your compliance with each EP. There are three scoring criterion categories: A, B, and C (described below). Please note that for each EP scoring criterion category, your hospital must meet the performance requirement itself and the track record achievements (*see* "Track Record Achievements").

Category A
These EPs relate to the presence or absence of the requirement(s) and are scored either yes (2) or no (0); however, score 1 for partial compliance is also possible based on track record achievements.

If an A EP has multiple components designated by bullets, your hospital must be compliant with all the bullets to receive a score of 2. If your hospital does not meet one or more requirements in the bullets, you will receive a score of 0.

Category B
Category B EPs are scored in two steps:
1. As with category A EPs, category B EPs relate to the presence or absence of the requirement(s). If your hospital *does not meet* the requirement(s), the EP is scored 0; there is no need to assess your compliance with the principles of good process design.
2. If your hospital *does meet* the requirement(s), but there is concern about the quality or comprehensiveness of the effort, then and only then should you assess the qualitative aspect of the EP. That is, review the applicable principles of good process design and ask how the principles were applied in the situation under

---

* **Track record** The amount of time that an organization has been in compliance with a standard, element of performance, or other requirement.

discussion. Good process design has the following characteristics:
- Is consistent with your hospital's mission, values, and goals
- Meets the needs of patients
- Reflects the use of currently accepted practices (doing the right thing, using resources responsibly, using practice guidelines)
- Incorporates current safety information and knowledge such as sentinel event data and National Patient Safety Goals
- Incorporates relevant performance improvement results

This two-part evaluation applies to both simple and bulleted B EPs. First, the EPs are assessed to determine if the requirements are present. If the EP has multiple components designated by bullets, as with the category A EPs, your hospital must meet the requirements in *all* the bulleted items to get a score of 2. If your hospital meets *none* of the requirements in the bullets, it receives a score of 0. If your hospital meets *at least one, but not all*, of the bulleted requirements, it will receive a score of 1 for the EPs.

Use the following rules to determine your EP score:
- Your EP score is 0 if your hospital does not meet the requirement(s); you *do not* need to assess your compliance with the preceding applicable principles of good process design
- Your EP score is 1 if your hospital does meet the requirement(s), but considered only *some* of the preceding applicable principles of good process design
- Your EP score is 2 if your hospital does meet the requirement(s) *and* considered *all* the preceding principles of good process design

Category C
C EPs are scored 0, 1, or 2 based on the number of times your hospital does not meet the EP. These EPs are frequency based and require totaling the number of occurrences (that is, results of performance or nonperformance) related to a particular EP. Each situation discovered by a surveyor(s) will be counted as a separate occurrence.

Note: *Multiple events of the same type related to a single patient and single practitioner/staff member are counted as* one occurrence only.

Use the following rules to determine your EP score:
- Your EP score is 2 if you find one or fewer occurrences of noncompliance with the EP
- Your EP score is 1 if you find two occurrences of noncompliance with the EP
- Your EP score is 0 if you find three or more occurrences of noncompliance with the EP

If an EP in the C category has multiple requirements designated by bullets, the following scoring guidelines apply:
- If there are fewer than 2 findings in all bullets, the EP is scored 2
- If there are three or more findings in all bullets, the EP is scored 0
- In all other combinations of findings, the EP is scored 1

Track Record Achievements

In addition to meeting the requirement(s) in each EP, regardless of category, your hospital must also meet the following track record achievements:

Score	Initial Survey	Full Survey
2	4 months or more	12 months or more
1	2 to 3 months	6 to 11 months
0	Fewer than 2 months	Fewer than 6 months

Sample Sizes

If during an onsite survey, your hospital has been found to be not compliant with one or more standards, you must demonstrate Evidence of Standards Compliance (ESC) for each standard that is not compliant. The ESC must address compliance at the EP level; when an EP within a noncompliant standard requires an MOS, your hospital must demonstrate achievement with the MOS when completing the ESC.

Note: *Not every EP requires an MOS. EPs that do require an MOS are clearly marked in this chapter. Organizations are required to demonstrate achievement with an MOS only for EPs within a noncompliant standard that require an MOS. Organizations do not need to demonstrate achievement with an MOS for any EP within a compliant standard.*

When demonstrating achievement with the MOS during the ESC process, your hospital is **required** to use the following sample sizes, which were established because of their statistical significance, their relative simplicity in application, and their sensitivity to an organization's population size:
- For a population size of fewer than 30 cases, sample 100% of available cases
- For a population size of 30 to 100 cases, sample 30 cases
- For a population size of 101 to 500 cases, sample 50 cases
- For a population size greater than 500 cases, sample 70 cases

Note: *Hospitals are encouraged, but not required, to follow this sample size when demonstrating achievement with an MOS for an EP within a noncompliant standard after conducting a full, Option 1, or Option 2 Periodic Performance Review (PPR).*

When conducting PPR (optional use) or demonstrating an ESC (mandatory use), use the following percentages to determine your score: 90% through 100% of your sample size is in compliance = score 2; 80% through 89% (two instances of noncompliance) of your sample size is in compliance = score 1; less than 80% (three or more instances of noncompliance) of your sample size is in compliance = score 0.

In addition, the following information should govern your hospital's selection of samples:
- The appropriate sample size should be determined by the specific population related to the survey findings
- The sampling approach should involve either systematic random sampling (for example, your hospital selects every second or third case for review) or simple random sampling (for example, your hospital uses a series of random numbers generated by a computer to identify the cases to be reviewed)

- If your hospital chooses not to use these sample sizes while conducting PPR options 1 or 2, you should make sure that your sample size is sufficiently large enough to ensure statistical significance
- When submitting a clarifying ESC, if your hospital selects records as part of its sample, the records should be from a period of no more than three months before the last date of the survey
- Assessment of MOS compliance is conducted for a four-month period following the date of ESC approval. Your hospital should select records as a part of your sample following the date of ESC approval and use the required sample sizes. MOS percentage compliance rates are derived from the average of all four months.

Step 2: Use Your EP Scores to Gauge Your Compliance with the Standards

Now that you have evaluated and scored each EP for a particular standard, use these simple rules to determine your compliance with the standard itself:
- Your hospital is not in compliance (that is, "not compliant") with the standard if any EP is scored 0
- Otherwise, your hospital is in compliance with a standard if 65% or more of its EPs are scored 2

Standards, Rationales, Elements of Performance, and Scoring

Patient-Specific Information

Standard MM.1.10
Patient-specific information is readily accessible to those involved in the medication management system.

Rationale for MM.1.10
A major cause of medication-related sentinel events and medication errors is a lack of information. Licensed independent practitioners, appropriate health care professionals, and staff who participate in the medication management system need access to important information about each patient in order to do the following:
- Facilitate continuity of care, treatment, and service
- Create an accurate medication history and a current list of medications (also known as a drug profile)
- Safely order, prepare, dispense, administer, and monitor medications, as appropriate

Elements of Performance for MM.1.10
B   1. A written policy describes the minimum amount of information about the patient that is to be available to those involved in medication management.

         Note: *The hospital defines who has access to this information; see standard IM.2.10.*

A   2. At a minimum, the information includes the following:
- The patient's age
- The patient's sex
- The patient's current medications
- The patient's diagnoses, comorbidities, and concurrently occurring conditions
- The patient's relevant laboratory values
- The patient's allergies and past sensitivities

         As appropriate to the patient, the hospital also includes information regarding the following:
- Weight and height
- Pregnancy and lactation status
- Any other information required by the hospital for safe medication management

Medication Management

C Ⓜ 3. The information is accessible when needed (except in emergency situations when time does not permit) to licensed independent practitioners, appropriate health care professionals, and staff.

Selection and Procurement

Standard MM.2.10
Medications available for dispensing or administration are selected, listed, and procured based on criteria.

Note: *The formulary is synonymous with the list of medications available for use.*

Elements of Performance for MM.2.10

B   1. Members of the medical staff, licensed independent practitioners, appropriate health care professionals, and staff involved in ordering, dispensing, administering, and/or monitoring effects of medications develop written criteria for determining what medications are available for dispensing or administration.

A   2. At a minimum, the criteria include the indication for use, effectiveness, risks (including propensity for medication errors, abuse potential, and sentinel events), and costs.

A   3. A list of medications for dispensing or administration (including strength and dosage form) is maintained and readily available.

Note: *Sample medications are not required to be on this list.*

B   4. Processes and mechanisms are established to monitor patient responses to a newly added medication before the medication is made available for dispensing or administration within the hospital.

B   5. Medications designated as available for dispensing or administration are reviewed at least annually based on emerging safety and efficacy information.

B   6. The hospital has processes to approve and procure medications that are not on the hospital's medication list.

B   7. The hospital has processes to address medication shortages and outages, including the following:
- Communicating with appropriate prescribers and staff
- Developing approved substitution protocols
- Educating appropriate licensed independent practitioners, appropriate health care professionals, and staff about these protocols
- Obtaining medications in the event of a disaster

Storage

Standard MM.2.20
Medications are properly and safely stored throughout the hospital.

Note: *The following elements of performance also apply to emergency medications. Additional requirements for emergency medications are addressed at standard MM.2.30.*

Elements of Performance for MM.2.20

A Ⓜ 1. Only approved medications are routinely stocked or stored.*

A Ⓜ 2. Medications are stored under necessary conditions to ensure stability.

A 3. Medications are secured in accordance with the hospital's policy and law and regulation so that unauthorized persons cannot obtain access to them.

   Note: *The Centers for Medicare & Medicaid Services' (CMS') definition of "secured" states that all medications including nonprescription medications are in locked containers in a room or are under constant surveillance.*

A 4. Controlled substances are stored to prevent diversion and according to state and federal laws and regulations.

A 5. All expired, damaged, and/or contaminated medications are segregated until they are removed from the hospital.

B 6. Medications that are easy to confuse (for example, sound-alike and look-alike drugs or reagents and chemicals that may be mistaken for medications) are segregated.

A 7. Medications and chemicals used to prepare medications are accurately labeled with contents, expiration dates, and appropriate warnings.

A 8. Drug concentrations available in the hospital are standardized and limited in number.

A Ⓜ 9. Concentrated electrolytes are removed from care units or areas, unless patient safety is at risk if the concentrated electrolyte is not immediately available on a specific care unit or area and specific precautions are taken to prevent inadvertent administration.

B 10. Medications in care areas are maintained in the most ready-to-administer forms available from the manufacturer or if feasible, in unit-doses that have been repackaged by the pharmacy or a licensed repackager.

11. Not applicable

---

* **Note:** See *standard MM.2.40 for the exception to this standard: The hospital has a process to safely manage medications brought in by the patient or the patient's family.*

Medication Management

      12. Not applicable

C Ⓜ 13. All medication storage areas are periodically inspected according to the hospital's policy to make sure medications are stored properly.

Standard MM.2.30

Emergency medications and/or supplies, if any, are consistently available, controlled, and secure in the hospital's patient care areas.

Note: *The following requirements for emergency medications are in addition to the requirements at standard MM.2.20, which are also applicable to emergency medications.*

Elements of Performance for MM.2.30

      1. Not applicable

B   2. Hospital leadership, in conjunction with members of the medical staff and licensed independent practitioners, decides which emergency medications and/or supplies will be readily available in patient care areas.

B   3. Emergency medications are available in unit-dose, age-specific, and ready-to-administer forms whenever possible.

      4. Not applicable

      5. Not applicable

A Ⓜ 6. Emergency medications are stored in sealed or in locked containers; in a locked room; or under constant supervision (per CMS requirements).

B   7. Emergency medications and supplies are replaced as soon as possible after their use in accordance with the hospital's policies and procedures.

Standard MM.2.40

A process is established to safely manage medications brought into the hospital by patients or their families.

Rationale for MM.2.40

A number of valid reasons exist for allowing patients to use their own medications in a health care organization, including avoidance of interruption in therapy; a patient's use of a nonformulary medication; or a lack of alternatives to a patient's personal medication. The hospital defines its responsibilities for the safe use of these medications.

Elements of Performance for MM.2.40

The hospital develops a policy that addresses the use of medications brought into the hospital by patients or their families. The policy specifies the following:

B   1. When such medications can be used or administered

B   2. A process for the identification of the medication and the visual evaluation of its integrity if medications brought in by the patient or family are allowed

A   3. A process to inform the prescriber and patient if medications brought into the hospital by patients or their families are not permitted

Ordering and Transcribing

Standard MM.3.10
Only medications needed to treat the patient's condition are ordered.

Element of Performance for MM.3.10
C Ⓜ   1. There is a documented diagnosis, condition, or indication-for-use for each medication ordered.

Standard MM.3.20
Medication orders are written clearly and transcribed accurately.

Rationale for MM.3.20
Many medication errors occur while communicating or transcribing medication orders. The hospital should take steps to reduce the potential for error or misinterpretation when orders are written or verbally communicated.

Elements of Performance for MM.3.20
Written policy(ies) address the following:

B   1. The required elements of a complete medication order

A   2. When generic or brand names are acceptable or required as part of a medication order

A   3. Whether or when indication for use is required on a medication order

B   4. Any special precautions or procedures for ordering drugs with look-alike or sound-alike names

B   5. Actions to take when medication orders are incomplete, illegible, or unclear

B   6. The hospital specifies the required elements of any of the following types of orders that it deems acceptable for use:
- "As needed" (PRN) orders
- Standing orders

- Hold orders
- Automatic stop orders
- Resume orders*
- Titrating orders—orders in which the dose is either progressively increased or decreased in response to the patient's status
- Taper orders—orders in which the dose is decreased by a particular amount with each dosing interval
- Range orders—orders in which the dose or dosing interval varies over a prescribed range, depending on the situation or patient's status
- Orders for compounded drugs or drug mixtures not commercially available
- Orders for medication-related devices, for example, nebulizers and catheters
- Orders for investigational medications
- Orders for herbal products
- Orders for medications at discharge

In addition, the hospital does the following:

B   7. Minimizes the use of verbal and telephone orders

B   8. Reviews and updates preprinted order sheets as needed

A   9. Specifies that blanket reinstatement of previous orders for medications are not acceptable

B   10. Defines in writing when weight-based dosing for pediatric populations is required

Preparing and Dispensing

Standard MM.4.10
All prescriptions or medication orders are reviewed for appropriateness.

Elements of Performance for MM.4.10
C Ⓜ 1. Before dispensing, removal from floor stock, or removal from an automated storage and distribution device, a pharmacist reviews all prescription or medication orders unless a licensed independent practitioner controls the ordering, preparation, and administration of the medication; or in urgent situations when the resulting delay would harm the patient, including situations in which the patient experiences a sudden change in clinical status (for example, new onset of nausea).

     2. Not applicable

---

* **Note:** See *EP 9—A blanket reinstatement of previous orders for medications is not acceptable.*

A 3. When an onsite licensed pharmacy is not open 24 hours a day, 7 days a week, a health care professional determined to be qualified by the hospital reviews the medication order in the pharmacist's absence.

C Ⓜ 4. When the pharmacy is not open 24 hours a day, 7 days a week, the pharmacist conducts a retrospective review of the order as soon as the pharmacist is available or the pharmacy opens.

B 5. The hospital has a process to review all prescriptions for the following:
- The appropriateness of the drug, dose, frequency, and route of administration
- Therapeutic duplication
- Real or potential allergies or sensitivities
- Real or potential interactions between the prescription and other medications, food, and laboratory values
- Other contraindications
- Variation from organizational criteria for use
- Other relevant medication-related issues or concerns

B 6. All concerns, issues, or questions are clarified with the individual prescriber before dispensing the medication.

Standard MM.4.20
Medications are prepared safely.

Elements of Performance for MM.4.20
B 1. When an onsite, licensed pharmacy is available, only the pharmacy compounds or admixes all sterile medications, intravenous admixtures, or other drugs except in emergencies or when not feasible (for example, when the product's stability is short).

C Ⓜ 2. Wherever medications are prepared, staff use safety materials and equipment while preparing hazardous medications.

C Ⓜ 3. Wherever medications are prepared, staff use techniques to assure accuracy in medication preparation.

C Ⓜ 4. Wherever medications are prepared, staff use appropriate techniques to avoid contamination during medication preparation, which include but are not limited to the following:
- Using clean or sterile technique as appropriate
- Maintaining clean, uncluttered, and functionally separate areas for product preparation to minimize the possibility of contamination
- Using a laminar airflow hood or other class 100 environment while preparing any intravenous (IV) admixture in the pharmacy, any sterile product made from non-sterile ingredients, or any sterile product that will not be used within 24 hours
- Visually inspecting the integrity of the medications

Standard MM.4.30
Medications are appropriately labeled.

Rationale for MM.4.30
A standardized method for labeling all medications will minimize errors.

Elements of Performance for MM.4.30

B   1. Medications are labeled in a standardized manner according to hospital policy, applicable law and regulation, and standards of practice.

B   2. Any time one or more medications are prepared but are not administered immediately, the medication container* must be appropriately labeled.

A   3. At a minimum, all medications are labeled with the following:
- Drug name, strength, amount (if not apparent from the container)
- Expiration date† when not used within 24 hours
- Expiration time when expiration occurs in less than 24 hours
- The date prepared and the diluent for all compounded IV admixtures and parenteral nutrition solutions

A   4. When preparing individualized medications for multiple specific patients or when the person preparing the individualized medications is not the person administering the medication, the label also includes the following:
- Patient name
- Patient location
- Directions for use and any applicable cautionary statements either on the label or attached as an accessory label (for example, "requires refrigeration," "for IM use only")

Standard MM.4.40
Medications are dispensed safely.

Elements of Performance for MM.4.40

B   1. Quantities of medications are dispensed which minimize diversion yet are still consistent with the patient's needs.

B   2. Dispensing adheres to law, regulation, licensure, and professional standards of practice, including record keeping.

C Ⓜ   3. Medications are dispensed in a timely manner to meet patient needs.

---

* A container can be any storage device such as a plastic bag, syringe, bottle, or box which can be labeled and secured in such a way that it can be readily determined that the contents are intact and have not expired.

† Expiration date, also called the "beyond use date," refers to the last date that the product should be used by the patient.

C Ⓜ 4. Medications are dispensed in the most ready-to-administer forms available from the manufacturer or if feasible, in unit-doses that have been repackaged by the pharmacy or licensed repackager.

B 5. The hospital consistently uses the same dose packaging system, or if a different system is used, provides education about the use of the dose packaging system to the appropriate patients.

Standard MM.4.50

The hospital has a system for safely providing medications to meet patient needs when the pharmacy is closed.

Note: *This standard only applies when a hospital has an on-site pharmacy and patients present in the hospital.*

Rationale for MM.4.50

If an urgent or emergent patient need occurs, the hospital must be able to provide medications to the patients in its facility.

Elements of Performance for MM.4.50

B 1. The hospital has a process for providing medications to meet patient needs when the pharmacy is closed.

B 2. When nonpharmacist health care professionals are allowed by law and regulation to obtain medications after the pharmacy is closed, the following safeguards are applied:
- Access is limited to a set of medications that has been approved by the hospital. These medications can be stored in a night cabinet, automated storage and distribution device, or a limited section of the pharmacy.
- Only trained, designated prescribers and nurses are permitted access to medications.
- Quality control procedures (such as an independent second check by another individual or a secondary verification built into the system, such as bar coding) are in place to prevent medication retrieval errors.
- The hospital arranges for a qualified pharmacist to be available either on-call or at another location (for example, at another organization that has 24-hour pharmacy service) to answer questions or provide medications beyond those accessible to nonpharmacy staff.

B 3. This process is evaluated on an ongoing basis to determine the medications accessed routinely and the causes of accessing the pharmacy after hours.

C Ⓜ 4. Changes are implemented as appropriate to reduce the amount of times nonpharmacist health care professionals are obtaining medications after the pharmacy is closed.

Medication Management

Standard MM.4.60
Not applicable

Standard MM.4.70
Medications dispensed by the hospital are retrieved when recalled or discontinued by the manufacturer or the Food and Drug Administration for safety reasons.

Elements of Performance for MM.4.70

A 1. When the hospital has been informed of a medication recall or discontinuation by the manufacturer or the Food and Drug Administration (FDA) for safety reasons, medications within the hospital are retrieved* and appropriately handled per hospital policy and law and regulation.

A 2. When the hospital has been informed of a medication recall or discontinuation by the manufacturer or the FDA for safety reasons, all those ordering, dispensing, and/or administering recalled or discontinued medications are notified.

A 3. When the hospital has been informed of a medication recall or discontinuation by the manufacturer or the FDA for safety reasons, patients who may have received the medication are identified and informed of the recall or discontinuation.

Standard MM.4.80
Medications returned to the pharmacy are appropriately managed.

Rationale for MM.4.80
Medications may be returned when allowed under law and regulation and hospital policy. Previously dispensed but unused, expired, or returned medications in the hospital must be accounted for and controlled. The pharmacy is responsible for controlling and accounting for all unused medications returned to the pharmacy.

Elements of Performance for MM.4.80

B 1. The hospital has a process in place that addresses if and when unused, expired, or returned medications will be managed by the pharmacy.

B 2. The hospital has a process in place that addresses how medications can be returned to the pharmacy's control, including procedures that address preventing diversion of medications and account for all unused, expired, or returned medications.

B 3. The hospital has a process in place that addresses how outside sources, if any, are used for destruction of medications.

C Ⓜ 4. These processes are implemented.

---
* Although recalls are generally by lot number, an organization may retrieve all lots of a recalled medication instead of recording and identifying medications by their lot number.

Administering

Standard MM.5.10
Medications are safely and accurately administered.

Elements of Performance for MM.5.10
Policies and procedures address the following:

    1. Not applicable

B   2. Guidelines for prescriber notification in the event of an adverse drug reaction or medication error

Before administering a medication, the licensed independent practitioner or appropriate health care professional administering the medication does the following:

C Ⓜ 3. Verifies that the medication selected for administration is the correct one based on the medication order and product label

C Ⓜ 4. Verifies that the medication is stable based on visual examination for particulates or discoloration and that the medication has not expired

C Ⓜ 5. Verifies that there is no contraindication for administering the medication

C Ⓜ 6. Verifies that the medication is being administered at the proper time, in the prescribed dose, and by the correct route

C Ⓜ 7. Advises the patient or, if appropriate, the patient's family, about any potential clinically significant adverse reaction or other concerns about administering a new medication

C Ⓜ 8. Discusses any unresolved, significant concerns about the medication with the patient's physician, prescriber (if different from the physician), and/or relevant staff involved with the patient's care, treatment, and service

Standard MM.5.20
Self-administered medications are safely and accurately administered.

Elements of Performance for MM.5.20

B   1. If self administration is allowed, procedures guide the safe and accurate self administration* of medications or administration of medications by a person who is not a staff member and address training, supervision, and administration documentation.

C Ⓜ 2. Persons who administer medications but are not staff members (for example, the patient if self-administering) receive training and appropriate information about the following:

---

* Self administration includes those instances where a patient independently uses a medication, including medications that may be held by the hospital for the independent use by the patient.

Medication Management

- The nature of the medications to be administered
- How to administer medications, such as the appropriate frequency, route of administration, and dose
- The expected actions and side effects of the medications to be administered
- How to monitor the effects of the medications on the patient

C Ⓜ 3. Persons who administer medications but are not staff members (including the patient if self-administering) are determined to be competent at medication administration before being allowed to administer medications.

Monitoring

Standard MM.6.10
The effects of medication(s) on patients are monitored.

Rationale for MM.6.10
Monitoring the effects of medications on patients helps to assure that medication therapy is appropriate and minimizes the occurrence of adverse events.

Elements of Performance for MM.6.10

C Ⓜ 1. Each patient's response to his or her medication is monitored according to the clinical needs of the patient and addresses the patient's response to the prescribed medication and actual or potential medication-related problems.

C Ⓜ 2. Monitoring a medication's effect on a patient includes the following:
- Gathering the patient's own perceptions about side effects, and when appropriate, perceived efficacy
- Referring to information from the patient's medical record, relevant laboratory results, clinical response, and medication profile

B 3. The hospital has a process for monitoring the patient's response to the first dose(s) of a medication new to a patient while he or she is under the direct care of the hospital.

Standard MM.6.20
The hospital responds appropriately to actual or potential adverse drug events and medication errors.

Elements of Performance for MM.6.20

B 1. The hospital has a process to respond to actual or potential adverse drug events and medication errors.

C Ⓜ 2. Appropriate action is taken when an actual or potential adverse drug event is identified (this may be limited to calling for outside assistance depending upon the hospital's services).

C Ⓜ 3. The hospital or responsible individual complies with internal and external reporting requirements for actual or potential adverse drug events (for example, to the United States Pharmacopoeia [USP], the FDA, and the Institute for Safe Medication Practices [ISMP]).

High-Risk Medications

High-risk or high-alert drugs are those drugs involved in a high percentage of medication errors and/or sentinel events and medications that carry a higher risk for abuse, errors, or other adverse outcomes. Lists of high-risk or high-alert drugs are available from such organizations as the ISMP, the USP, and so forth, based on national data about medication use. However, the hospital needs to develop its own list of high-risk or high-alert drugs based on its unique utilization patterns or drugs and its own internal data about medication errors and sentinel events. Examples of high-risk drugs may include investigational drugs, controlled medications, medications not on the approved FDA list, medications with a narrow therapeutic range, psychotherapeutic medications, and look-alike/sound-alike medications. Medications that are new to the market or new to the hospital should also be considered.

Standard MM.7.10
The hospital develops processes for managing high-risk or high-alert medications.

Elements of Performance for MM.7.10

A 1. The hospital identifies the high-risk or high-alert medications used within the hospital, if any.

B 2. As appropriate to the services provided, the hospital develops processes for procuring, storing, ordering, transcribing, preparing, dispensing, administering, and/or monitoring high-risk or high-alert medications.

Standard MM.7.20
Not applicable

Standard MM.7.30
Not applicable

Standard MM.7.40
Investigational medications are safely controlled and administered.

Rationale for MM.7.40
The hospital protects the safety of patients participating in investigational or clinical medication studies by ensuring that these activities are adequately controlled and supported. In addition, the hospital should be sensitive to the use of particular populations for experimentation and research, and review all investigational medications to evaluate safety (*see* standard RI.2.180).

Element of Performance for MM.7.40
B   1. Procedures for the use of investigational medications, when used, are implemented and maintained including the following:
- Having a written process for reviewing, approving, supervising, and monitoring investigational medications use
- Specifying that when an investigational medication protocol is being conducted independent of the hospital, the hospital will review and accommodate, as appropriate, the patient's continued participation in the protocol (*see* standard RI.2.180)
- Specifying that when pharmacy services are provided, the pharmacy controls the storage, dispensing, labeling, and distribution of the investigational medication

Evaluation

Standard MM.8.10
The hospital evaluates its medication management system.

Elements of Performance for MM.8.10
B   1. The hospital evaluates its medication management system for risk points and identifies areas to improve safety.

B   2. The hospital routinely evaluates the literature for new technologies or successful practices that have been demonstrated to enhance safety in other hospitals to determine if it can improve its own medication management system.

B   3. The hospital should also review internally generated reports to identify trends or issues in its own system (*see* standards PI.2.10 and PI.2.20).

Surveillance, Prevention, and Control of Infection*

Overview

Prevention of health care–associated infections (HAIs) represents one of the major safety initiatives a hospital can undertake, making the effective evaluation and possible redesign of existing infection prevention and control programs (hereafter referred to as the "IC program") a priority. The Centers for Disease Control and Prevention (CDC, 2000)[†] estimates that each year, approximately 2 million patients admitted to acute care hospitals in the United States acquire infections that were not related to the condition for which they were hospitalized. These infections result in approximately 90,000 deaths and add between $4.5 to $5.7 billion per year to patient care costs (CDC, 1992).[‡] While the precise causes of HAIs are difficult to identify, it has been estimated that approximately one third of HAIs could be prevented using current recommendations.[§||]

Effective infection prevention and control requires an integrated, responsive process involving collaboration by many programs, services, and settings throughout the hospital to develop, implement, and evaluate the IC program. The design and scope of the IC program are based on the risk that the hospital faces related to the acquisition and transmission of infectious disease.

The goal of an effective IC program is to reduce the risk of acquisition and transmission of HAIs. Hospitals must do the following to achieve this goal:
1. The hospital incorporates its infection control program as a major component of its safety and performance improvement programs
2. The hospital performs an ongoing assessment to identify its risks for the acquisition and transmission of infectious agents

---

* Revised standards, rationales, and elements of performance, effective January 1, 2005. However, beginning July 1, 2004, surveyors will explore a hospital's progress toward meeting this standard and its EPs and provide education on the findings as necessary. Findings will not be included in the survey report, nor will they influence the final accreditation decision.

[†] Monitoring hospital-acquired infections to promote patient safety—United States, 1990–1999. *MMWR Morb Mortal Wkly Rep* 49:149–153, Mar. 10, 2000.

[‡] Public Health Focus: surveillance, prevention and control of nosocomial infections. *MMWR Morb Mortal Wkly Rep* 41:783–787, Oct. 23, 1992.

[§] Harbarth S., Sax H., Gastmeier P.: The preventable proportion of nosocomial infections: an overview of published reports. *J Hosp Infect* 54:258–256, Aug. 2003.

[||] Haley R.W., et al.: The efficacy of infection surveillance and control programs in preventing nosocomial infections in U.S. hospitals. *Am J Epidemiol* 121:182–205, Feb. 1985.

3. The hospital uses an epidemiological approach that consists of surveillance, data collection, and trend identification
4. The hospital effectively implements infection prevention and control processes
5. The hospital educates and collaborates with hospitalwide leaders to effectively participate in the design and implementation of the IC program
6. The hospital integrates its efforts with health care and community leaders to the extent practicable, recognizing that infection prevention and control is a communitywide effort
7. To remain a viable community resource, the hospital must plan for responding to infections that potentially overwhelm its resources

A program with aims of such broad scope and depth requires the direct involvement of hospital leaders. Only with the ongoing attention and direction of hospital leadership can the appropriate scope of the IC program be determined and adequately resourced.

The standards in this chapter, which focus on development and implementation of plans to prevent and control infections, are supported by standards in other chapters, such as "Management of the Environment of Care," "Management of Human Resources," "Improving Organization Performance," and "Leadership," to produce a comprehensive approach to IC.

Standards

The following is a list of all standards for this function. They are presented here for your convenience without footnotes or other explanatory text. If you have a question about a term used here, please check the Glossary.

Note: *A revised standard numbering system is being used with the reformatted standards. The revised numbering system will allow for more flexibility to add standards while maintaining the current number for each standard.*

The IC Program and Its Components

IC.1.10 The risk of development of a health care–associated infection is minimized through a hospitalwide infection control program.

IC.2.10 The infection control program identifies risks for the acquisition and transmission of infectious agents on an ongoing basis.

IC.3.10 Based on risks, the hospital establishes priorities and sets goals for preventing the development of health care–associated infections within the hospital.

IC.4.10 Once the hospital has prioritized its goals, strategies must be implemented to achieve those goals.

IC.5.10 The infection control program evaluates the effectiveness of the infection control interventions and, as necessary, redesigns the infection control interventions.

IC.6.10 As part of emergency management activities, the hospital prepares to respond to an influx, or the risk of an influx, of infectious patients.

Structure and Resources for the IC Program

IC.7.10 The infection control program is managed effectively.

IC.8.10 Representatives from relevant components/functions within the hospital collaborate to implement the infection control program.

IC.9.10 Hospital leaders allocate adequate resources for the infection control program.

Understanding the Parts of This Chapter

To help you navigate this reformatted standards chapter, it may be helpful to think of its parts this way:
- The **standard** is the "goal."
- The **rationale** explains why it's important to achieve this goal.
- The **elements of performance** identify the step(s) needed to achieve this goal.

These parts are defined as follows.

Standard A statement that defines the performance expectations and/or structures or processes that must be in place in order for a hospital to provide safe, high-quality care, treatment, and services. A hospital is either "compliant" or "not compliant" with a standard.

Accreditation decisions are based on simple counts of the standards that are determined to be "not compliant."

Rationale A statement that provides background, justification, or additional information about a standard. A standard's rationale is not scored. In some instances, the rationale for a standard is self-evident. Therefore, not every standard has a written rationale.

Elements of performance (EPs) The specific performance expectations and/or structures or processes that must be in place in order for a hospital to provide safe, high-quality care, treatment, and services. The scoring of EP compliance determines a hospital's overall compliance with a standard. EPs are evaluated on the following scale:

  0   Insufficient compliance
  1   Partial compliance
  2   Satisfactory compliance
  NA Not applicable

You will find a **measure of success** icon—Ⓜ—next to some EPs. Measures of success (MOS) need to be developed for certain EPs when a standard is judged to be out of compliance through either the Periodic Performance Review (PPR) or the onsite survey. An MOS is defined as a quantifiable measure, usually related to an audit, that can be used to determine whether an action has been effective and is being sustained.*

Assessing Your Compliance

Once you are familiar with the parts of this chapter, you can begin to assess your compliance with its requirements. The scoring category for each EP is noted next to the EP. If you would like to assess your hospital's performance, mark your scores for the EPs and the standards by following the simple steps described below.

---

* For more information about measures of success, *see* the "The New Joint Commission Accreditation Process" chapter in this book.

Two components are scored for each EP: (1) compliance with the requirement itself **and** (2) compliance with the track record* for that requirement. Scoring has been simplified, and track record achievements (which have always been part of the scoring) have been appropriately modified.

Note: *Some standards and EPs do not apply to a particular type of organization; these standards and EPs are marked "not applicable" and the related text is not included. Your hospital is not expected to comply with standards and EPs marked "not applicable."*

In addition, some standards and EPs that do apply to organizations may not apply to the specific care, treatment, and services that your individual hospital provides. Although these standards and EPs are included in the manual, you are not expected to comply with them. If you are unsure about the standards or EPs that apply to your hospital, please contact the Joint Commission's Standards Interpretation Group at 630/792-5900.

Step 1: Score Your Compliance with Each Element of Performance

Before you can determine your compliance with the standards, you must score your compliance with each EP. There are three scoring criterion categories: A, B, and C (described below). Please note that for each EP scoring criterion category, your hospital must meet the performance requirement itself and the track record achievements (*see* "Track Record Achievements").

Category A
These EPs relate to the presence or absence of the requirement(s) and are scored either yes (2) or no (0); however, score 1 for partial compliance is also possible based on track record achievements.

If an A EP has multiple components designated by bullets, your hospital must be compliant with all the bullets to receive a score of 2. If your hospital does not meet one or more requirements in the bullets, you will receive a score of 0.

Category B
Category B EPs are scored in two steps:
1. As with category A EPs, category B EPs relate to the presence or absence of the requirement(s). If your hospital *does not meet* the requirement(s), the EP is scored 0; there is no need to assess your compliance with the principles of good process design.
2. If your hospital *does meet* the requirement(s), but there is concern about the quality or comprehensiveness of the effort, then and only then should you assess the qualitative aspect of the EP. That is, review the applicable principles of good process design and ask how the principles were applied in the situation under discussion. Good process design has the following characteristics:

---

* **Track record** The amount of time that an organization has been in compliance with a standard, element of performance, or other requirement.

- Is consistent with your hospital's mission, values, and goals
- Meets the needs of patients
- Reflects the use of currently accepted practices (doing the right thing, using resources responsibly, using practice guidelines)
- Incorporates current safety information and knowledge such as sentinel event data and National Patient Safety Goals
- Incorporates relevant performance improvement results

This two-part evaluation applies to both simple and bulleted B EPs. First, the EPs are assessed to determine if the requirements are present. If the EP has multiple components designated by bullets, as with the category A EPs, your hospital must meet the requirements in *all* the bulleted items to get a score of 2. If your hospital meets *none* of the requirements in the bullets, it receives a score of 0. If your hospital meets *at least one, but not all*, of the bulleted requirements, it will receive a score of 1 for the EPs.

Use the following rules to determine your EP score:
- Your EP score is 0 if your hospital does not meet the requirement(s); you *do not* need to assess your compliance with the preceding applicable principles of good process design
- Your EP score is 1 if your hospital does meet the requirement(s), but considered only *some* of the preceding applicable principles of good process design
- Your EP score is 2 if your hospital does meet the requirement(s) *and* considered *all* the preceding principles of good process design

Category C

C EPs are scored 0, 1, or 2 based on the number of times your hospital does not meet the EP. These EPs are frequency based and require totaling the number of occurrences (that is, results of performance or nonperformance) related to a particular EP. Each situation discovered by a surveyor(s) will be counted as a separate occurrence.

Note: *Multiple events of the same type related to a single patient and single practitioner/staff member are counted as* one occurrence only.

Use the following rules to determine your EP score:
- Your EP score is 2 if you find one or fewer occurrences of noncompliance with the EP
- Your EP score is 1 if you find two occurrences of noncompliance with the EP
- Your EP score is 0 if you find three or more occurrences of noncompliance with the EP

If an EP in the C category has multiple requirements designated by bullets, the following scoring guidelines apply:
- If there are fewer than 2 findings in all bullets, the EP is scored 2
- If there are three or more findings in all bullets, the EP is scored 0
- In all other combinations of findings, the EP is scored 1

Surveillance, Prevention, and Control of Infection

Track Record Achievements
In addition to meeting the requirement(s) in each EP, regardless of category, your hospital must also meet the following track record achievements:

Score	Initial Survey	Full Survey
2	4 months or more	12 months or more
1	2 to 3 months	6 to 11 months
0	Fewer than 2 months	Fewer than 6 months

Sample Sizes
If during an onsite survey, your hospital has been found to be not compliant with one or more standards, you must demonstrate Evidence of Standards Compliance (ESC) for each standard that is not compliant. The ESC must address compliance at the EP level; when an EP within a noncompliant standard requires an MOS, your hospital must demonstrate achievement with the MOS when completing the ESC.

Note: *Not every EP requires an MOS. EPs that do require an MOS are clearly marked in this chapter. Organizations are required to demonstrate achievement with an MOS only for EPs within a noncompliant standard that require an MOS. Organizations do not need to demonstrate achievement with an MOS for any EP within a compliant standard.*

When demonstrating achievement with the MOS during the ESC process, your hospital is **required** to use the following sample sizes, which were established because of their statistical significance, their relative simplicity in application, and their sensitivity to an organization's population size:
- For a population size of fewer than 30 cases, sample 100% of available cases
- For a population size of 30 to 100 cases, sample 30 cases
- For a population size of 101 to 500 cases, sample 50 cases
- For a population size greater than 500 cases, sample 70 cases

Note: *Hospitals are encouraged, but not required, to follow this sample size when demonstrating achievement with an MOS for an EP within a noncompliant standard after conducting a full, Option 1, or Option 2 Periodic Performance Review (PPR).*

When conducting PPR (optional use) or demonstrating an ESC (mandatory use), use the following percentages to determine your score: 90% through 100% of your sample size is in compliance = score 2; 80% through 89% (two instances of noncompliance) of your sample size is in compliance = score 1; less than 80% (three or more instances of noncompliance) of your sample size is in compliance = score 0.

In addition, the following information should govern your hospital's selection of samples:
- The appropriate sample size should be determined by the specific population related to the survey findings
- The sampling approach should involve either systematic random sampling (for example, your hospital selects every second or third case for review) or simple random sampling (for example, your hospital uses a series of random numbers generated by a computer to identify the cases to be reviewed)

- If your hospital chooses not to use these sample sizes while conducting PPR options 1 or 2, you should make sure that your sample size is sufficiently large enough to ensure statistical significance
- When submitting a clarifying ESC, if your hospital selects records as part of its sample, the records should be from a period of no more than three months before the last date of the survey
- Assessment of MOS compliance is conducted for a four-month period following the date of ESC approval. Your hospital should select records as a part of your sample following the date of ESC approval and use the required sample sizes. MOS percentage compliance rates are derived from the average of all four months.

Step 2: Use Your EP Scores to Gauge Your Compliance with the Standards

Now that you have evaluated and scored each EP for a particular standard, use these simple rules to determine your compliance with the standard itself:
- Your hospital is not in compliance (that is, "not compliant") with the standard if any EP is scored 0
- Otherwise, your hospital is in compliance with a standard if 65% or more of its EPs are scored 2

Standards, Rationales, Elements of Performance, and Scoring

The IC Program and Its Components

Standard IC.1.10
The risk of development of a health care–associated infection is minimized through a hospitalwide infection control program.

Rationale for IC.1.10
The risk of HAIs exists throughout the hospital. An effective IC program that can systematically identify risks and respond appropriately must involve all relevant programs and settings within the hospital.

Elements of Performance for IC.1.10

B   1. A hospitalwide IC program is implemented.

B   2. Individuals and/or positions with the authority to take steps to prevent or control the acquisition and transmission of infectious agents are identified.

B   3. All applicable organizational components and functions are integrated into the IC program.

B   4. Systems are in place to communicate with licensed independent practitioners, staff, students/trainees, volunteers, and as appropriate, visitors, patients, and families about infection prevention and control issues, including their responsibilities in preventing the spread of infection within the hospital.

B   5. The hospital has systems for reporting infection surveillance, prevention, and control information to the following:
- The appropriate staff within the hospital
- Federal, state, and local public health authorities in accordance with law and regulation
- Accrediting bodies (*see* Sentinel Event Reporting, pages SE-10–SE-11, and National Patient Safety Goals, page NPSG-4)
- The referring or receiving organization when a patient was transferred or referred and the presence of an HAI was not known at the time of transfer or referral

B   6. Systems for the investigation of outbreaks of infectious diseases are in place.

B   7. Applicable policies and procedures are in place throughout the hospital.

8. Not applicable

B 9. The hospital has a written IC plan* that includes the following:
- A description of prioritized risks
- A statement of the goals of the IC program
- A description of the hospital's strategies to minimize, reduce, or eliminate the prioritized risks
- A description of how the strategies will be evaluated

Standard IC.2.10
The infection control program identifies risks for the acquisition and transmission of infectious agents on an ongoing basis.

Rationale for IC.2.10
A hospital's risks of infection will vary based on the hospital's geographic location, the community environment, the types of programs/services provided, and the characteristics and behaviors of the population served. As these risks change over time—sometimes rapidly—risk assessment must be an ongoing process.

Elements of Performance for IC.2.10
B 1. The hospital identifies risks for the transmission and acquisition of infectious agents throughout the hospital based on the following factors:
- The geographic location and community environment of the hospital, program/services provided, and the characteristics of the population served
- The results of the analysis of the hospital's infection prevention and control data
- The care, treatment, and services provided

A 2. The risk analysis is formally reviewed at least annually and whenever significant changes occur in any of the above factors.

B 3. Surveillance activities, including data collection and analysis, are used to identify infection prevention and control risks pertaining to the following:
- Patients
- Licensed independent practitioners, staff, volunteers, and student/trainees
- Visitors and families, as warranted

Standard IC.3.10
Based on risks, the hospital establishes priorities and sets goals for preventing the development of health care–associated infections within the hospital.

---
* **Written plan** A succinct, useful document, formulated beforehand, that identifies needs, lists strategies to meet those needs, and sets goals and objectives. The format of the "plan" may include narratives, policies and procedures, protocols, practice guidelines, clinical paths, care maps, or a combination of these.

Surveillance, Prevention, and Control of Infection

Rationale for IC.3.10
The risks of HAIs within a hospital are many while resources are limited. An effective IC program requires a thoughtful prioritization of the most important risks to be addressed. Priorities and goals related to the identified risks guide the choice and design of strategies for infection prevention and control in a hospital. These priorities and goals provide a framework for evaluating the strategies.

Elements of Performance for IC.3.10

B   1. Priorities are established and goals related to preventing the acquisition and transmission of potentially infectious agents are developed based on the risks identified.

These goals include, but are not limited to, the following:

A   2. Limiting unprotected exposure to pathogens throughout the hospital

A   3. Enhancing hand hygiene

       4. Not applicable

A   5. Minimizing the risk of transmitting infections associated with the use of procedures, medical equipment, and medical devices

Standard IC.4.10
Once the hospital has prioritized its goals, strategies must be implemented to achieve those goals.

Rationale for IC.4.10
The hospital plans and implements interventions to address the IC issues that it finds important based on prioritized risks and associated surveillance data.

Elements of Performance for IC.4.10

B   1. Interventions are designed to incorporate relevant guidelines* for infection prevention and control activities.

Interventions are implemented which include the following (EPs 2 and 3):

A   2. A hospitalwide hand hygiene program that complies with current Centers for Disease Control and Prevention (CDC) hand hygiene guidelines (National Patient Safety Goal 7, requirement 7.a)

B   3. Methods to reduce the risks associated with procedures, medical equipment,† and medical devices, including the following:
- Appropriate storage, cleaning, disinfection, sterilization, and/or disposal of supplies and equipment

---

* Examples of guidelines include those offered by the CDC, Healthcare Infection Control Practices Advisory Committee (HICPAC), and National Quality Forum (NQF).

† **Medical equipment** Fixed and portable equipment used for the diagnosis, treatment, monitoring, and direct care of individuals.

- Reuse of equipment designated by the manufacturer as disposable in a manner that is consistent with regulatory and professional standards
- The appropriate use of personal protective equipment

B   4. Implementation of applicable precautions, as appropriate, is based on the following:
- The potential for transmission
- The mechanism of transmission
- The care, treatment, and service setting
- The emergence and reemergence of pathogens in the community that could affect the hospital

Interventions are implemented which include the following (EPs 5–7):

C Ⓜ   5. Screening for exposure and/or immunity to infectious diseases that licensed independent practitioners, staff, student/trainees, and volunteers may come in contact with in their work is available as warranted

C Ⓜ   6. Referral for assessment, potential testing, immunization and/or prophylaxis/treatment, and counseling as appropriate of licensed independent practitioners, staff, students/trainees, and volunteers who are identified as potentially having an infectious disease or risk of infectious disease that may put the population they serve at risk

C Ⓜ   7. Referral for assessment, potential testing, immunization and/or prophylaxis/treatment, and counseling as appropriate of patients, students/trainees, and volunteers who have been exposed to infectious disease(s) at the hospital and licensed independent practitioners or staff who are occupationally exposed

B   8. Reduction of risks associated with animals brought into the hospital

Standard IC.5.10
The infection control program evaluates the effectiveness of the infection control interventions and, as necessary, redesigns the infection control interventions.

Rationale for IC.5.10
The evaluation of the effectiveness of interventions helps to identify which activities of the IC program are effective and which activities need to be changed to improve outcomes.

Elements of Performance for IC.5.10

A   1. The hospital formally evaluates and revises the goals and program (or portions of the program) at least annually and whenever risks significantly change.

Surveillance, Prevention, and Control of Infection

B   2.   The evaluation addresses changes in the scope of the IC program (for example, resulting from the introduction of new services or new sites of care).

B   3.   The evaluation addresses changes in the results of the IC program risk analysis.

B   4.   The evaluation addresses emerging and reemerging problems in the health care community that potentially affect the hospital (for example, highly infectious agents).

B   5.   The evaluation addresses the assessment of the success or failure of interventions for preventing and controlling infection.

B   6.   The evaluation addresses responses to concerns raised by leadership and others within the hospital.

B   7.   The evaluation addresses the evolution of relevant infection prevention and control guidelines that are based on evidence or, in the absence of evidence, expert consensus.

Standard IC.6.10

As part of emergency management activities, the hospital prepares to respond to an influx, or the risk of an influx, of infectious patients.

Rationale for IC.6.10

The health care organization is an important resource for the continued functioning of a community. A hospital's ability to deliver care, treatment, and services is threatened when it is ill-prepared to respond to an epidemic or infections likely to require expanded or extended care capabilities over a prolonged period. Therefore, it is important for a hospital to plan how to prevent the introduction of the infection into the hospital, how to quickly recognize that this type of infection has been introduced, and/or how to contain the spread of the infection if it is introduced.

This planned response may include a broad range of options including the temporary halting of services and/or admissions, delaying transfer or discharge, limiting visitors within a hospital, or fully activating the hospital's emergency management plan. The actual response depends upon issues such as the extent to which the community is affected by the spread of the infection, the types of services offered, and the hospital's capabilities.

The concepts included in these standards are supported by standards found elsewhere in the book, including standard EC.4.10.

Elements of Performance for IC.6.10

B   1.   The hospital plans its response to an influx or risk of an influx of infectious patients.

B   2.   The hospital has a plan for managing an ongoing influx of potentially infectious patients over an extended period.

B   3. The hospital does the following:
- Determines how it will keep abreast of current information about the emergence of epidemics or new infections which may result in the hospital activating its response
- Determines how it will disseminate critical information to staff and other key practitioners
- Identifies resources in the community (through local, state, and/or federal public health systems) for obtaining additional information

Structure and Resources for the IC Program

Standard IC.7.10
The infection control program is managed effectively.

Rationale for IC.7.10
The IC program requires management by an individual (or individuals) with knowledge that is appropriate to the risks identified by the hospital, as well as knowledge of the analysis of infection risks, principles of infection prevention and control, and data analysis. This individual may be employed by the hospital or the hospital may contract with this individual. The number of individuals and their qualifications are based on the hospital's size, complexity, and needs.

Elements of Performance for IC.7.10

A   1. The hospital assigns responsibility for managing IC program activities to one or more individuals whose number, competency, and skill mix are determined by the goals and objectives of the IC activities.

B   2. Qualifications of the individual(s) responsible for managing the IC program are determined by the risks entailed in the care, treatment, and services provided, the hospital's patient population(s), and the complexity of the activities that will be carried out.

> **Note:** *Qualifications may be met through ongoing education, training, experience, and/or certification (such as that offered by the Certification Board for Infection Control [CBIC]) in the prevention and control of infections.*

B   3. This individual(s) coordinates all infection prevention and control activities within the hospital.

B   4. This individual(s) facilitates ongoing monitoring of the effectiveness of prevention and/or control activities and interventions.

Standard IC.8.10
Representatives from relevant components/functions within the hospital collaborate to implement the infection control program.

Rationale for IC.8.10
The successful creation of a hospitalwide IC program requires collaboration with all relevant components/functions. This collaboration is vital to successful data gathering and interpretation, design of interventions, and effective implementation of interventions. Individuals within the hospital who have the power to implement plans and make decisions about interventions related to infection prevention and control participate in the IC program. While a formal committee consisting of leadership and other components is not required as evidence of this collaboration, the hospital may want to consider this option.

Elements of Performance for IC.8.10

B 1. Hospital leaders, with licensed independent practitioners, medical staff, and other direct and indirect patient care staff (including, when applicable, administration, building maintenance/engineering, food services, housekeeping, laboratory, pharmacy, and sterilization services, collaborate on an ongoing basis with the qualified individual(s) managing the IC program.

B 2. These representatives participate in the following:
- Development of strategies for each component's/function's role in the IC program
- Assessment of the adequacy of the human, information, physical, and financial resources allocated to support infection prevention and control activities
- Assessment of the overall failure or success of key processes for preventing and controlling infection
- The review and revision of the IC program as warranted to improve outcomes

Standard IC.9.10
Hospital leaders allocate adequate resources for the infection control program.

Rationale for IC.9.10
Adequate resources are needed to effectively plan and successfully implement a program of this scope.

Elements of Performance for IC.9.10

A 1. The effectiveness of the hospital's infection prevention and control activities is reviewed on an ongoing basis, and findings are reported to the integrated patient safety program at least annually.

B   2. Adequate systems to access information are provided to support infection prevention and control activities.

B   3. Adequate laboratory support is provided to support infection prevention and control activities.

B   4. Adequate equipment and supplies are provided to support infection prevention and control activities.

Improving Organization Performance

Overview

Performance improvement (PI) is a continuous process. It involves measuring the functioning of important processes and services, and, when indicated, identifying changes that enhance performance. These changes are incorporated into new or existing work processes, products or services, and performance is monitored to ensure that the improvements are sustained.

Performance improvement focuses on outcomes of care, treatment, and services. Leaders establish a planned, systematic, and organizationwide approach(es) to performance improvement. They set priorities for performance improvement and ensure that the disciplines representing the scope of care, treatment, and services across the hospital work collaboratively to plan and implement improvement activities. The leaders' responsibilities are described in the "Leadership" chapter (standards LD.4.10 through LD.4.70) of this book.

An important aspect of improving organization performance is effectively reducing factors that contribute to unanticipated adverse events and/or outcomes. Unanticipated adverse events and/or outcomes may be caused by poorly designed systems, system failures, or errors. Reducing unanticipated adverse events and/or unanticipated outcomes requires an environment in which patients, their families, and hospital staff and leaders can identify and manage actual and potential risks to safety. Such an environment encourages the following:
- Recognizing and acknowledging risks and unanticipated adverse events
- Initiating actions to reduce these risks and unanticipated adverse events
- Reporting internally on risk reduction initiatives and their effectiveness
- Focusing on processes and systems
- Minimizing individual blame or retribution for involvement in an unanticipated adverse event
- Investigating factors that contribute to unanticipated adverse events and sharing that acquired knowledge both internally and with other hospitals

The leaders are responsible for fostering such an environment through their personal example and by supporting effective responses to actual occurrences of unanticipated adverse events; ongoing proactive reduction of safety risks to patients; and integration of safety priorities into the design and redesign of all relevant organization processes, functions, and services. (*See* standard LD.4.50.)

This chapter focuses on the following fundamental components of performance improvement:
- Measuring performance through data collection
- Assessing current performance
- Improving performance

Standards

The following is a list of all standards for this function. They are presented here for your convenience without footnotes or other explanatory text. If you have a question about a term used here, please check the Glossary.

Note: *A revised standard numbering system is being used with the standards. This revised numbering system will allow for more flexibility to add standards while maintaining the current label for each standard.*

PI.1.10 The hospital collects data to monitor its performance.

PI.2.10 Data are systematically aggregated and analyzed.

PI.2.20 Undesirable patterns or trends in performance are analyzed.

PI.2.30 Processes for identifying and managing sentinel events are defined and implemented.

PI.3.10 Information from data analysis is used to make changes that improve performance and patient safety and reduce the risk of sentinel events.

PI.3.20 An ongoing, proactive program for identifying and reducing unanticipated adverse events and safety risks to patients is defined and implemented.

Improving Organization Performance

Understanding the Parts of This Chapter

To help you navigate this reformatted standards chapter, it may be helpful to think of its parts this way:
- The **standard** is the "goal."
- The **rationale** explains why it's important to achieve this goal.
- The **elements of performance** identify the step(s) needed to achieve this goal.

These parts are defined as follows.

Standard A statement that defines the performance expectations and/or structures or processes that must be in place in order for a hospital to provide safe, high-quality care, treatment, and services. A hospital is either "compliant" or "not compliant" with a standard.

Accreditation decisions are based on simple counts of the standards that are determined to be "not compliant."

Rationale A statement that provides background, justification, or additional information about a standard. A standard's rationale is not scored. In some instances, the rationale for a standard is self-evident. Therefore, not every standard has a written rationale.

Elements of performance (EPs) The specific performance expectations and/or structures or processes that must be in place in order for a hospital to provide safe, high-quality care, treatment, and services. The scoring of EP compliance determines a hospital's overall compliance with a standard. EPs are evaluated on the following scale:

- 0 Insufficient compliance
- 1 Partial compliance
- 2 Satisfactory compliance
- NA Not applicable

You will find a **measure of success** icon—Ⓜ—next to some EPs. Measures of success (MOS) need to be developed for certain EPs when a standard is judged to be out of compliance through either the Periodic Performance Review (PPR) or the onsite survey. An MOS is defined as a quantifiable measure, usually related to an audit, that can be used to determine whether an action has been effective and is being sustained.*

Assessing Your Compliance

Once you are familiar with the parts of this chapter, you can begin to assess your compliance with its requirements. The scoring category for each EP is noted next to the EP. If you would like to assess your hospital's performance, mark your scores for the EPs and the standards by following the simple steps described below.

---

* For more information about measures of success, *see* the "The New Joint Commission Accreditation Process" chapter in this book.

2005 Hospital Accreditation Standards

Two components are scored for each EP: (1) compliance with the requirement itself **and** (2) compliance with the track record* for that requirement. Scoring has been simplified, and track record achievements (which have always been part of the scoring) have been appropriately modified.

Note: *Some standards and EPs do not apply to a particular type of organization; these standards and EPs are marked "not applicable" and the related text is not included. Your hospital is not expected to comply with standards and EPs marked "not applicable."*

In addition, some standards and EPs that do apply to organizations may not apply to the specific care, treatment, and services that your individual hospital provides. Although these standards and EPs are included in the manual, you are not expected to comply with them. If you are unsure about the standards or EPs that apply to your hospital, please contact the Joint Commission's Standards Interpretation Group at 630/792-5900.

Step 1: Score Your Compliance with Each Element of Performance

Before you can determine your compliance with the standards, you must score your compliance with each EP. There are three scoring criterion categories: A, B, and C (described below). Please note that for each EP scoring criterion category, your hospital must meet the performance requirement itself and the track record achievements (*see* "Track Record Achievements").

PI

Category A

These EPs relate to the presence or absence of the requirement(s) and are scored either yes (2) or no (0); however, score 1 for partial compliance is also possible based on track record achievements.

If an A EP has multiple components designated by bullets, your hospital must be compliant with all the bullets to receive a score of 2. If your hospital does not meet one or more requirements in the bullets, you will receive a score of 0.

Category B

Category B EPs are scored in two steps:
1. As with category A EPs, category B EPs relate to the presence or absence of the requirement(s). If your hospital *does not meet* the requirement(s), the EP is scored 0; there is no need to assess your compliance with the principles of good process design.
2. If your hospital *does meet* the requirement(s), but there is concern about the quality or comprehensiveness of the effort, then and only then should you assess the qualitative aspect of the EP. That is, review the applicable principles of good process design and ask how the principles were applied in the situation under discussion. Good process design has the following characteristics:

---
* **Track record** The amount of time that an organization has been in compliance with a standard, element of performance, or other requirement.

- Is consistent with your hospital's mission, values, and goals
- Meets the needs of patients
- Reflects the use of currently accepted practices (doing the right thing, using resources responsibly, using practice guidelines)
- Incorporates current safety information and knowledge such as sentinel event data and National Patient Safety Goals
- Incorporates relevant performance improvement results

This two-part evaluation applies to both simple and bulleted B EPs. First, the EPs are assessed to determine if the requirements are present. If the EP has multiple components designated by bullets, as with the category A EPs, your hospital must meet the requirements in *all* the bulleted items to get a score of 2. If your hospital meets *none* of the requirements in the bullets, it receives a score of 0. If your hospital meets *at least one, but not all*, of the bulleted requirements, it will receive a score of 1 for the EPs.

Use the following rules to determine your EP score:
- Your EP score is 0 if your hospital does not meet the requirement(s); you *do not* need to assess your compliance with the preceding applicable principles of good process design
- Your EP score is 1 if your hospital does meet the requirement(s), but considered only *some* of the preceding applicable principles of good process design
- Your EP score is 2 if your hospital does meet the requirement(s) *and* considered *all* the preceding principles of good process design

Category C

C EPs are scored 0, 1, or 2 based on the number of times your hospital does not meet the EP. These EPs are frequency based and require totaling the number of occurrences (that is, results of performance or nonperformance) related to a particular EP. Each situation discovered by a surveyor(s) will be counted as a separate occurrence.

Note: *Multiple events of the same type related to a single patient and single practitioner/staff member are counted as* one occurrence only.

Use the following rules to determine your EP score:
- Your EP score is 2 if you find one or fewer occurrences of noncompliance with the EP
- Your EP score is 1 if you find two occurrences of noncompliance with the EP
- Your EP score is 0 if you find three or more occurrences of noncompliance with the EP

If an EP in the C category has multiple requirements designated by bullets, the following scoring guidelines apply:
- If there are fewer than 2 findings in all bullets, the EP is scored 2
- If there are three or more findings in all bullets, the EP is scored 0
- In all other combinations of findings, the EP is scored 1

Track Record Achievements

In addition to meeting the requirement(s) in each EP, regardless of category, your hospital must also meet the following track record achievements:

Score	Initial Survey	Full Survey
2	4 months or more	12 months or more
1	2 to 3 months	6 to 11 months
0	Fewer than 2 months	Fewer than 6 months

Sample Sizes

If during an onsite survey, your hospital has been found to be not compliant with one or more standards, you must demonstrate Evidence of Standards Compliance (ESC) for each standard that is not compliant. The ESC must address compliance at the EP level; when an EP within a noncompliant standard requires an MOS, your hospital must demonstrate achievement with the MOS when completing the ESC.

Note: *Not every EP requires an MOS. EPs that do require an MOS are clearly marked in this chapter. Organizations are required to demonstrate achievement with an MOS only for EPs within a noncompliant standard that require an MOS. Organizations do not need to demonstrate achievement with an MOS for any EP within a compliant standard.*

When demonstrating achievement with the MOS during the ESC process, your hospital is **required** to use the following sample sizes, which were established because of their statistical significance, their relative simplicity in application, and their sensitivity to an organization's population size:

- For a population size of fewer than 30 cases, sample 100% of available cases
- For a population size of 30 to 100 cases, sample 30 cases
- For a population size of 101 to 500 cases, sample 50 cases
- For a population size greater than 500 cases, sample 70 cases

Note: *Hospitals are encouraged, but not required, to follow this sample size when demonstrating achievement with an MOS for an EP within a noncompliant standard after conducting a full, Option 1, or Option 2 Periodic Performance Review (PPR).*

When conducting PPR (optional use) or demonstrating an ESC (mandatory use), use the following percentages to determine your score: 90% through 100% of your sample size is in compliance = score 2; 80% through 89% (two instances of noncompliance) of your sample size is in compliance = score 1; less than 80% (three or more instances of noncompliance) of your sample size is in compliance = score 0.

In addition, the following information should govern your hospital's selection of samples:

- The appropriate sample size should be determined by the specific population related to the survey findings
- The sampling approach should involve either systematic random sampling (for example, your hospital selects every second or third case for review) or simple random sampling (for example, your hospital uses a series of random numbers generated by a computer to identify the cases to be reviewed)

- If your hospital chooses not to use these sample sizes while conducting PPR options 1 or 2, you should make sure that your sample size is sufficiently large enough to ensure statistical significance
- When submitting a clarifying ESC, if your hospital selects records as part of its sample, the records should be from a period of no more than three months before the last date of the survey
- Assessment of MOS compliance is conducted for a four-month period following the date of ESC approval. Your hospital should select records as a part of your sample following the date of ESC approval and use the required sample sizes. MOS percentage compliance rates are derived from the average of all four months.

Step 2: Use Your EP Scores to Gauge Your Compliance with the Standards

Now that you have evaluated and scored each EP for a particular standard, use these simple rules to determine your compliance with the standard itself:

- Your hospital is not in compliance (that is, "not compliant") with the standard if any EP is scored 0
- Otherwise, your hospital is in compliance with a standard if 65% or more of its EPs are scored 2

Standards, Rationales, Elements of Performance, and Scoring

Standard PI.1.10
The hospital collects data to monitor its performance.

Rationale for PI.1.10
Data help determine performance improvement priorities. The data collected for high priority and required areas are used to monitor the stability of existing processes, identify opportunities for improvement, identify changes that lead to improvement, or sustain improvement. Data collection helps identify specific areas that require further study. These areas are determined by considering the information provided by the data about process stability, risks, and sentinel events, and priorities set by the leaders. In addition, the hospital identifies those areas needing improvement and identifies desired changes. Performance measures are used to determine whether the changes result in desired outcomes. The hospital identifies the frequency and detail of data collection.

Note: *The hospital also collects data on the following areas that will be scored in their respective chapters:*
- *Evaluation and improvement of conditions in the environment (see "Management of the Environment of Care" chapter)*
- *Staffing effectiveness (see "Management of Human Resources" chapter)*

Elements of Performance for PI.1.10

B   1. The hospital collects data for priorities identified by leaders (*see* standard LD.4.50).

A   2. The hospital considers collecting data in the following areas:
- Staff opinions and needs
- Staff perceptions of risks to individuals and suggestions for improving patient safety
- Staff willingness to report unanticipated adverse events

B   3. The hospital collects data on the perceptions of care, treatment, and services* of patients, including the following:
- Their specific needs and expectations
- How well the hospital meets these needs and expectations
- How the hospital can improve patient safety
- The effectiveness of pain management, when applicable

---

* The Joint Commission is moving from the phrase *satisfaction with care, treatment, and services* toward the more inclusive phrase *perception of care, treatment, and services* to better measure the performance of organizations meeting the needs, expectations and concerns of clients. By using this term, the organization will be prompted to assess not only patients' and/or families' satisfaction with care, treatment, or services, but also whether the organization meets their needs and expectations.

Improving Organization Performance

The hospital collects data that measure the performance of each of the following potentially high-risk processes, when provided:

A 4. Medication management
A 5. Blood and blood product use
A 6. Restraint use
A 7. Seclusion use
A 8. Behavior management and treatment
    9. Not applicable
A 10. Operative and other invasive procedures
    11. Not applicable
A 12. Resuscitation and its outcomes

Relevant information developed from the following activities is integrated into performance improvement initiatives. This occurs in a way consistent with any hospital policies or procedures intended to preserve any confidentiality or privilege of information established by applicable law.

B 13. Risk management
B 14. Utilization management
B 15. Quality control
B 16. Infection control surveillance and reporting
B 17. Research, as applicable
B 18. Autopsies, when performed

Standard PI.2.10
Data are systematically aggregated and analyzed.

Rationale for PI.2.10
Aggregating and analyzing data means transforming data into information. Aggregating data at points in time enables the hospital to judge a particular process's stability or a particular outcome's predictability in relation to performance expectations. Accumulated data are analyzed in such a way that current performance levels, patterns, or trends can be identified.

Elements of Performance for PI.2.10
B 1. Collected data are aggregated and analyzed.
B 2. Data are aggregated at the frequency appropriate to the activity or process being studied.

B	3.	Statistical tools and techniques are used to analyze and display data.
B	4.	Data are analyzed and compared internally over time and externally* with other sources of information when available.
B	5.	Comparative data are used to determine if there is excessive variability or unacceptable levels of performance when available.

Standard PI.2.20

Undesirable patterns or trends in performance are analyzed.

Elements of Performance for PI.2.20

B	1.	Analysis is performed when data comparisons indicate that levels of performance, patterns, or trends vary substantially from those expected.
B	2.	Analysis occurs for those topics chosen by leaders as performance improvement priorities.
B	3.	Analysis is performed when undesirable variation occurs which changes priorities.

An analysis is performed for the following:

A	4.	All confirmed transfusion reactions, if applicable to the hospital
A	5.	All serious adverse drug events, if applicable and as defined by the hospital
A	6.	All significant medication errors, if applicable and as defined by the hospital
A	7.	All major discrepancies between preoperative and postoperative (including pathologic) diagnoses
A	8.	Adverse events or patterns of adverse events during moderate or deep sedation and anesthesia use
A	9.	Hazardous conditions
A	10.	Staffing effectiveness issues

Standard PI.2.30

Processes for identifying and managing sentinel events are defined and implemented.

---

* External sources of information include recent scientific, clinical, and management literature, including sentinel event alerts; well-formulated practice guidelines or parameters; performance measures; reference databases; other organizations with similar processes, and standards that are periodically reviewed and revised.

Improving Organization Performance

Rationale for PI.2.30
Identifying, reporting, analyzing, and managing sentinel events can help the hospital to prevent such incidents. Leaders define and implement such a program as part of the process to measure, assess, and improve the hospital's performance.

Elements of Performance for PI.2.30
Processes for identifying and managing sentinel events include the following:

A   1. Defining "sentinel event" and communicating this definition throughout the hospital (At a minimum, the hospital's definition includes those events subject to review under the Joint Commission's Sentinel Event Policy as published in this manual and may include any process variation which does not affect the outcome or result in an adverse event, but for which a recurrence carries significant chance of a serious adverse outcome or result in an adverse event, often referred to as a "near miss.")

A   2. Reporting sentinel events through established channels in the hospital and, as appropriate, to external agencies in accordance with law and regulation

B   3. Conducting thorough and credible root cause analyses that focus on process and system factors

B   4. Creating, documenting, and implementing a risk-reduction strategy and action plan that includes measuring the effectiveness of process and system improvements to reduce risk

B   5. The processes are implemented.

Standard PI.3.10
Information from data analysis is used to make changes that improve performance and patient safety and reduce the risk of sentinel events.

Elements of Performance for PI.3.10

B   1. The hospital uses the information from data analysis to identify and implement changes that will improve the quality of care, treatment, and services.

B   2. The hospital identifies and implements changes that will reduce the risk of sentinel events.

B   3. The hospital uses the information from data analysis to identify changes that will improve patient safety.

B   4. Changes made to improve processes or outcomes are evaluated to ensure that they achieve the expected results.

B   5. Appropriate actions are undertaken when planned improvements are not achieved or sustained.

Standard PI.3.20

An ongoing, proactive program for identifying and reducing unanticipated adverse events and safety risks to patients is defined and implemented.

Rationale for PI.3.20

Hospitals should proactively seek to identify and reduce risks to the safety of patients. Such initiatives have the obvious advantage of *preventing* adverse events rather than simply *reacting* when they occur. This approach also avoids the barriers to understanding created by hindsight bias and the fear of disclosure, embarrassment, blame, and punishment that can happen after an event.

Elements of Performance for PI.3.20

The following proactive activities to reduce risks to patients are conducted:

A   1. Selecting a high-risk process* to be analyzed (at least one high-risk process is chosen annually—the choice should be based in part on information published periodically by the Joint Commission about the most frequent sentinel events and risks)

B   2. Describing the chosen process (for example, through the use of a flowchart)

B   3. Identifying the ways in which the process could break down† or fail to perform its desired function

B   4. Identifying the possible effects that a breakdown or failure of the process could have on patients and the seriousness of the possible effects

B   5. Prioritizing the potential process breakdowns or failures

B   6. Determining why the prioritized breakdowns or failures could occur, which may include performing a hypothetical root cause analysis

B   7. Redesigning the process and/or underlying systems to minimize the risk of the effects on patients

B   8. Testing and implementing the redesigned process

B   9. Monitoring the effectiveness of the redesigned process

---

* **High-risk process** A process that if not planned and/or implemented correctly, has a significant potential for impacting the safety of the patient.

† The ways in which processes could break down or fail to perform its desired function are many times referred to as "the failure modes."

Leadership

Overview

A hospital's leaders provide the framework for planning, directing, coordinating, providing, and improving care, treatment, and services to respond to community and patient needs and improve health care outcomes.

Effective leadership depends on the following processes and tools:
- **Governance.** The governance of a hospital sets the framework for supporting quality patient care, treatment, and services.
- **Management.** Leaders create an environment that enables a hospital to fulfill its mission and meet or exceed its goals. They provide for a well-managed hospital with clear lines of responsibility and accountability.
- **Planning, designing, and providing services.** Leaders develop a mission that is reflected in long-range, strategic, and operational plans; service design; resource allocation; and organizational policies. They provide organization, direction, and staffing for care, treatment, and services. Leaders also communicate objectives and coordinate efforts to integrate care, treatment, and services throughout the hospital.
- **Improving safety and quality of care.** Leaders plan and implement a safety management program. They are ultimately responsible for the safety of all patients and staff. Leaders also establish expectations, plans, and priorities and manage the performance improvement process. They ensure that a process is in place to measure, assess, and improve the hospital's governance, management, clinical, and support functions.
- **Use of clinical practice guidelines.** The standards do not require the leaders to use clinical practice guidelines; however, they do provide a framework for developing and using clinical practice guidelines if the leaders choose to do so. A guideline provides an effective way to improve processes by reducing variance. A hospital's success in implementing and using clinical practice guidelines on an ongoing basis depends on the processes for reviewing, revising, and implementing the guidelines.
- **Teaching and coaching staff.** To realize the hospital's vision and values, leaders are involved in teaching and coaching staff; thus, staff education is an essential leadership function.

Standards

The following is a list of all standards for this function. They are presented here for your convenience without footnotes or other explanatory text. If you have a question about a term used here, please check the Glossary.

Note: *A revised standard numbering system is being used with the reformatted standards. This revised numbering system will allow for more flexibility to add standards while maintaining the current label for each standard.*

LD.1.10   The hospital identifies how it is governed.

LD.1.20   Governance responsibilities are defined in writing, as applicable.

LD.1.30   The hospital complies with applicable law and regulation.

LD.2.10   An individual(s) or designee(s) is responsible for operating the hospital according to the authority conferred by governance.

LD.2.20   Each organizational program, service, site, or department has effective leadership.

LD.2.30   Not applicable

LD.2.40   Not applicable

LD.2.50   The leaders develop and monitor an annual operating budget and, as appropriate, a long-term capital expenditure plan.

LD.3.10   The leaders engage in both short-term and long-term planning.

LD.3.15   The leaders develop and implement plans to identify and mitigate impediments to efficient patient flow throughout the hospital.

LD.3.20   Patients with comparable needs receive the same standard of care, treatment, and services throughout the hospital.

LD.3.30   A hospital demonstrates a commitment to its community by providing essential services in a timely manner.

LD.3.40   Not applicable

LD.3.50   Services provided by consultation, contractual arrangements, or other agreements are provided safely and effectively.

LD.3.60	Communication is effective throughout the hospital.
LD.3.70	The leaders define the required qualifications and competence of those staff who provide care, treatment, and services and recommend a sufficient number of qualified and competent staff to provide care, treatment, and services.
LD.3.80	The leaders provide for adequate space, equipment, and other resources.
LD.3.90	The leaders develop and implement policies and procedures for care, treatment, and services.
LD.3.100	Not applicable
LD.3.110	The hospital implements policies and procedures developed with the medical staff's participation for procuring and donating organs and other tissues.
LD.3.120	The leaders plan for and support the provision and coordination of patient education activities.
LD.3.130	Academic education is arranged for children and youth, when appropriate.
LD.3.140	In hospitals that do not primarily provide psychiatric or substance abuse services, a written plan clearly defines the care, treatment, and services or appropriate referral of patients who are emotionally ill, who become emotionally ill while in the hospital, or who suffer the results of alcoholism or drug abuse.
LD.3.150	The hospital plans for the appropriate care, treatment, and services of patients under legal or correctional restrictions.
LD.4.10	The leaders set expectations, plan, and manage processes to measure, assess, and improve the hospital's governance, management, clinical, and support activities.
LD.4.20	New or modified services or processes are designed well.
LD.4.30	Not applicable
LD.4.40	The leaders ensure that an integrated patient safety program is implemented throughout the hospital.

LD.4.50 The leaders set performance improvement priorities and identify how the hospital adjusts priorities in response to unusual or urgent events.

LD.4.60 The leaders allocate adequate resources for measuring, assessing, and improving the hospital's performance and improving patient safety.

LD.4.70 The leaders measure and assess the effectiveness of the performance improvement and safety improvement activities.

LD.5.10 The hospital considers clinical practice guidelines when designing or improving processes, as appropriate.

LD.5.20 When clinical practice guidelines are used, the leaders identify criteria for their selection and implementation.

LD.5.30 Appropriate leaders, practitioners, and health care professionals in the hospital review and approve clinical practice guidelines selected for implementation.

LD.5.40 The leaders evaluate the outcomes related to use of clinical practice guidelines and determine steps to improve processes.

Leadership

Understanding the Parts of This Chapter

To help you navigate this reformatted standards chapter, it may be helpful to think of its parts this way:
- The **standard** is the "goal."
- The **rationale** explains why it's important to achieve this goal.
- The **elements of performance** identify the step(s) needed to achieve this goal.

These parts are defined as follows.

Standard A statement that defines the performance expectations and/or structures or processes that must be in place in order for a hospital to provide safe, high-quality care, treatment, and services. A hospital is either "compliant" or "not compliant" with a standard.

Accreditation decisions are based on simple counts of the standards that are determined to be "not compliant."

Rationale A statement that provides background, justification, or additional information about a standard. A standard's rationale is not scored. In some instances, the rationale for a standard is self-evident. Therefore, not every standard has a written rationale.

Elements of performance (EPs) The specific performance expectations and/or structures or processes that must be in place in order for a hospital to provide safe, high-quality care, treatment, and services. The scoring of EP compliance determines a hospital's overall compliance with a standard. EPs are evaluated on the following scale:

- **0** Insufficient compliance
- **1** Partial compliance
- **2** Satisfactory compliance
- **NA** Not applicable

You will find a **measure of success** icon—Ⓜ—next to some EPs. Measures of success (MOS) need to be developed for certain EPs when a standard is judged to be out of compliance through either the Periodic Performance Review (PPR) or the onsite survey. An MOS is defined as a quantifiable measure, usually related to an audit, that can be used to determine whether an action has been effective and is being sustained.*

Assessing Your Compliance

Once you are familiar with the parts of this chapter, you can begin to assess your compliance with its requirements. The scoring category for each EP is noted next to the EP. If you would like to assess your hospital's performance, mark your scores for the EPs and the standards by following the simple steps described below.

---

* For more information about measures of success, *see* the "The New Joint Commission Accreditation Process" chapter in this book.

Two components are scored for each EP: (1) compliance with the requirement itself **and** (2) compliance with the track record* for that requirement. Scoring has been simplified, and track record achievements (which have always been part of the scoring) have been appropriately modified.

Note: *Some standards and EPs do not apply to a particular type of organization; these standards and EPs are marked "not applicable" and the related text is not included. Your hospital is not expected to comply with standards and EPs marked "not applicable."*

In addition, some standards and EPs that do apply to organizations may not apply to the specific care, treatment, and services that your individual hospital provides. Although these standards and EPs are included in the manual, you are not expected to comply with them. If you are unsure about the standards or EPs that apply to your hospital, please contact the Joint Commission's Standards Interpretation Group at 630/792-5900.

Step 1: Score Your Compliance with Each Element of Performance

Before you can determine your compliance with the standards, you must score your compliance with each EP. There are three scoring criterion categories: A, B, and C (described below). Please note that for each EP scoring criterion category, your hospital must meet the performance requirement itself and the track record achievements (see "Track Record Achievements").

Category A

These EPs relate to the presence or absence of the requirement(s) and are scored either yes (2) or no (0); however, score 1 for partial compliance is also possible based on track record achievements.

If an A EP has multiple components designated by bullets, your hospital must be compliant with all the bullets to receive a score of 2. If your hospital does not meet one or more requirements in the bullets, you will receive a score of 0.

Category B

Category B EPs are scored in two steps:
1. As with category A EPs, category B EPs relate to the presence or absence of the requirement(s). If your hospital *does not meet* the requirement(s), the EP is scored 0; there is no need to assess your compliance with the principles of good process design.
2. If your hospital *does meet* the requirement(s), but there is concern about the quality or comprehensiveness of the effort, then and only then should you assess the qualitative aspect of the EP. That is, review the applicable principles of good process design and ask how the principles were applied in the situation under discussion. Good process design has the following characteristics:

---

* **Track record** The amount of time that an organization has been in compliance with a standard, element of performance, or other requirement.

- Is consistent with your hospital's mission, values, and goals
- Meets the needs of patients
- Reflects the use of currently accepted practices (doing the right thing, using resources responsibly, using practice guidelines)
- Incorporates current safety information and knowledge such as sentinel event data and National Patient Safety Goals
- Incorporates relevant performance improvement results

This two-part evaluation applies to both simple and bulleted B EPs. First, the EPs are assessed to determine if the requirements are present. If the EP has multiple components designated by bullets, as with the category A EPs, your hospital must meet the requirements in *all* the bulleted items to get a score of 2. If your hospital meets *none* of the requirements in the bullets, it receives a score of 0. If your hospital meets *at least one, but not all*, of the bulleted requirements, it will receive a score of 1 for the EPs.

Use the following rules to determine your EP score:
- Your EP score is 0 if your hospital does not meet the requirement(s); you *do not* need to assess your compliance with the preceding applicable principles of good process design
- Your EP score is 1 if your hospital does meet the requirement(s), but considered only *some* of the preceding applicable principles of good process design
- Your EP score is 2 if your hospital does meet the requirement(s) *and* considered *all* the preceding principles of good process design

Category C

C EPs are scored 0, 1, or 2 based on the number of times your hospital does not meet the EP. These EPs are frequency based and require totaling the number of occurrences (that is, results of performance or nonperformance) related to a particular EP. Each situation discovered by a surveyor(s) will be counted as a separate occurrence.

Note: *Multiple events of the same type related to a single patient and single practitioner/staff member are counted as* one occurrence only.

Use the following rules to determine your EP score:
- Your EP score is 2 if you find one or fewer occurrences of noncompliance with the EP
- Your EP score is 1 if you find two occurrences of noncompliance with the EP
- Your EP score is 0 if you find three or more occurrences of noncompliance with the EP

If an EP in the C category has multiple requirements designated by bullets, the following scoring guidelines apply:
- If there are fewer than 2 findings in all bullets, the EP is scored 2
- If there are three or more findings in all bullets, the EP is scored 0
- In all other combinations of findings, the EP is scored 1

Track Record Achievements

In addition to meeting the requirement(s) in each EP, regardless of category, your hospital must also meet the following track record achievements:

Score	Initial Survey	Full Survey
2	4 months or more	12 months or more
1	2 to 3 months	6 to 11 months
0	Fewer than 2 months	Fewer than 6 months

Sample Sizes

If during an onsite survey, your hospital has been found to be not compliant with one or more standards, you must demonstrate Evidence of Standards Compliance (ESC) for each standard that is not compliant. The ESC must address compliance at the EP level; when an EP within a noncompliant standard requires an MOS, your hospital must demonstrate achievement with the MOS when completing the ESC.

Note: *Not every EP requires an MOS. EPs that do require an MOS are clearly marked in this chapter. Organizations are required to demonstrate achievement with an MOS only for EPs within a noncompliant standard that require an MOS. Organizations* do not *need to demonstrate achievement with an MOS for any EP within a compliant standard.*

When demonstrating achievement with the MOS during the ESC process, your hospital is **required** to use the following sample sizes, which were established because of their statistical significance, their relative simplicity in application, and their sensitivity to an organization's population size:

- For a population size of fewer than 30 cases, sample 100% of available cases
- For a population size of 30 to 100 cases, sample 30 cases
- For a population size of 101 to 500 cases, sample 50 cases
- For a population size greater than 500 cases, sample 70 cases

Note: *Hospitals are encouraged, but not required, to follow this sample size when demonstrating achievement with an MOS for an EP within a noncompliant standard after conducting a full, Option 1, or Option 2 Periodic Performance Review (PPR).*

When conducting PPR (optional use) or demonstrating an ESC (mandatory use), use the following percentages to determine your score: 90% through 100% of your sample size is in compliance = score 2; 80% through 89% (two instances of noncompliance) of your sample size is in compliance = score 1; less than 80% (three or more instances of noncompliance) of your sample size is in compliance = score 0.

In addition, the following information should govern your hospital's selection of samples:
- The appropriate sample size should be determined by the specific population related to the survey findings
- The sampling approach should involve either systematic random sampling (for example, your hospital selects every second or third case for review) or simple random sampling (for example, your hospital uses a series of random numbers generated by a computer to identify the cases to be reviewed)

Leadership

- If your hospital chooses not to use these sample sizes while conducting PPR options 1 or 2, you should make sure that your sample size is sufficiently large enough to ensure statistical significance
- When submitting a clarifying ESC, if your hospital selects records as part of its sample, the records should be from a period of no more than three months before the last date of the survey
- Assessment of MOS compliance is conducted for a four-month period following the date of ESC approval. Your hospital should select records as a part of your sample following the date of ESC approval and use the required sample sizes. MOS percentage compliance rates are derived from the average of all four months.

Step 2: Use Your EP Scores to Gauge Your Compliance with the Standards

Now that you have evaluated and scored each EP for a particular standard, use these simple rules to determine your compliance with the standard itself:

- Your hospital is not in compliance (that is, "not compliant") with the standard if any EP is scored 0
- Otherwise, your hospital is in compliance with a standard if 65% or more of its EPs are scored 2

Standards, Rationales, Elements of Performance, and Scoring

Standard LD.1.10
The hospital identifies how it is governed.

Rationale for LD.1.10
The hospital has governance with ultimate responsibility and legal authority for the safety and quality of care, treatment, and services. Governance establishes policy, promotes performance improvement, and provides for organizational management and planning.

Elements of Performance for LD.1.10
- **A** 1. The hospital identifies how it is governed.
- **A** 2. The hospital identifies lines of authority for key planning, management, and operations activities.
- **A** 3. The hospital identifies those responsible for governance.
- **B** 4. The governance provides for appropriate medical staff participation in governance.
- **A** 5. The medical staff has the right to representation (through attendance and voice), by one or more medical staff members selected by the medical staff, at governing body meetings.
- **A** 6. Medical staff members are eligible for full membership in the hospital's governance, unless legally prohibited.

Standard LD.1.20
Governance responsibilities are defined in writing, as applicable.

Elements of Performance for LD.1.20
- **A** 1. Governance defines its responsibilities in writing, as applicable.
- **A** 2. If the hospital is part of a larger corporate structure, the scope and degree of leaders' involvement, authority, and responsibility in corporate policy decisions are described in writing.
- **B** 3. Governance provides for organizational management and planning.
- **A** 4. The hospital's scope of services is defined in writing and approved by the governance.
- **A** 5. Governance either selects the individual(s) responsible for operating the hospital or approves one selected by corporate management or another group.

Leadership

B   6. Governance provides for coordination and integration among the hospital's leaders to establish policy, maintain quality care and patient safety, and provide for necessary resources.

A   7. Governance annually evaluates the hospital's performance in relation to its vision, mission, and goals.

       8. Through 11. Not applicable

B   12. Governance provides a system for resolving conflicts among leaders and the individuals under their leadership.

Standard LD.1.30
The hospital complies with applicable law and regulation.

Elements of Performance for LD.1.30
A   1. The hospital provides all care, treatment, and services in accordance with applicable licensure requirements, law, rules, and regulation.

A   2. The hospital acts upon any reports and/or recommendations from authorized agencies, as appropriate.

A   3. The hospital possesses a license, certificate, or permit, as required by applicable law and regulation, to provide the health care services for which the hospital is seeking accreditation.

Standard LD.2.10
An individual(s) or designee(s) is responsible for operating the hospital according to the authority conferred by governance.

Elements of Performance for LD.2.10
B   1. The individual(s) designated by governance is responsible for establishing internal controls to effectively operate the hospital including the following:
- Establishing and maintaining information and support systems
- Recruiting and retaining staff
- Conserving physical and financial assets

A   2. When this individual(s) is absent from the hospital, an appropriately qualified individual(s) is designated to perform the duties of that position.

       3. Not applicable

B   4. As appropriate, reports are provided to governance.

Standard LD.2.20
Each hospital program, service, site, or department has effective leadership.

Rationale for LD.2.20
Effective leaders at the site or department level help to create an environment or culture that enables a hospital to fulfill its mission and meet or exceed its goals. They support staff and instill in them a sense of ownership of their work processes. Although it may be appropriate for leaders to delegate work to qualified staff, the leaders are ultimately responsible for care, treatment, or services provided in their area.

Elements of Performance for LD.2.20
B 1. The program, service, site, or department leaders ensure that operations are effective and efficient.

B 2. Leaders hold staff accountable for their responsibilities.

B 3. Programs, services, sites, or departments providing patient care are directed by one or more qualified professionals with appropriate training and experience or by a qualified licensed independent practitioner with appropriate clinical privileges.

B 4. Responsibility for administrative and clinical direction of these programs, services, sites, or departments is defined in writing.

B 5. Leaders ensure that a process is in place to coordinate care, treatment, and service processes among programs, services, sites, or departments.

Standard LD.2.30
Not applicable

Standard LD.2.40
Not applicable

Standard LD.2.50
The leaders develop and monitor an annual operating budget and, as appropriate, a long-term capital expenditure plan.

Elements of Performance for LD.2.50
A 1. An operating budget is developed annually and approved by the governance.

A 2. The budget reflects the hospital's goals and objectives and, at a minimum, meets applicable law and regulation.

B 3. The leaders include staff input when developing the budget.

A   4. The governing body or authority approves a long-term capital expenditure plan, as appropriate.

A   5. An independent public accountant conducts an annual audit of the hospital's finances, unless otherwise provided by law.

Standard LD.3.10
The leaders engage in both short-term and long-term planning.

Elements of Performance for LD.3.10
A   1. Leaders create vision, mission, and goal statements.

A   2. The hospital's plan for services specifies which care, treatment, or services are provided directly and which through consultation, contract, or other agreement.

A   3. Anesthesia services are available if surgery or obstetrical services are provided.

     4. Through 25. Not applicable

B   26. Planning for care, treatment, and services addresses the following:
- The needs and expectations of patients and, as appropriate, families and referral sources
- Staff needs
- The scope of care, treatment, and services needed by patients at all of the hospital's locations
- Resources (financial and human) for providing care and support services
- Recruitment, retention, development, and continuing education needs of all staff
- Data for measuring the performance of processes and outcomes of care

Standard LD.3.15*
The leaders develop and implement plans to identify and mitigate impediments to efficient patient flow throughout the hospital.

Rationale for LD.3.15
Managing the flow of patients through their care is essential to the prevention of patient crowding, a problem that can lead to lapses in patient safety and quality of care. The emergency department is particularly vulnerable to experiencing negative effects of inefficiency in the management of this process. For this reason, while emergency departments have little control over the volume and type of patient arrivals and most hospitals have lost the "surge capacity" that existed at one time to

---

* This standard and its EPs will become effective January 1, 2005. However, beginning July 1, 2004, surveyors will explore a hospital's progress toward meeting this standard and its EPs and provide education on the findings as necessary. Findings will not be included in the survey report, nor will they influence the final accreditation decision. **Note:** *This standard is numbered LD.3.11 until January 1, 2005.*

manage the elastic nature of emergency admissions, other opportunities for improvement do exist. Improved management of processes can ensure the wise use of limited resources and thereby reduce the risk to patients of negative outcomes from delays in the delivery of care, treatment, or services.

To understand the system implications of the issues, leadership should identify all of the processes critical to patient flow through the hospital system from the time the patient arrives, through admitting, patient assessment and treatment, and discharge. Supporting processes are included if identified by leadership as impacting patient flow, for example, diagnostic, communication, and patient transportation procedures. Relevant measurements are selected and implemented to enable monitoring of each process and supporting process(es) by the hospital leaders. These critical processes should be modified for the purposes of improving patient flow.

Elements of Performance for LD.3.15

B 1. Leaders assess patient flow issues within the hospital, the impact on patient safety, and plan to mitigate that impact.

B 2. Planning encompasses the delivery of appropriate and adequate care to admitted patients who must be held in temporary bed locations, for example, postanesthesia care unit and emergency department areas.

B 3. Leaders and medical staff share accountability to develop processes that support efficient patient flow.

B 4. Planning includes the delivery of adequate care, treatment, and services to those patients who are placed in overflow locations, such as corridors.

B 5. Specific indicators are used to measure components of the patient flow process and address the following:
- Available supply of patient bed space
- Efficiency of patient care, treatment, and service areas
- Safety of patient care, treatment, and service areas
- Support service processes that impact patient flow

B 6. Indicator results are available to those individuals who are accountable for processes that support patient flow.

A 7. Indicator results are reported to leadership on a regular basis to support planning.

B 8. The hospital improves inefficient or unsafe processes identified by leadership as essential to the efficient movement of patients through the hospital.

B 9. Criteria are defined to guide decisions about initiating diversion.

Standard LD.3.20
Patients with comparable needs receive the same standard of care, treatment, and services throughout the hospital.

Leadership

Rationale for LD.3.20
Factors such as different individuals providing care, treatment, and services; different payment sources; or different settings of care do not intentionally negatively influence the outcome.

Elements of Performance for LD.3.20
B   1.   Patients with comparable needs receive the same standard of care, treatment, and services throughout the hospital.

B   2.   The hospital plans, designs, and monitors care, treatment, and services so they are consistent with the mission, vision, and goals.

Standard LD.3.30
A hospital demonstrates a commitment to its community by providing essential services in a timely manner.

Rationale for LD.3.30
Through the planning process, the leaders determine, first, what diagnostic, therapeutic, rehabilitative and other services are essential to the community; second, which of these services the hospital will provide directly and which through referral, consultation, contractual arrangements, or other agreements; and third, time frames for providing patient care.

Elements of Performance for LD.3.30
A   1.   Essential services include at least the following:
- Diagnostic radiology
- Dietetic
- Emergency
- Nuclear medicine*
- Nursing care
- Pathology and clinical laboratory
- Pharmaceutical
- Physical rehabilitation*
- Respiratory care*
- Social work

A   2.   In addition, the hospital has at least one of the following acute care clinical services:
- Medicine
- Obstetrics and gynecology[†]
- Pediatrics
- Surgery[†]
- Child, adolescent, or adult psychiatry
- Substance abuse treatment

---

* Not required for hospitals that provide only psychiatric and substance abuse services.

[†] When the hospital provides surgical or obstetric services, anesthesia services are also available.

Standard LD.3.40
Not applicable

Standard LD.3.50
Services provided by consultation, contractual arrangements, or other agreements are provided safely and effectively.

Elements of Performance for LD.3.50

A   1. The leaders approve sources for the hospital's services that are provided by consultation, contractual arrangements, or other agreements.

A   2. The medical staff advises the hospital's leaders on the sources of clinical services to be provided by consultation, contractual arrangements, or other agreements.

       3. Not applicable

A   4. The nature and scope of services provided by consultation, contractual arrangements, or other agreements are defined in writing.*

B   5. Services provided by consultation, contractual arrangements, or other agreements meet applicable Joint Commission standards.

B   6. The hospital evaluates the contracted care, treatment, and services to determine whether they are being provided according to the contract and the level of safety and quality that the hospital expects.

A   7. The hospital retains overall responsibility and authority for services furnished under a contract.

A   8. All reference and contract laboratory services† meet the applicable federal regulations for clinical laboratories and maintain evidence of the same.

---

* When a hospital contracts for patient care, treatment, and services rendered outside the hospital but under the control of a Joint Commission-accredited organization, the primary organization can do the following:
- Specify in the contract that the contracting entity will ensure that all services provided by contracted individuals who are licensed independent practitioners will be within the scope of his or her privileges

or
- Verify that all contracted individuals who are licensed independent practitioners and who will be providing patient care, treatment, and services have appropriate privileges, for example by obtaining a copy of the list of privileges

When a hospital contracts for patient care, treatment, and services rendered outside the hospital and under the control of a non-Joint Commission-accredited organization, all licensed independent practitioners who will be providing services are privileged by the Joint Commission-accredited organization through the process described in the "Medical Staff" chapter in this manual.

† A written agreement (such as a formal contract) is not required for reference laboratories; however, it is required for a contract service where a major portion of laboratory testing is provided by an outside laboratory.

Standard LD.3.60
Communication is effective throughout the hospital.

Elements of Performance for LD.3.60
B   1. The leaders ensure processes are in place for communicating relevant information throughout the hospital in a timely manner.

B   2. Effective communication occurs in the hospital, among the hospital's programs, among related hospitals, with outside organizations, and with patients and families, as appropriate.

B   3. The leaders communicate the hospital's mission and appropriate policies, plans, and goals to all staff.

Standard LD.3.70
The leaders define the required qualifications and competence of those staff who provide care, treatment, and services, and recommend a sufficient number of qualified and competent staff to provide care, treatment, and services.

Rationale for LD.3.70
The determination of competence and qualifications of staff is based on the following:
- The hospital's mission
- The hospital's care, treatment, and services
- The complexity of care, treatment, and services needed by patients
- The technology used
- The health status of staff, as required by law and regulation

Elements of Performance for LD.3.70
B   1. The leaders provide for the allocation of competent qualified staff.

B   2. The leaders ensure that physician assistants and advanced practice registered nurses who practice within the hospital are credentialed and privileged and reprivileged through the medical staff process or an equivalent process that has been approved by the governing body. An equivalent process at a minimum does the following:
   - Evaluates the applicant's credentials
   - Evaluates the applicant's current competence
   - Includes peer recommendations
   - Involves communication with and input from individuals and committees, including the Medical Staff Executive Committee, to make an informed decision regarding the applicant's request for privileges

Standard LD.3.80
The leaders provide for adequate space, equipment, and other resources.

Elements of Performance for LD.3.80

B   1. The leaders provide for the arrangement and allocation of space to facilitate efficient, effective delivery of care, treatment, and services.

B   2. The leaders provide for the appropriateness of interior and exterior space for the care, treatment, and services offered and for the ages and other characteristics of the patients.

B   3. The leaders provide for the safe use, maintenance, accessibility, and supervision of grounds, equipment, and special activity areas.

B   4. The leaders provide for adequate equipment and other resources.

Standard LD.3.90

The leaders develop and implement policies and procedures for care, treatment, and services.

Elements of Performance for LD.3.90

B   1. The leaders develop policies and procedures that guide and support patient care, treatment, and services.

C Ⓜ   2. Policies and procedures are consistently implemented.

Standard LD.3.100

Not applicable

Standard LD.3.110

The hospital implements policies and procedures developed with the medical staff's participation for procuring and donating organs and other tissues.

Elements of Performance for LD.3.110

A   1. The hospital has an agreement with an appropriate organ procurement organization (OPO) and follows its rules and regulations.

A   2. The hospital's policies and procedures identify the OPO with which it is affiliated.

A   3. The hospital has an agreement with at least one tissue bank and at least one eye bank (as long as the process does not interfere with organ procurement) to cooperate in retrieving, processing, preserving, storing, and distributing tissues and eyes.

A   4. The hospital notifies the OPO in a timely manner of patients who have died or whose death is imminent.

A   5. In Department of Defense hospitals, Veterans Affairs medical centers, and other federally administered health care agencies, this notification is done according to procedures approved by the respective agency.

Leadership

A   6. The OPO determines medical suitability for organ donation and, in the absence of alternative arrangements by the hospital, for tissue and eye donation.

A   7. The hospital has procedures, developed in collaboration with the designated OPO, for notifying the family of each potential donor of the option to donate—or decline to donate—organs, tissues, or eyes.

A   8. This notification is made by an organ procurement representative or the hospital's designated requester.

A   9. Written documentation by the hospital's designated requester shows that the patient or family accepts or declines the opportunity for the patient to become an organ or tissue donor.

A   10. The hospital's staff exercises discretion and sensitivity to the circumstances, beliefs, and desires of the families of potential donors.

A   11. The hospital maintains records of potential donors whose names have been sent to the OPO and tissue and eye banks.

A   12. The hospital works with the OPO and tissue and eye banks as follows:
- In reviewing death records to improve identification of potential donors
- To maintain potential donors while the necessary testing and placement of potential donated organs, tissues, and eyes takes place
- In educating staff about donation issues

Additional Elements of Performance for Hospitals Performing Transplant Services

A   13. A hospital transplanting human organs must belong to the organ procurement and transplantation network (OPTN) established under section 372 of the Public Health Service Act and must abide by its rules.

A   14. If requested, the hospital provides all organ transplant-related data to the OPTN, the Scientific Registry, or the hospital's designated OPO.

Standard LD.3.120

The leaders plan for and support the provision and coordination of patient education activities.

Elements of Performance for LD.3.120

B   1. The leaders plan and support patient education activities appropriate to the hospital's mission and scope of services.

B   2. The leaders identify and provide the resources necessary for achieving educational objectives.

Standard LD.3.130

Academic education is arranged for children and youth, when appropriate.

Rationale for LD.3.130

Educational resources are selected based on identified patient needs. The hospital makes educational resources available that do the following:
- Help maintain the educational and intellectual development of patients
- Address opportunities to catch up for those patients who have fallen behind in their education because of their condition

Element of Performance for LD.3.130

A   1. Academic education is arranged for children and youth either through direct provision of services or community resources, such as tutors or attendance at classes in public schools, when appropriate.

Standard LD.3.140

In hospitals that do not primarily provide psychiatric or substance abuse services, a written plan clearly defines the care, treatment, and services or appropriate referral of patients who are emotionally ill, who become emotionally ill while in the hospital, or who suffer the results of alcoholism or drug abuse.

Elements of Performance for LD.3.140

B   1. In hospitals that do not primarily provide psychiatric or substance abuse services, a written plan defines the care, treatment, and services or appropriate referral of patients who are emotionally ill or who suffer the results of alcoholism or drug abuse.

B   2. Patient care, treatment, and services or appropriate referral is consistent with this written plan.

Standard LD.3.150

The hospital plans for the appropriate care, treatment, and services of patients under legal or correctional restrictions.

Elements of Performance for LD.3.150

Administrative and clinical decisions are coordinated on at least the following issues:

B   1. Use of seclusion and restraint for nonclinical purposes

B   2. Imposition of disciplinary restrictions

B   3. Length of stay

B   4. Restriction of rights

B   5. Plan for discharge and continuing care, treatment, and services

Leadership

Standard LD.4.10
The leaders set expectations, plan, and manage processes to measure, assess, and improve the hospital's governance, management, clinical, and support activities.

Elements of Performance for LD.4.10
- **B** 1. The leaders set expectations for performance improvement.
- **B** 2. The leaders develop plans for performance improvement.
- **B** 3. The leaders manage processes to improve hospital performance.
- **B** 4. The leaders participate in performance improvement activities.
- **B** 5. Appropriate individuals and professions from each relevant site or department participate collaboratively in hospitalwide performance improvement activities.

Standard LD.4.20
New or modified services or processes are designed well.

Elements of Performance for LD.4.20
The design of new or modified services or processes incorporates the following:
- **B** 1. The needs and expectations of patients, staff, and others
- **B** 2. The results of performance improvement activities, when available
- **B** 3. Information about potential risks to patients, when available
- **B** 4. Current knowledge, when available and relevant (for example, practice guidelines, successful practices, information from relevant literature and clinical standards)
- **B** 5. Information about sentinel events, when available and relevant
- **B** 6. Testing and analysis to determine whether the proposed design or redesign is an improvement
- **B** 7. The leaders collaborate with staff and appropriate stakeholders to design services.

Standard LD.4.30
Not applicable

Standard LD.4.40
The leaders ensure that an integrated patient safety program is implemented throughout the hospital.

Rationale for LD.4.40

The leaders should work to foster a safe environment throughout the hospital by integrating safety priorities into all relevant hospital processes, functions, and services. In pursuit of this effort, a patient safety program can work to improve safety by reducing the risk of system or process failures. As part of its responsibility to communicate objectives and coordinate efforts to integrate patient care and support services throughout the hospital and with contracted services, leadership takes the lead in developing, implementing, and overseeing a patient safety program.

The standard does not require the creation of new structures or "offices" in the hospital; rather, the standard emphasizes the need to integrate all patient-safety activities, both existing and newly created, with the hospital's leadership identified as accountable for this integration.

Elements of Performance for LD.4.40

The patient safety program includes the following:

A 1. One or more qualified individuals or an interdisciplinary group assigned to manage the hospitalwide safety program

B 2. Definition of the scope of the program's oversight, typically ranging from no-harm, frequently occurring "slips" to sentinel events with serious adverse outcomes

B 3. Integration into and participation of all components of the hospital into the hospitalwide program

B 4. Procedures for immediately responding to system or process failures, including care, treatment, or services for the affected individual(s), containing risk to others, and preserving factual information for subsequent analysis

B 5. Clear systems for internal and external reporting of information about system or process failures

B 6. Defined responses to various types of unanticipated adverse events and processes for conducting proactive risk assessment/risk reduction activities

B 7. Defined support systems* for staff members who have been involved in a sentinel event

A 8. Reports, at least annually, to the hospital's governance or authority on system or process failures and actions taken to improve safety, both proactively and in response to actual occurrences

---

* Support systems provide individuals with additional help and support as well as additional resources through the human resources function or an employee assistance program. Support systems recognize that conscientious health care workers who are involved in sentinel events are themselves victims of the event and require support. Support systems also focus on the process rather than blaming the involved individuals.

Standard LD.4.50
The leaders set performance improvement priorities and identify how the hospital adjusts priorities in response to unusual or urgent events.

Elements of Performance for LD.4.50
B   1. The leaders set priorities for performance improvement for hospital-wide activities, staffing effectiveness, and patient health outcomes.

B   2. The leaders give high priority to high-volume, high-risk, or problem-prone processes.

B   3. Performance improvement activities are reprioritized in response to significant changes in the internal or external environment.

Standard LD.4.60
The leaders allocate adequate resources for measuring, assessing, and improving the hospital's performance and improving patient safety.

Elements of Performance for LD.4.60
B   1. Sufficient staff is assigned to conduct activities for performance improvement and safety improvement.

B   2. Adequate time is provided for staff to participate in activities for performance improvement and safety improvement.

B   3. Adequate information systems are provided to support activities for performance improvement and safety improvement.

B   4. Staff is trained in performance improvement and safety improvement approaches and methods.

Standard LD.4.70
The leaders measure and assess the effectiveness of the performance improvement and safety improvement activities.

Elements of Performance for LD.4.70
B   1. Leaders continually monitor the effectiveness of the performance improvement and safety improvement activities.

B   2. The leaders develop and implement improvements for these activities.

B   3. The leaders assess the adequacy of the human, information, physical, and financial resources allocated to support performance improvement and safety improvement activities.

Standard LD.5.10

The hospital considers clinical practice guidelines when designing or improving processes, as appropriate.

Rationale for LD.5.10

Clinical practice guidelines can improve the quality, utilization, and value of health care services. Clinical practice guidelines help practitioners and patients in making decisions about preventing, diagnosing, treating, and managing selected conditions. Clinical practice guidelines can also be used in designing clinical processes or checking the design of existing processes. The leaders may consider sources of clinical practice guidelines such as the Agency for Healthcare Research and Quality, National Guideline Clearinghouse, and professional organizations.

Element of Performance for LD.5.10

A 1. The leaders have considered the use of clinical practice guidelines in designing or improving processes.

Standard LD.5.20

When clinical practice guidelines are used, the leaders identify criteria for their selection and implementation.

Rationale for LD.5.20

Selecting and implementing clinical practice guidelines that are appropriate to the hospital are critical. The leaders set criteria to guide the selection and implementation of clinical practice guidelines that are consistent with the hospital's mission and priorities. The leaders also consider the steps and changes or variations needed to encourage use, dissemination, and implementation of chosen guidelines throughout the hospital. This includes staff communication, training, implementation, feedback, and evaluation.

Elements of Performance for LD.5.20

B 1. When guidelines are used, the leaders have identified criteria to guide the selection and implementation of guidelines.

B 2. The hospital manages, evaluates, and learns from variation.

Standard LD.5.30

Appropriate leaders, practitioners, and health care professionals in the hospital review and approve clinical practice guidelines selected for implementation.

Rationale for LD.5.30

To be successfully implemented, clinical practice guidelines should be reviewed, revised, or adapted by the providers using them and approved by the hospital's leaders.

Element of Performance for LD.5.30
A   1. Appropriate hospital leaders have reviewed and approved the clinical practice guidelines selected for use.

Standard LD.5.40
The leaders evaluate the outcomes related to use of clinical practice guidelines and determine steps to improve processes.

Rationale for LD.5.40
To fully benefit from the use of clinical practice guidelines, the outcomes of patients treated using clinical practice guidelines are evaluated, and refinements are made to how the guidelines are used, if necessary.

Element of Performance for LD.5.40
A   1. Clinical practice guidelines are monitored and reviewed for effectiveness and are modified as necessary.

Management of the Environment of Care

Overview

The **goal** of this function is to provide a safe, functional, supportive, and effective environment for patients, staff members, and other individuals in the hospital. This is crucial to providing quality patient care, achieving good outcomes, and improving patient safety. Achieving this goal depends on performing the following processes:
- Performing strategic and ongoing master planning by hospital leaders for the space, clear circulation of occupants, equipment, supportive environment, and resources needed to safely and effectively support the services provided. Planning and designing of the environment is consistent with the hospital's mission and vision, and the patient's physical condition/health, cultural background, age, and cognitive abilities.
- Educating staff about the role of the environment in safely, sensitively, and effectively supporting patient care. The hospital educates staff about the physical characteristics necessary for attaining such an environment, and the processes for monitoring, maintaining, and reporting on the hospital's environment of care.
- Developing standards to measure staff and hospital performance in managing and improving the environment of care.
- Implementing plans to create and manage the hospital's environment of care. An Information Collection and Evaluation System (ICES) is developed and used to continuously measure, assess, and improve the status of the environment of care.

The "environment of care" is made up of three basic components: building(s), equipment, and people. A variety of key elements and issues can contribute in creating the way the space feels and works for patients, families, staff, and others experiencing the health care delivery system. In addition, they can be significant in their ability to positively influence patient outcomes, satisfaction, and improve patient safety. These elements include the following:
- Light (both natural and artificial)
- Privacy (visual and auditory)
- Space size and configuration that are appropriate and consistent with the clinical philosophy
- Security
- Orientation and access to nature and the outside
- Clarity of access (both exterior and interior circulation)
- Color
- Efficient layouts that support staffing and overall functional operation

When appropriately designed into and managed as part of the physical environment, these elements create safe, welcoming, and comfortable environments that support and maintain patient dignity and personhood, allow ease of interaction, reduce stressors, and encourage family participation in the delivery of care.

These key elements and issues need to be incorporated into both inpatient sites (such as acute care hospitals, psychiatric hospitals, hospice facilities, subacute care facilities, or nursing homes), as well as outpatient settings (such as clinics, counseling centers, preadmission testing offices, infirmaries, same-day surgery centers, dialysis centers, or imaging centers). Effective management of the environment of care includes using processes and activities to do the following:

- Reduce and control environmental hazards and risks
- Prevent accidents and injuries
- Maintain safe conditions for patients, staff, and others coming to the hospital's facilities
- Maintain an environment that is sensitive to patient needs for comfort, social interaction, and positive distraction
- Maintain an environment that minimizes unnecessary environmental stresses for patients, staff, and others coming to the hospital's facilities

The standards in this chapter focus on how everyone in the hospital participates in the processes and activities that make the care environment safe and effective. They also address department leaders' responsibility for identifying and communicating the care environment needs to the hospital and allocating appropriate space, equipment, and resources to safely and effectively support the hospital's services.

Some of the standards in this chapter recognize that certain settings where care, treatment, and services are provided have more risk than others. Therefore, some of the requirements are noted as being applicable to only certain "occupancy* types." The following occupancy definitions are used in this chapter:

- **Health care occupancy.** An occupancy used for purposes of medical or other treatment or care of four or more persons who are mostly incapable of self-preservation due to age or physical or mental disability, or because of security measures not under the occupant's control. Health care occupancies include hospitals, nursing homes, and limited care facilities.
- **Ambulatory health care occupancy.** An occupancy used to provide to four or more patients at the same time either (1) outpatient services or treatment that render them incapable of taking actions for self-preservation under emergency conditions without the assistance of others; or (2) anesthesia that renders them incapable of taking actions for self-preservation under emergency conditions without the assistance of others.
- **Business occupancy.** An occupancy used to provide outpatient services or treatment that does not meet the criteria in the ambulatory health care occupancy definition.

---

* **Occupancy** The purpose for which a building or portion thereof is used or intended to be used.

Note 1: *The standards in this chapter do not prescribe any particular structure (such as a safety committee), specific individual (such as one employee hired to be a safety officer), or format for the required designs and planning activities.*

Note 2: *The standards do not require the Statement of Conditions™ compliance document to be completed by anyone other than an employee of the hospital. This statement is the basis for corrective actions needed to make the environment compliant with the requirements of the* Life Safety Code® *(LSC), NFPA 101®.*

Note 3: *The standards in this chapter require each hospital to develop a written plan for the following:*
1. *Safety management (EC.1.10)*
2. *Security management (EC.2.10)*
3. *Hazardous materials and waste management (EC.3.10)*
4. *Emergency management (EC.4.10)*
5. *Fire safety (EC.5.10)*
6. *Medical equipment management (EC.6.10)*
7. *Utilities management (EC.7.10)*

If a hospital has multiple sites, it may have separate management plans for each of its locations, or it may choose to have one comprehensive set of plans. In either case, the hospital must address specific risks and the unique conditions at each of its sites.

Standards

The following is a list of all standards for this function. They are presented here for your convenience without footnotes or other explanatory text. If you have a question about a term used here, please check the Glossary.

Note: *A revised standard numbering system is being used with the reformatted standards. The revised numbering system will allow for more flexibility to add standards while maintaining the current number for each standard.*

Planning and Implementation Activities

EC.1.10 The hospital manages safety risks.

EC.1.20 The hospital maintains a safe environment.

EC.1.30 The hospital develops and implements a policy to prohibit smoking except in specified circumstances.

EC.2.10 The hospital identifies and manages its security risks.

EC.3.10 The hospital manages its hazardous materials and waste risks.

EC.4.10 The hospital addresses emergency management.

EC.4.20 The hospital conducts drills regularly to test emergency management.

EC.5.10 The hospital manages fire safety risks.

EC.5.20 Newly constructed and existing environments of care are designed and maintained to comply with the *Life Safety Code*®.

EC.5.30 The hospital conducts fire drills regularly.

EC.5.40 The hospital maintains fire-safety equipment and building features.

EC.5.50 The hospital develops and implements activities to protect occupants during periods when a building does not meet the applicable provisions of the *Life Safety Code*®.

EC.6.10 The hospital manages medical equipment risks.

EC.6.20 Medical equipment is maintained, tested, and inspected.

EC.7.10 The hospital manages its utility risks.

EC.7.20 The hospital provides a reliable emergency electrical power source.

EC.7.30 The hospital maintains, tests, and inspects its utility systems.

EC.7.40 The hospital maintains, tests, and inspects its emergency power systems.

EC.7.50 The hospital maintains, tests, and inspects its medical gas and vacuum systems.

EC.8.10 The hospital establishes and maintains an appropriate environment.

EC.8.20 Not applicable

EC.8.30 The hospital manages the design and building of the environment when it is renovated, altered, or newly created (*see* also standard EC.5.50).

Measuring and Improving Activities

EC.9.10 The hospital monitors conditions in the environment.

EC.9.20 The hospital analyzes identified environment issues and develops recommendations for resolving them.

EC.9.30 The hospital improves the environment.

Understanding the Parts of This Chapter

To help you navigate this reformatted standards chapter, it may be helpful to think of its parts this way:
- The **standard** is the "goal."
- The **rationale** explains why it's important to achieve this goal.
- The **elements of performance** identify the step(s) needed to achieve this goal.

These parts are defined as follows.

Standard A statement that defines the performance expectations and/or structures or processes that must be in place in order for a hospital to provide safe, high-quality care, treatment, and services. A hospital is either "compliant" or "not compliant" with a standard.

Accreditation decisions are based on simple counts of the standards that are determined to be "not compliant."

Rationale A statement that provides background, justification, or additional information about a standard. A standard's rationale is not scored. In some instances, the rationale for a standard is self-evident. Therefore, not every standard has a written rationale.

Elements of performance (EPs) The specific performance expectations and/or structures or processes that must be in place in order for a hospital to provide safe, high-quality care, treatment, and services. The scoring of EP compliance determines a hospital's overall compliance with a standard. EPs are evaluated on the following scale:

0	Insufficient compliance
1	Partial compliance
2	Satisfactory compliance
NA	Not applicable

You will find a **measure of success** icon—Ⓜ—next to some EPs. Measures of success (MOS) need to be developed for certain EPs when a standard is judged to be out of compliance through either the Periodic Performance Review (PPR) or the onsite survey. An MOS is defined as a quantifiable measure, usually related to an audit, that can be used to determine whether an action has been effective and is being sustained.*

Assessing Your Compliance

Once you are familiar with the parts of this chapter, you can begin to assess your compliance with its requirements. The scoring category for each EP is noted next to the EP. If you would like to assess your hospital's performance, mark your scores for the EPs and the standards by following the simple steps described below.

---

* For more information about measures of success, *see* the "The New Joint Commission Accreditation Process" chapter in this book.

Management of the Environment of Care

Two components are scored for each EP: (1) compliance with the requirement itself **and** (2) compliance with the track record* for that requirement. Scoring has been simplified, and track record achievements (which have always been part of the scoring) have been appropriately modified.

Note: *Some standards and EPs do not apply to a particular type of organization; these standards and EPs are marked "not applicable" and the related text is not included. Your hospital is not expected to comply with standards and EPs marked "not applicable."*

In addition, some standards and EPs that do apply to organizations may not apply to the specific care, treatment, and services that your individual hospital provides. Although these standards and EPs are included in the manual, you are not expected to comply with them. If you are unsure about the standards or EPs that apply to your hospital, please contact the Joint Commission's Standards Interpretation Group at 630/792-5900.

Step 1: Score Your Compliance with Each Element of Performance

Before you can determine your compliance with the standards, you must score your compliance with each EP. There are three scoring criterion categories: A, B, and C (described below). Please note that for each EP scoring criterion category, your hospital must meet the performance requirement itself and the track record achievements (*see* "Track Record Achievements").

Category A

These EPs relate to the presence or absence of the requirement(s) and are scored either yes (2) or no (0); however, score 1 for partial compliance is also possible based on track record achievements.

If an A EP has multiple components designated by bullets, your hospital must be compliant with all the bullets to receive a score of 2. If your hospital does not meet one or more requirements in the bullets, you will receive a score of 0.

Category B

Category B EPs are scored in two steps:
1. As with category A EPs, category B EPs relate to the presence or absence of the requirement(s). If your hospital *does not meet* the requirement(s), the EP is scored 0; there is no need to assess your compliance with the principles of good process design.
2. If your hospital *does meet* the requirement(s), but there is concern about the quality or comprehensiveness of the effort, then and only then should you assess the qualitative aspect of the EP. That is, review the applicable principles of good process design and ask how the principles were applied in the situation under discussion. Good process design has the following characteristics:

---

* **Track record** The amount of time that an organization has been in compliance with a standard, element of performance, or other requirement.

- Is consistent with your hospital's mission, values, and goals
- Meets the needs of patients
- Reflects the use of currently accepted practices (doing the right thing, using resources responsibly, using practice guidelines)
- Incorporates current safety information and knowledge such as sentinel event data and National Patient Safety Goals
- Incorporates relevant performance improvement results

This two-part evaluation applies to both simple and bulleted B EPs. First, the EPs are assessed to determine if the requirements are present. If the EP has multiple components designated by bullets, as with the category A EPs, your hospital must meet the requirements in *all* the bulleted items to get a score of 2. If your hospital meets *none* of the requirements in the bullets, it receives a score of 0. If your hospital meets *at least one, but not all*, of the bulleted requirements, it will receive a score of 1 for the EPs.

Use the following rules to determine your EP score:
- Your EP score is 0 if your hospital does not meet the requirement(s); you *do not* need to assess your compliance with the preceding applicable principles of good process design
- Your EP score is 1 if your hospital does meet the requirement(s), but considered only *some* of the preceding applicable principles of good process design
- Your EP score is 2 if your hospital does meet the requirement(s) *and* considered *all* the preceding principles of good process design

Category C

C EPs are scored 0, 1, or 2 based on the number of times your hospital does not meet the EP. These EPs are frequency based and require totaling the number of occurrences (that is, results of performance or nonperformance) related to a particular EP. Each situation discovered by a surveyor(s) will be counted as a separate occurrence.

Note: *Multiple events of the same type related to a single patient and single practitioner/staff member are counted as* one occurrence only.

Use the following rules to determine your EP score:
- Your EP score is 2 if you find one or fewer occurrences of noncompliance with the EP
- Your EP score is 1 if you find two occurrences of noncompliance with the EP
- Your EP score is 0 if you find three or more occurrences of noncompliance with the EP

If an EP in the C category has multiple requirements designated by bullets, the following scoring guidelines apply:
- If there are fewer than 2 findings in all bullets, the EP is scored 2
- If there are three or more findings in all bullets, the EP is scored 0
- In all other combinations of findings, the EP is scored 1

Management of the Environment of Care

Track Record Achievements

In addition to meeting the requirement(s) in each EP, regardless of category, your hospital must also meet the following track record achievements:

Score	Initial Survey	Full Survey
2	4 months or more	12 months or more
1	2 to 3 months	6 to 11 months
0	Fewer than 2 months	Fewer than 6 months

Sample Sizes

If during an onsite survey, your hospital has been found to be not compliant with one or more standards, you must demonstrate Evidence of Standards Compliance (ESC) for each standard that is not compliant. The ESC must address compliance at the EP level; when an EP within a noncompliant standard requires an MOS, your hospital must demonstrate achievement with the MOS when completing the ESC.

Note: *Not every EP requires an MOS. EPs that do require an MOS are clearly marked in this chapter. Organizations are required to demonstrate achievement with an MOS only* for EPs within a noncompliant standard that require an MOS. Organizations do not *need to demonstrate achievement with an MOS for any EP within a compliant standard.*

When demonstrating achievement with the MOS during the ESC process, your hospital is **required** to use the following sample sizes, which were established because of their statistical significance, their relative simplicity in application, and their sensitivity to an organization's population size:
- For a population size of fewer than 30 cases, sample 100% of available cases
- For a population size of 30 to 100 cases, sample 30 cases
- For a population size of 101 to 500 cases, sample 50 cases
- For a population size greater than 500 cases, sample 70 cases

Note: *Hospitals are encouraged, but not required, to follow this sample size when demonstrating achievement with an MOS for an EP within a noncompliant standard after conducting a full, Option 1, or Option 2 Periodic Performance Review (PPR).*

When conducting PPR (optional use) or demonstrating an ESC (mandatory use), use the following percentages to determine your score: 90% through 100% of your sample size is in compliance = score 2; 80% through 89% (two instances of noncompliance) of your sample size is in compliance = score 1; less than 80% (three or more instances of noncompliance) of your sample size is in compliance = score 0.

In addition, the following information should govern your hospital's selection of samples:
- The appropriate sample size should be determined by the specific population related to the survey findings
- The sampling approach should involve either systematic random sampling (for example, your hospital selects every second or third case for review) or simple random sampling (for example, your hospital uses a series of random numbers generated by a computer to identify the cases to be reviewed)

- If your hospital chooses not to use these sample sizes while conducting PPR options 1 or 2, you should make sure that your sample size is sufficiently large enough to ensure statistical significance
- When submitting a clarifying ESC, if your hospital selects records as part of its sample, the records should be from a period of no more than three months before the last date of the survey
- Assessment of MOS compliance is conducted for a four-month period following the date of ESC approval. Your hospital should select records as a part of your sample following the date of ESC approval and use the required sample sizes. MOS percentage compliance rates are derived from the average of all four months.

Step 2: Use Your EP Scores to Gauge Your Compliance with the Standards

Now that you have evaluated and scored each EP for a particular standard, use these simple rules to determine your compliance with the standard itself:

- Your hospital is not in compliance (that is, "not compliant") with the standard if any EP is scored 0
- Otherwise, your hospital is in compliance with a standard if 65% or more of its EPs are scored 2

Management of the Environment of Care

Standards, Rationales, Elements of Performance, and Scoring

Planning and Implementation Activities

No hospital can ensure that patients, staff, and others coming to the hospital's facilities will never suffer an accidental injury. However, hospitals can minimize avoidable risks and injuries through sound planning, resource allocation (*see* "Leadership" chapter), effective training (*see* "Management of Human Resources" chapter), implementation, and ongoing monitoring and improvement of risk reduction activities. These activities can be accomplished through the management process, staff activities, and/or technology.

Standard EC.1.10
The hospital manages safety risks.

Rationale for EC.1.10
Each hospital has inherent safety risks associated with providing services for patients, the performance of daily activities by staff, and the physical environment in which services occur. It is important that each hospital identifies these risks and plans and implements processes to minimize the likelihood of those risks causing incidents.

Elements of Performance for EC.1.10

B   1. The hospital develops and maintains a written management plan describing the processes it implements to effectively manage the environmental safety of patients, staff, and other people coming to the hospital's facilities.

A   2. The hospital identifies a person(s), as designated by leadership, to coordinate the development, implementation, and monitoring of the safety management activities.

A   3. The hospital identifies a person(s) to intervene whenever conditions immediately threaten life or health or threaten damage to equipment or buildings.

B   4. The hospital conducts comprehensive, proactive risk assessments that evaluate the potential adverse impact of buildings, grounds, equipment, occupants, and internal physical systems on the safety and health of patients, staff, and other people coming to the hospital's facilities.

C Ⓜ   5. The hospital uses the risks identified to select and implement procedures and controls to achieve the lowest potential for adverse impact on the safety and health of patients, staff, and other people coming to the hospital's facilities.

C Ⓜ 6. The hospital establishes safety policies and procedures that are distributed, practiced, and reviewed as frequently as necessary, but at least every three years.

7. Not applicable

B 8. The hospital ensures that a process exists for responding to product safety recalls by appropriate hospital staff.

B 9. The hospital ensures that all grounds and equipment are maintained appropriately.

Standard EC.1.20
The hospital maintains a safe environment.

Rationale for EC.1.20
It is essential that the hospital conduct periodic environmental tours to determine if its current processes for managing patient, public, and staff safety risks are being practiced correctly and are effective. These tours can also be used to assess staff knowledge and behaviors, identify new or altered risks in areas where construction or changes in services have occurred, and identify opportunities to improve the environment.

Elements of Performance for EC.1.20

B 1. The hospital conducts environmental tours to identify environmental deficiencies, hazards, and unsafe practices.

C Ⓜ 2. The hospital conducts environmental tours at least every six months in all areas where individuals are served.

C Ⓜ 3. The hospital conducts environmental tours at least annually in areas where individuals are not served.

Standard EC.1.30
The hospital develops and implements a policy to prohibit smoking except in specified circumstances.

Rationale for EC.1.30
This standard is intended to reduce the following risks:
- To people who smoke, including possible adverse effects on care, treatment, and services
- Of passive smoking for others
- Of fire

The standard prohibits smoking in all areas of all building(s) under the hospital's control, except for patients in circumstances specified in the EPs below.

Management of the Environment of Care

Elements of Performance for EC.1.30

B   1. The hospital develops a policy regarding smoking in all areas of all building(s) under the hospital's control.

B   2. The hospital's policy prohibits smoking in all areas of all building(s) under the hospital's control (no medical exceptions allowed) for the following:
- All hospital-based outpatients
- All children or youth patients

B   3. The hospital's policy may permit patients to smoke in the hospital's buildings under the following circumstance(s):
- A patient is residing in long term care settings (that is, longer than 30 days' length of stay); or
- A patient is granted permission that has been authorized by a licensed independent practitioner, based on criteria developed by the medical staff

B   4. When patients are permitted to smoke in the hospital's buildings, they smoke only under the following circumstance(s):
- In designated locations environmentally separate from care, treatment, and service areas*
- After the hospital has taken measures to minimize fire risks

C Ⓜ   5. Patients who do smoke in the hospital's buildings are provided education, including information about options for smoking cessation.

B   6. The hospital identifies and implements a process(es) for monitoring compliance with the policy.

B   7. The hospital develops strategies to eliminate the incidence of policy violations when identified.

A   8. Smoking is not permitted in the laboratory and areas under the control of the laboratory.

Standard EC.2.10
The hospital identifies and manages its security risks.

Rationale for EC.2.10
It is essential that a hospital manages the physical and personal security of patients, staff (including addressing the risks of violence in the workplace), and individuals coming to the hospital's facilities. In addition, security of the established environment, equipment, supplies, and information is also important.

---

* Note: This does not require that a designated smoking area be a specific distance from care, treatment, and service areas. A physically separate, well-ventilated room (a designated area for authorized smoking by patients that is exhausted to the outside) is acceptable.

Elements of Performance for EC.2.10

B 1. The hospital develops and maintains a written management plan describing the processes it implements to effectively manage the security of patients, staff, and other people coming to the hospital's facilities.

A 2. The hospital identifies a person(s), as designated by leadership, to coordinate the development, implementation, and monitoring of the security management activities.

B 3. The hospital conducts proactive risk assessments that evaluate the potential adverse impact of the external environment and the services provided on the security of patients, staff, and other people coming to the hospital's facilities.*

C Ⓜ 4. The hospital uses the risks identified to select and implement procedures and controls to achieve the lowest potential for adverse impact on security.

B 5. The hospital identifies, as appropriate, patients, staff, and other people entering the hospital's facilities.

C Ⓜ 6. The hospital controls access to and egress from security-sensitive areas, as determined by the hospital.

B 7. The hospital identifies and implements security procedures that address actions taken in the event of a security incident.

B 8. The hospital identifies and implements security procedures that address handling of an infant or pediatric abduction, as applicable.

B 9. The hospital identifies and implements security procedures that address handling of situations involving VIPs or the media.

B 10. The hospital identifies and implements security procedures that address vehicular access to emergency care areas.

Standard EC.3.10

The hospital manages its hazardous materials and waste† risks.

Rationale for EC.3.10

Hospitals must identify materials they use that need special handling and implement processes to minimize the risks of their unsafe use and improper disposal.

---

* The potential for workplace violence is considered during the risk assessment.

† **Hazardous materials (HAZMAT) and waste** Materials whose handling, use, and storage are guided or regulated by local, state, or federal regulation. Examples include OSHA's Regulations for Bloodborne Pathogens (regarding the blood, other infectious materials, contaminated items which would release blood or other infectious materials, or contaminated sharps), the Nuclear Regulatory Commission's regulations for handling and disposal of radioactive waste, management of hazardous vapors (such as glutaraldehyde, ethylene oxide, and nitrous oxide), chemicals regulated by the EPA, Department of Transportation requirements, and hazardous energy sources (for example, ionizing or non-ionizing radiation, lasers, microwaves, and ultrasound).

Elements of Performance for EC.3.10

B 1. The hospital develops and maintains a written management plan describing the processes it implements to effectively manage hazardous materials and waste.

B 2. The hospital creates and maintains an inventory that identifies hazardous materials and waste used, stored, or generated using criteria consistent with applicable law and regulation (for example, the Environmental Protection Agency [EPA] and the Occupational Safety and Health Administration [OSHA]).

The hospital establishes and implements processes for selecting, handling, storing, transporting, using, and disposing of hazardous materials and waste from receipt or generation through use and/or final disposal, including managing the following (EPs 3–6):

C Ⓜ 3. Chemicals

A 4. Chemotherapeutic materials

A 5. Radioactive materials

C Ⓜ 6. Infectious and regulated medical waste, including sharps

B 7. The hospital provides adequate and appropriate space and equipment for safely handling and storing hazardous materials and waste.

B 8. The hospital monitors and disposes of hazardous gases and vapors.

B 9. The hospital identifies and implements emergency procedures that include the specific precautions, procedures, and protective equipment used during hazardous materials and waste spills or exposures.

A 10. The hospital maintains documentation, including required permits, licenses, and adherence to other regulations.

C Ⓜ 11. The hospital maintains required manifests for handling hazardous materials and waste.

C Ⓜ 12. The hospital properly labels hazardous materials and waste.

B 13. The hospital effectively separates hazardous materials and waste storage and processing areas from other areas of the facility.

Standard EC.4.10

The hospital addresses emergency management.

2005 Hospital Accreditation Standards

Rationale for EC.4.10

An emergency* in the hospital or its community could suddenly and significantly affect the need for the hospital's services or its ability to provide those services. Therefore, a hospital needs to have an emergency management plan that comprehensively describes its approach to emergencies in the hospital or in its community.

Elements of Performance for EC.4.10

A 1. The hospital conducts a hazard vulnerability analysis[†] to identify potential emergencies that could affect the need for its services or its ability to provide those services.

A 2. The hospital establishes the following with the community:
- Priorities among the potential emergencies identified in the hazard vulnerability analysis
- The hospital's role in relation to a communitywide emergency management program
- An "all-hazards" command structure within the hospital that links with the community's command structure

B 3. The hospital develops and maintains a written emergency management plan describing the process for disaster readiness and emergency management, and implements it when appropriate.

A 4. At a minimum, an emergency management plan is developed with the involvement of the hospital's leaders including those of the medical staff.

B 5. The plan identifies specific procedures that describe mitigation,[‡] preparedness,[§] response, and recovery strategies, actions, and responsibilities for each priority emergency.

B 6. The plan provides processes for initiating the response and recovery phases of the plan, including a description of how, when, and by whom the phases are to be activated.

---

* **Emergency** A natural or manmade event that significantly disrupts the environment of care (for example, damage to the hospital's building[s] and grounds due to severe winds, storms, or earthquakes) that significantly disrupts care, treatment, and services (for example, loss of utilities such as power, water, or telephones due to floods, civil disturbances, accidents, or emergencies within the hospital or in its community); or that results in sudden, significantly changed, or increased demands for the hospital's services (for example, bioterrorist attack, building collapse, plane crash in the hospital's community). Some emergencies are called "disasters" or "potential injury creating events" (PICEs).

[†] **Hazard vulnerability analysis** The identification of potential emergencies and the direct and indirect effects these emergencies may have on the hospital's operations and the demand for its services.

[‡] **Mitigation activities** Those activities a hospital undertakes in attempting to lessen the severity and impact of a potential emergency.

[§] **Preparedness activities** Those activities a hospital undertakes to build capacity and identify resources that may be used if an emergency occurs.

B   7. The plan provides processes for notifying staff when emergency response measures are initiated.

B   8. The plan provides processes for notifying external authorities of emergencies, including possible community emergencies identified by the hospital (for example, evidence of a possible bioterrorist attack).

B   9. The plan provides processes for identifying and assigning staff to cover all essential staff functions under emergency conditions.

B   10. The plan provides processes for managing the following under emergency conditions:
- Activities related to care, treatment, and services (for example, scheduling, modifying, or discontinuing services; controlling information about patients; referrals; transporting patients)
- Staff support activities (for example, housing, transportation, incident stress debriefing)
- Staff family support activities
- Logistics relating to critical supplies (for example, pharmaceuticals, supplies, food, linen, water)
- Security (for example, access, crowd control, traffic control)
- Communication with the news media
- Communication with patients

   11. Not applicable

B   12. The plan provides processes for evacuating the entire facility (both horizontally and, when applicable, vertically) when the environment cannot support adequate care, treatment, and services.

B   13. The plan provides processes for establishing an alternate care site(s) that has the capabilities to meet the needs of patients when the environment cannot support adequate care, treatment, and services including processes for the following:
- Transporting patients, staff, and equipment to the alternative care site(s)
- Transferring to and from the alternative care site(s), the necessities of patients (for example, medications, medical records)
- Tracking of patients
- Interfacility communication between the hospital and the alternative care site(s)

B   14. The plan provides processes for identifying care providers and other personnel during emergencies.

B   15. The plan provides processes for cooperative planning with health care organizations that together provide services to a contiguous geographic area (for example, among hospitals serving a town or borough) to facilitate the timely sharing of information about the following:

- Essential elements of their command structures and control centers for emergency response
- Names and roles of individuals in their command structures and command center telephone numbers
- Resources and assets that could potentially be shared in an emergency response
- Names of patients and deceased individuals brought to their hospitals to facilitate identifying and locating victims of the emergency

16. Not applicable

17. Not applicable

B 18. The plan identifies backup internal and external communication systems in the event of failure during emergencies.

B 19. The plan identifies alternate roles and responsibilities of staff during emergencies, including to whom they report in the hospital's command structure and, when activated, in the community's command structure.

B 20. The plan identifies an alternative means of meeting essential building utility needs when the hospital is designated by its emergency management plan to provide continuous service during an emergency (for example, electricity, water, ventilation, fuel sources, medical gas/vacuum systems).

B 21. The plan identifies means for radioactive, biological, and chemical isolation and decontamination.

Standard EC.4.20

The hospital conducts drills regularly to test emergency management.

Elements of Performance for EC.4.20

A 1. The hospital tests the response phase of its emergency management plan twice a year, either in response to an actual emergency or in planned drills.*

Note 1: *Staff in each freestanding building classified as a business occupancy (as defined by the LSC) that does not offer emergency services nor is community-designated as a disaster-receiving station need to participate in only one emergency management drill annually. Staff in areas of the building that the hospital occupies must participate in this drill.*

Note 2: *Tabletop exercises, though useful in planning or training, are only acceptable substitutes for communitywide practice drills.*

---

* **Note:** *Drills that involve packages of information that simulate patients, their families, and the public are acceptable.*

A   2. Drills are conducted at least four months apart and no more than eight months apart.

A   3. Hospitals that offer emergency services or are community-designated disaster receiving stations must conduct at least one drill a year that includes an influx of volunteers or simulated patients.

A   4. The hospital participates in at least one communitywide practice drill a year (where applicable) relevant to the priority emergencies identified in its hazard vulnerability analysis. The drill assesses the communication, coordination, and effectiveness of the hospital's and community's command structures.

> **Note 1:** *"Communitywide" may range from a contiguous geographic area served by the same health care providers, to a large borough, town, city, or region.*
>
> **Note 2:** *Tests of EPs 3 and 4 may be separate, simultaneous, or combined.*

      5. Not applicable

B   6. All drills are critiqued to identify deficiencies and opportunities for improvement.

Standard EC.5.10
The hospital manages fire safety risks.

Rationale for EC.5.10
All facilities are designed, constructed, maintained, and operated to minimize the possibility of a fire emergency requiring the evacuation of occupants. Because the safety of occupants cannot be ensured adequately by dependence on evacuation of the building, their protection from fire shall be provided by appropriate arrangement of facilities; adequate, trained staff; and development of operating and maintenance procedures composed of the following:
- Design, construction, and compartmentation
- Provision for detection, alarm, and extinguishment
- Fire prevention and the planning, training, and drilling programs for the isolation of fire, transfer of occupants to areas of refuge, or evacuation of the building

Elements of Performance for EC.5.10

B   1. The hospital develops and maintains a written management plan describing the processes it implements to effectively manage fire safety.

B   2. The hospital identifies proactive processes for protecting patients, staff, and others coming to the hospital's facilities, as well as protecting property from fire, smoke, and other products of combustion.

B 3. The hospital identifies processes for regularly inspecting, testing, and maintaining fire protection and fire safety systems, equipment, and components.

B 4. The hospital develops and implements a fire response plan that addresses the following:
   - Facilitywide fire response
   - Area-specific needs including fire evacuation routes
   - Specific roles and responsibilities of staff, licensed independent practitioners, and volunteers at a fire's point of origin
   - Specific roles and responsibilities of staff, licensed independent practitioners, and volunteers away from a fire's point of origin
   - Specific roles and responsibilities of staff, licensed independent practitioners, and volunteers in preparing for building evacuation

B 5. The hospital reviews proposed acquisitions of bedding, window draperies, and other curtains, furnishings, decorations, and other equipment for fire safety.

Standard EC.5.20

Newly constructed and existing environments are designed and maintained to comply with the *Life Safety Code®*.*

Rationale for EC.5.20

The *Life Safety Code®* (*LSC*) requires that a building is designed, constructed, and maintained with the capability of being fire safe. When undertaking the design of a newly-remodeled building, the hospital should also satisfy any requirements of others (local, state, or federal) that may be more stringent than the *LSC*.

Note 1: *This standard does not apply to the following facilities:*
- *Classified as a business occupancy by the LSC that are freestanding buildings*
- *Classified as a business occupancy by the LSC that are connected to a health care occupancy, but are separated by a two-hour rated fire barrier and do not serve as a required means of egress from the health care occupancy*
- *Housing three or fewer patients*

Note 2: *All hospitals seeking accreditation for Medicare certification purposes replace all existing roller latches on corridor doors with positive latching devices by March 13, 2006 (see Question 21.3 of Statement of Conditions™, Part 2).*

Elements of Performance for EC.5.20

B 1. Each building in which patients are housed or receive care, treatment, and services complies with the *LSC*, NFPA 101® 2000;

   or

---

* *Life Safety Code®* is a registered trademark of the National Fire Protection Association, Quincy, Massachusetts.

Management of the Environment of Care

Each building in which patients are housed or receive care, treatment, and services does not comply with the *LSC*, but the resolution of all deficiencies is evidenced through the following:

- An equivalency approved by the Joint Commission

or

- Continued progress in completing an acceptable Plan For Improvement (Statement of Conditions™, Part 4)

A   2.   A current, hospitalwide Statement of Conditions™ (SOC) compliance document* has been prepared.

Note: *You can obtain a copy of the SOC from our Web site at http://www.jcaho.org or by calling Customer Service at 630/792-5800. You may make as many copies of the SOC as you wish. However, remember to keep the original blank for future copying.*

3. Not applicable

4. Not applicable

A   5.   The hospital is making sufficient progress† toward the corrective actions described in a previously approved SOC.

Standard EC.5.30

The hospital conducts fire drills regularly.

Rationale for EC.5.30

The development of a fire response plan is an important part of achieving a fire-safe environment (*see* standard EC.5.10). It is important that this plan be regularly evaluated during implementations (in drill scenarios or actual fire situations) for performance of the fire safety equipment and staff.

Implementation of the plan should be realistic and held at varied times. An implementation held at shift change may present an unrealistic picture as to the number of staff likely available any time a fire occurs. Actual evacuation of patients during the drills is not required.

---

* **Statement of Conditions™ (SOC) compliance document**   A proactive document that helps a hospital perform a critical self-assessment of its current level of compliance and describe how to resolve any *LSC* deficiencies. The SOC was created to be a living, ongoing management tool that should be used in a management process that continually identifies, assesses, and resolves *LSC* deficiencies.

† **Sufficient progress**   Failure to make sufficient progress toward the corrective actions described in an approved Statement of Conditions™, Part 4, Plan For Improvement, would result in a recommendation of Conditional Accreditation (*see* Conditional Accreditation rule CON04).

Elements of Performance for EC.5.30

C Ⓜ 1. Fire drills are conducted quarterly on all shifts in each building defined by the *LSC* as the following:
- Ambulatory health care occupancy
- Health care occupancy

A 2. Fire drills are conducted annually in all freestanding buildings classified as a business occupancy as defined by the *LSC* where patients are seen or treated.

Note: *In leased or rented facilities, only staff in areas of the building that the hospital occupies must participate in such drills.*

3. Not applicable

C Ⓜ 4. At least 50% of the required drills are unannounced.

B 5. Staff in all areas of every building where patients are housed or treated participates in drills to the extent called for in the facility's fire plan (*see standard EC.5.10 for required content of fire response plan*).*

B 6. All fire drills are critiqued to identify deficiencies and opportunities for improvement.

A 7. The effectiveness of fire response training according to the fire plan is evaluated at least annually.

B 8. During fire drills, staff knowledge is evaluated including the following:
- When and how to sound fire alarms (where such alarms are available)
- When and how to transmit for offsite fire responders
- Containment of smoke and fire
- Transfer of patients to areas of refuge
- Fire extinguishment
- Specific fire response duties
- Preparation for building evacuation

Standard EC.5.40

The hospital maintains fire-safety equipment and building features.

Note 1: *This standard does not require hospitals to have the types of fire-safety equipment and building features discussed below. However, if these types of equipment or features exist within the hospital, then the following maintenance, testing, and inspection requirements apply.*

Note 2: *Hospitals that offer care, treatment, and services in leased facilities need to communicate maintenance expectations for building equipment not under their control to their landlord through contractual language, lease agreements, memos, and so forth. These hospitals are not required to possess maintenance documentation,*

---

* When drills are conducted between 9:00 P.M. and 6:00 A.M., a coded announcement will be permitted to be used instead of audible alarms.

Management of the Environment of Care

but must only have access to such documentation as needed and during survey. It is also important that the landlord communicate to the hospital any building equipment problems identified that could negatively affect the safety or health of patients, staff, and other people coming to the hospital, as well as the landlord's plan to resolve such issues.

Elements of Performance for EC.5.40

C Ⓜ 1. Initiating devices and fire detection and alarm equipment are tested as follows:*
- All supervisory signal devices (except valve tamper switches) are tested at least quarterly
- All valve tamper switches and water flow devices are tested at least semiannually
- All duct detectors, electromechanical releasing devices, heat detectors, manual fire alarm boxes, and smoke detectors are tested at least annually

C Ⓜ 2. Occupant alarm notification devices, including all audible devices, speakers, and visible devices, are tested at least annually.†

A 3. Off-premises emergency services notification transmission equipment is tested at least quarterly.†

C Ⓜ 4. For water-based automatic fire-extinguishing systems, all fire pumps are tested at least weekly under no-flow condition.‡

C Ⓜ 5. For water-based automatic fire-extinguishing systems, all water-storage tank high- and low-water level alarms are tested at least semiannually.

C Ⓜ 6. For water-based automatic fire-extinguishing systems, all water-storage tank low-water temperature alarms (during cold weather only) are tested at least monthly.

C Ⓜ 7. For water-based automatic fire-extinguishing systems, main drain tests are conducted at least annually at all system risers.

C Ⓜ 8. For water-based automatic fire-extinguishing systems, all fire department connections are inspected quarterly.

A 9. For water-based automatic fire-extinguishing systems, all fire pumps are tested at least annually under flow.

A 10. Kitchen automatic fire-extinguishing systems are inspected for proper operation at least semiannually (actual discharge of the fire-extinguishing system is not required).

---

* For additional guidance, see NFPA 72-1999 edition (Table 7-3.2).

† For additional guidance, see NFPA 72-1999 edition (Table 7-3.2).

‡ For additional guidance, see NFPA 25-1998 edition.

C Ⓜ 11. Carbon dioxide and other gaseous automatic fire-extinguishing systems are tested for proper operation at least annually (actual discharge of the fire-extinguishing system is not required).

C Ⓜ 12. All portable fire extinguishers* are clearly identified, inspected at least monthly, and maintained at least annually.

C Ⓜ 13. All standpipe occupant hoses are hydrostatically tested five years after installation and at least every three years thereafter;[†] and systems receive water-flow tests at least every five years.[‡]

C Ⓜ 14. All fire and smoke dampers are operated at least every four years (with fusible links removed where applicable) to verify that they fully close.[§]

A 15. All automatic smoke-detection shutdown devices for air-handling equipment are tested at least annually.[ǁ]

C Ⓜ 16. All horizontal and vertical sliding and rolling fire doors are tested for proper operation and full closure at least annually.[#]

Standard EC.5.50

The hospital develops and implements activities to protect occupants during periods when a building does not meet the applicable provisions of the *Life Safety Code*®.

Note: *This standard does not apply to facilities classified as a business occupancy by the LSC.*

Rationale for EC.5.50

When building code deficiencies are identified and cannot be immediately corrected or during renovation or construction activities, the safety of patients, staff, and other people coming to the hospital's facilities is diminished. Hospitals need to proactively identify administrative actions (for example, additional training, additional inspections, additional fire drills, and so on) to be taken if these scenarios arise.

---

* For additional guidance, see NFPA 10-1998 edition (sections 1-6, 4-3, and 4-4).

[†] For additional guidance, see NFPA 1962-1998 edition (section 2-3).

[‡] For additional guidance, see NFPA 25-1998 edition.

[§] For additional guidance, see NFPA 90A-1999 edition (section 3-4.7).

[ǁ] For additional guidance, see NFPA 90A-1999 edition (section 4-4.1).

[#] For additional guidance, see NFPA 80-1999 edition (section 15-2.4).

Management of the Environment of Care

Elements of Performance for EC.5.50

B   1. Each hospital develops a policy for using interim life safety measures (ILSMs).

B   2. The policy includes written criteria for evaluating various deficiencies and construction hazards to determine when and to what extent one or more of the following measures apply:
- Ensuring free and unobstructed exits. Staff receives additional information/communication when alternative exits are designated. Buildings or areas under construction must maintain escape routes for construction workers at all times, and the means of exiting construction areas are inspected daily.
- Ensuring free and unobstructed access to emergency services and for fire, police, and other emergency forces
- Ensuring that fire alarm, detection, and suppression systems are in good working order. A temporary but equivalent system must be provided when any fire system is impaired. Temporary systems must be inspected and tested monthly.*
- Ensuring that temporary construction partitions are smoke-tight and built of noncombustible or limited combustible materials that will not contribute to the development or spread of fire
- Providing additional fire-fighting equipment and training staff in its use
- Prohibiting smoking throughout the hospital's buildings and in and near construction areas
- Developing and enforcing storage, housekeeping, and debris-removal practices that reduce the building's flammable and combustible fire load to the lowest feasible level
- Conducting a minimum of two fire drills per shift per quarter
- Increasing surveillance of buildings, grounds, and equipment, with special attention to excavations, construction areas, construction storage, and field offices
- Training staff to compensate for impaired structural or compartmentalization[†] features of fire safety
- Conducting hospitalwide safety education programs to promote awareness of fire-safety building deficiencies, construction hazards, and ILSMs

A   3. Each hospital implements ILSMs as defined in its policy.

---

* The *Life Safety Code*®, NFPA 101-2000 edition, requires that the municipal fire department is notified (or applicable emergency forces group) and a fire watch is provided whenever an approved fire alarm or automatic sprinkler system is out of service for more than four hours in a 24-hour period in an occupied building.

[†] **Compartmentalization** The concept of using various building components (fire walls and doors, smoke barriers, fire rated floor slabs, and so forth) to prevent the spread of fire and the production's combustion, and to provide a safe means of egress to an approved exit. The presence of these features varies depending upon the building occupancy classification.

Standard EC.6.10

The hospital manages medical equipment risks.

Rationale for EC.6.10

Medical equipment is a significant contributor to the quality of care. It is used in treatment, diagnostic activities and monitoring of the patient. It is essential that the equipment is appropriate for the intended use; that staff, including licensed independent practitioners, be trained to use the equipment safely and effectively; and it is essential that the equipment is maintained appropriately by qualified individuals.

Elements of Performance for EC.6.10

B   1. The hospital develops and maintains a written management plan describing the processes it implements to manage the effective, safe, and reliable operation of medical equipment.

B   2. The hospital identifies and implements a process(es) for selecting and acquiring medical equipment.*

B   3. The hospital establishes and uses risk criteria† for identifying, evaluating, and creating an inventory of equipment to be included in the medical equipment management plan before the equipment is used. These criteria address the following:
- Equipment function (diagnosis, care, treatment, life support, and monitoring)
- Physical risks associated with use
- Equipment incident history

B   4. The hospital identifies appropriate inspection and maintenance strategies for all equipment on the inventory for achieving effective, safe, and reliable operation of all equipment in the inventory.‡

B   5. The hospital defines intervals for inspecting, testing, and maintaining appropriate equipment on the inventory (that is, those pieces of equipment on the inventory benefiting from scheduled activities to minimize the clinical and physical risks) that are based upon criteria such as manufacturers' recommendations, risk levels, and current hospital experience.

B   6. The hospital identifies and implements processes for monitoring and acting on equipment hazard notices and recalls.

---

* **Note:** *The acquisition process includes initially evaluating the condition and function of the equipment when received and evaluating the training of users before use on patients.*

† **Note:** *The hospital may choose not to use risk criteria to limit the types of equipment to be included in the medical equipment management plan, rather include all medical equipment.*

‡ **Note:** *Hospitals may use different strategies for different items as appropriate. For example, strategies such as predictive maintenance, interval-based inspections, corrective maintenance, or metered maintenance may be selected to ensure reliable performance.*

Management of the Environment of Care

B   7. The hospital identifies and implements processes for monitoring and reporting incidents in which a medical device is suspected or attributed to the death, serious injury, or serious illness of any individual, as required by the Safe Medical Devices Act of 1990.

A   8. The hospital identifies and implements processes for emergency procedures that address the following:
- What to do in the event of equipment disruption or failure
- When and how to perform emergency clinical interventions when medical equipment fails
- Availability of back-up equipment
- How to obtain repair services

Standard EC.6.20
Medical equipment is maintained, tested, and inspected.

Elements of Performance for EC.6.20

C Ⓜ   1. The hospital documents a current, accurate, and separate inventory of all equipment identified in the medical equipment management plan, regardless of ownership.

A   2. The hospital documents performance and safety testing of all equipment identified in the medical equipment management program before initial use.

A   3. The hospital documents inspection and maintenance of equipment used for life support* that is consistent with maintenance strategies to minimize clinical and physical risks identified in the equipment management plan (*see* standard EC.6.10).

C Ⓜ   4. The hospital documents inspection and maintenance of non-life support equipment on the inventory that is consistent with maintenance strategies to minimize clinical and physical risks identified in the equipment management plan (*see* standard EC.6.10).

A Ⓜ   5. The hospital documents performance testing of all sterilizers used.

A Ⓜ   6. The hospital documents chemical and biological testing of water used in renal dialysis and other applicable tests based upon regulations, manufacturers' recommendations, and hospital experience.

Standard EC.7.10
The hospital manages its utility risks.

---

* **Life support equipment** Those devices intended to sustain life and whose failure to perform its primary function, when used according to manufacturer's instructions and clinical protocol, is expected to result in imminent death in the absence of immediate intervention (examples include ventilators, anesthesia machines, and heart-lung bypass machines).

Rationale for EC.7.10
Utility systems* are essential to the proper operation of the environment of care and significantly contribute to effective, safe, and reliable provision of care to patients in health care organizations. It is important that health care organizations establish and maintain a utility systems management program to promote a safe, controlled, and comfortable environment that does the following:
- Ensures operational reliability of utility systems
- Reduces the potential for organization-acquired illness to be transmitted through the utility systems
- Assesses the reliability and minimizes potential risks of utility system failures

Elements of Performance for EC.7.10
1. Through 6. Not applicable

B   7. The hospital develops and maintains a written management plan describing the processes it implements to manage the effective, safe, and reliable operation of utility systems.

B   8. The hospital designs and installs utility systems that meet the patient care and operational needs of the services in the hospital's buildings.

B   9. The hospital establishes risk criteria† for identifying, evaluating, and creating an inventory of operating components of systems before the equipment is used.

These criteria address the following:
- Life support
- Infection control
- Support of the environment
- Equipment support
- Communication

B   10. The hospital develops appropriate strategies for all utility systems equipment on the inventory for ensuring effective, safe, and reliable operation of all equipment in the inventory.‡

B   11. The hospital defines intervals for inspecting, testing, and maintaining appropriate utility systems equipment on the inventory (that is, those pieces of equipment on the inventory benefiting from scheduled activities to minimize the clinical and physical risks) that are based upon cri-

---

* **Utility systems** May include electrical distribution; emergency power; vertical and horizontal transport; heating, ventilating, and air conditioning; plumbing, boiler, and steam; piped gases; vacuum systems; or communication systems including data-exchange systems.

† **Note:** *The hospital may choose not to use risk criteria to limit the types of utility systems to be included in the utility management plan, but rather include all utility systems.*

‡ **Note:** *Hospitals may use different strategies as appropriate. For example, strategies such as predictive maintenance, interval-based inspections, corrective maintenance, or metered maintenance may be selected to ensure reliable performance.*

Management of the Environment of Care

teria such as manufacturers' recommendations, risk levels, and current hospital experience.

B 12. The hospital identifies and implements emergency procedures for responding to utility system disruptions or failures that address the following:
- What to do if utility systems malfunction
- Identification of an alternative source of hospital-defined essential utilities
- Shutting off the malfunctioning systems and notifying staff in affected areas
- How and when to perform emergency clinical interventions when utility systems fail
- Obtaining repair services

B 13. The hospital maps the distribution of utility systems.

C Ⓜ 14. The hospital labels controls for a partial or complete emergency shutdown.*

B 15. The hospital identifies and implements processes to minimize pathogenic biological agents in cooling towers, domestic hot/cold water systems, and other aerosolizing water systems.

A 16. The hospital designs, installs, and maintains ventilation equipment to provide appropriate pressure relationships, air-exchange rates, and filtration efficiencies for ventilation systems serving areas specially designed† to control airborne contaminants (such as biological agents, gases, fumes, and dust).

Standard EC.7.20
The hospital provides an emergency electrical power source.

Rationale for EC.7.20
The hospital properly installs an emergency power source that is adequately sized, designed, and fueled, as required by the *LSC* occupancy requirements and the services provided.

---

* Effective January 1, 2005.

† **Areas specially designed** Include spaces such as operating rooms, special procedure rooms, delivery rooms for patients diagnosed or suspected of having airborne communicable diseases (for example, pulmonary or laryngeal tuberculosis), patients in "protective environment" rooms (for example, those receiving bone marrow transplants), laboratories, pharmacies, and sterile supply rooms.

EC – 29

Elements of Performance for EC.7.20

The hospital provides a reliable emergency power system,* as required by the *LSC* occupancy requirements, that supplies electricity to the following areas when normal electricity is interrupted:

- **A** 1. Alarm systems
- **C Ⓜ** 2. Exit route illumination
- **A** 3. Emergency communication systems
- **C Ⓜ** 4. Illumination of exit signs

The hospital provides a reliable emergency power system, as required by the services provided and patients served, that supplies electricity to the following areas when normal electricity is interrupted:

- **A** 5. Blood, bone, and tissue storage units
- 6. Not applicable
- **A** 7. Emergency/urgent care areas
- **A** 8. Elevators (at least one for nonambulatory patients)
- **A** 9. Medical air compressors
- **A** 10. Medical and surgical vacuum systems
- **A** 11. Areas where electrically powered life-support equipment is used
- 12. Not applicable
- 13. Not applicable
- **A** 14. Operating rooms
- **A** 15. Postoperative recovery rooms
- **A** 16. Obstetrical delivery rooms
- **A** 17. Newborn nurseries

Standard EC.7.30

The hospital maintains, tests, and inspects its utility systems.

Note: *Hospitals that offer care, treatment, and services in leased facilities need to communicate maintenance expectations for building equipment not under their control to their landlord through contractual language, lease agreements, memos, and so forth. These hospitals are not required to possess maintenance documentation, but must only have access to such documentation as needed and during survey. It is also important that the landlord communicate to the hospital any building equip-*

---

* **Reliable emergency power system** For guidance in establishing a reliable emergency power system (that is, an Essential Electrical Distribution System), *see* NFPA 99-2002 edition (Chapters 13 and 14).

Management of the Environment of Care

ment problems identified that could negatively affect the safety or health of patients, staff, and other people coming to the hospital, as well as the landlord's plan to resolve such issues.

Elements of Performance for EC.7.30

C Ⓜ 1. The hospital maintains documentation of a current, accurate, and separate inventory of utility components identified in the utility management plan.

A Ⓜ 2. The hospital maintains documentation of performance and safety testing of each critical component identified in the plan before initial use.

A Ⓜ 3. The hospital maintains documentation of maintenance of critical components of life support utility systems/equipment consistent with maintenance strategies identified in the utility management plan (*see* standard EC.7.10).

A Ⓜ 4. The hospital maintains documentation of maintenance of critical components of infection control utility systems/equipment for high-risk patients consistent with maintenance strategies identified in the utility management plan (*see* standard EC.7.10).

C Ⓜ 5. The hospital maintains documentation of maintenance of critical components of non-life support utility systems/equipment on the inventory consistent with maintenance strategies identified in the utility management plan (*see* standard EC.7.10).

Standard EC.7.40

The hospital maintains, tests, and inspects its emergency power systems.

Note: *This standard does not require hospitals to have the types of emergency power systems discussed below. However, if a hospital has these types of systems, then the following maintenance, testing, and inspection requirements apply.*

Elements of Performance for EC.7.40

C Ⓜ 1. The hospital tests each generator 12 times a year, with testing intervals not less than 20 days and not more than 40 days apart. These tests shall be conducted for at least 30 continuous minutes under a dynamic load that is at least 30% of the nameplate rating of the generator.

> **Note:** *Hospitals may choose to test to less than 30% of the emergency generator's nameplate. However, these hospitals shall (in addition to performing a test for 30 continuous minutes under operating temperature at the intervals described above) revise their existing documented management plan to conform to current NFPA 99 and NFPA 110 testing and maintenance activities. These activities shall include inspection procedures for assessing the prime movers' exhaust gas temperature against the minimum temperature recommended by the manufacturer.*

> If diesel-powered generators do not meet the minimum exhaust gas temperatures as determined during these tests, they shall be exercised for 30 continuous minutes at the intervals described above with available Emergency Power Supply Systems (EPSS) load, and exercised annually with supplemental loads of
> - 25% of name plate rating for 30 minutes, followed by
> - 50% of name plate rating for 30 minutes, followed by
> - 75% of name plate rating for 60 minutes for a total of two continuous hours

C Ⓜ 2. The hospital tests all automatic transfer switches 12 times a year, with testing intervals not less than 20 days and not more than 40 days apart.

C Ⓜ 3. The hospital tests all battery-powered lights required for egress. Testing includes (a) a functional test at 30-day intervals for a minimum of 30 seconds; and (b) an annual test for a duration of 1.5 hours.

C Ⓜ 4. The hospital tests Stored Emergency Power Supply Systems (SEPSS) whose malfunction may severely jeopardize the occupants' life and safety.* Testing includes (a) a quarterly functional test for 5 minutes or as specified for its class,† whichever is less; and (b) an annual test at full load for 60% of the full duration of its class.

Standard EC.7.50

The hospital maintains, tests, and inspects its medical gas and vacuum systems.

Note: *This standard does not require hospitals to have the medical gas and vacuum systems discussed below. However, if a hospital has these types of systems, then the following maintenance, testing, and inspection requirements apply.*

Elements of Performance for EC.7.50

A 1. The hospital inspects, tests, and maintains critical components of piped medical gas systems including master signal panels, area alarms, automatic pressure switches, shutoff valves, flexible connectors, and outlets.

---

* **Stored Emergency Power Supply Systems (SEPSS)** Are intended to automatically supply illumination or power to critical areas and equipment essential for safety to human life. Included are systems that supply emergency power for such functions as illumination for safe exiting, ventilation where it is essential to maintain life, fire detection and alarm systems, public safety communications systems, and processes where the current interruption would produce serious life safety or health hazards to patients, the public, or staff.
Note: *Other non-SEPSS battery back-up emergency power systems that a hospital has determined to be critical for operations during a power failure (for example, laboratory equipment, electronic medical records) should be properly tested and maintained in accordance with manufacturer's recommendations.*

† **Class** Defines the minimum time for which the SEPSS is designed to operate at its rated load without being recharged (for additional guidance, see NFPA 111 [1996 edition] *Standard on Stored Electrical Energy Emergency and Standby Power Systems*).

Management of the Environment of Care

A   2.   The hospital tests piped medical gas and vacuum systems when the systems are installed, modified, or repaired, including cross-connection testing, piping purity testing, and pressure testing.

A   3.   The hospital maintains the main supply valve and area shut-off valves of piped medical gas and vacuum systems to be accessible and clearly labeled.

Standard EC.8.10
The hospital establishes and maintains an appropriate environment.

Rationale for EC.8.10
It is important that the physical environment is functional and promotes healing and caring. Certain key physical elements in the environment can be significant in their ability to positively influence patient outcomes and satisfaction and improve patient safety. These elements can also contribute in creating the way the space feels and works for patients, families, visitors, and staff experiencing the care, treatment, and service delivery system.

Elements of Performance for EC.8.10

B   1.   Interior spaces should be the following:
- Appropriate to the care, treatment, and services provided and the needs of the patients related to age and other characteristics
- Include closet and drawer space provided for storing personal property and other items provided for use by patients. Lockers, drawers, or closet space is provided for patients who are in charge of their own personal grooming and who wear street clothes (for example, behavioral health care patients who wear street clothes and are expected to meet their personal grooming needs).
- For hospital settings that provide longer term care (more than 30 days), allow for good recreational interchange, consider personal preferences when feasible, and accommodate equipment, such as wheelchairs, that are necessary to activities of daily living
- For hospital settings that provide longer term care (more than 30 days), have equipment for rehabilitation and activities adequate to accomplish goals without compromising the environment's safety

B   2.   Furnishings and equipment should have the following characteristics:
- Be maintained to be safe and in good repair
- Reflect the patient's level of ability and needs
- For hospital settings that provide longer term care (more than 30 days), help to normalize the patient's living environment

B   3.   For hospital settings that provide longer term care (more than 30 days), outside areas are the following:
- Provided when required by the care, treatment, and services (for example, when certain patient groups, such as pediatric, experience long lengths of stay)

EC – 33

- Appropriate and safe considering the care, treatment, and services provided and the needs of the patients related to age and other characteristics

C Ⓜ 4. Areas used by the patient are safe, clean, functional, and comfortable.

B 5. Lighting is suitable for care, treatment, and services and the specific activities being conducted.

C Ⓜ 6. Lighting is controlled by patients, when appropriate.

B 7. Ventilation provides for acceptable levels of temperature and humidity and eliminates odors.

8. Not applicable

9. Not applicable

10. Not applicable

A 11. Door locks and other structural restraints used are consistent with the needs of patients, program policy, law, and regulation.

A 12. Emergency access provision is provided to all locked and occupied spaces.*

Standard EC.8.20
Not applicable

Standard EC.8.30
The hospital manages the design and building of the environment when it is renovated, altered, or newly created (*see also* standard EC.5.50).

Elements of Performance for EC.8.30

B 1. When planning for the size, configuration, and equipping of the space of renovated, altered, or new construction, the hospital uses one of the following: applicable state rules and regulations; *Guidelines for Design and Construction of Hospitals and Health Care Facilities*, 2001 edition, published by the American Institute of Architects; or standards or guidelines that provide design criteria.

B 2. When planning demolition, construction, or renovation, the hospital conducts a proactive risk assessment using risk criteria to identify hazards that could potentially compromise care, treatment, and services in occupied areas of the hospital's buildings. The scope and nature of the activities should determine the extent of risk assessment.

---

* Effective January 1, 2005.

B   3. When planning demolition, construction, or renovation, the hospital uses risk criteria that address the impact of demolition, renovation, or new construction on air quality requirements, infection control, utility requirements, noise, vibration, and emergency procedures.

B   4. When planning demolition, construction, or renovation, the hospital selects and implements proper controls, as required, to reduce risk and minimize impact of these activities.

Measuring and Improving Activities

Standard EC.9.10
The hospital monitors conditions in the environment.

Elements of Performance for EC.9.10
B   1. The hospital establishes and implements process(es) for reporting and investigating the following:*
- Injuries to patients or others coming to the hospital's facilities, as well as incidents of property damage
- Occupational illnesses and injuries to staff
- Security incidents involving patients, staff, or others coming to the hospital's facilities or property
- Hazardous materials and waste spills, exposures, and other related incidents
- Fire-safety management problems, deficiencies, and failures
- Equipment-management problems, failures, and user errors
- Utility systems management problems, failures, or user errors

B   2. The hospital's leaders assign a person(s) (hereafter referred to as the "assigned person[s]") to monitor and respond to conditions in the hospital's environment. The assigned individual performs the following tasks:
- Coordinates the ongoing, hospitalwide collection of information about deficiencies and opportunities for improvement in the environment of care
- Coordinates the ongoing collection and dissemination of other sources of information, such as published hazard notices or recall reports

---

* Hospitals have the flexibility to develop a single reporting method that addresses one or more of the items listed.

- Coordinates the preparation of summaries of deficiencies, problems, failures, and user errors related to managing the environment of care*
- Coordinates the preparation of summaries on findings, recommendations, actions taken, and results of performance improvement (PI) activities
- Participates in hazard surveillance and incident reporting
- Participates in developing safety policies and procedures

B   3. The hospital establishes and implements a process(es) for ongoing monitoring of performance regarding actual or potential risk(s) in each of the environment of care management plans.†

A   4. Each of the environment of care management plans is evaluated at least annually.

B   5. The objectives, scope, performance, and effectiveness of each of the environment of care management plans are evaluated at least annually.

6. Through 9. Not applicable

B   10. Environmental safety monitoring and response activities are communicated to the patient safety program required in the "Leadership" chapter of this book.

Standard EC.9.20

The hospital analyzes identified environment issues and develops recommendations for resolving them.

Elements of Performance for EC.9.20

B   1. The hospital establishes an ongoing process for resolving environment of care issues that involves representatives from clinical, administrative, and support services.

C Ⓜ   2. A multidisciplinary improvement team meets at least bimonthly to address environment of care issues.‡

B   3. The hospital analyzes environment of care issues in a timely manner.

---

* **Note:** *Incidents involving patients may be reported to appropriate staff such as staff in quality assessment, improvement, or other functions. However, at least a summary of incidents is shared with the person designated to coordinate safety management activities (see standard EC.1.10). Review of incident reports often requires that various legal processes be followed to preserve confidentiality. Opportunities to improve care, treatment, and services or to prevent future similar incidents are not lost as a result of the legal process followed.*

† *The environment of care plans are for managing safety, security, hazardous materials and waste, emergency management, fire safety, medical equipment, and utilities.*

‡ **Note:** *Meetings held less frequently than bimonthly are acceptable when supported by current hospital experience and the multidisciplinary improvement team's approval. Ongoing justification of meeting frequency depends on a satisfactory annual evaluation of performance as required by standard EC.9.10.*

Management of the Environment of Care

- **B** 4. Recommendations are developed and approved as appropriate.
- **B** 5. Appropriate staff establishes measurement guidelines.
- **B** 6. Environment of care issues are communicated to the hospital's leaders and person(s) responsible for PI activities.
-     7. Not applicable
- **A** 8. A recommendation for one or more PI activities is communicated at least annually to the hospital's leaders based on the ongoing performance monitoring of the environment of care management plans.
- **B** 9. Recommendations for resolving environmental safety issues are communicated, when appropriate, to those responsible for managing the patient safety program required in the "Leadership" chapter of this book.

Standard EC.9.30
The hospital improves the environment.

Elements of Performance for EC.9.30
- **B** 1. Appropriate staff participates in implementing recommendations.
- **B** 2. Appropriate staff monitors the effectiveness of the recommendation's implementation.
- **B** 3. Monitoring results are reported through appropriate channels, including the hospital's leaders.
- **B** 4. Monitoring results are reported to the multidisciplinary improvement team responsible for resolving environment of care issues.
- **B** 5. Results of monitoring are reported (when appropriate) to those responsible for managing the patient safety program required in the "Leadership" chapter of this book.

EC

Management of Human Resources

Overview

The **goal** of the human resources function is to ensure that the hospital determines the qualifications and competencies for all staff positions (individuals such as employees, contractors, or temporary agency personnel who provide services in the hospital) based on its mission, population(s), and care, treatment, and services. *Also see* standard LD.3.40 in the "Leadership" chapter. Hospitals must also provide the right number of competent staff to meet patients' needs. To meet this goal, the hospital carries out the following processes and activities:

- **Providing an adequate number of staff.** The hospital determines the appropriate level of staffing to fulfill its mission and meet the needs of the population(s) served. There is a sufficient number of staff based on the hospital's determination of the appropriate level of staffing.
- **Providing competent staff.** The hospital provides for competent staff either through traditional employer–employee arrangements or through contractual arrangements with other entities or persons. An initial review of credentials and qualifications is performed. Experience, education, and abilities are confirmed during orientation.
- **Orienting, training, and educating staff.** The hospital provides ongoing in-service and other education and training to increase staff knowledge of specific work-related issues.
- **Assessing, maintaining, and improving staff competence.** Ongoing, periodic competence assessment evaluates staff members' continuing abilities to perform throughout their association with the hospital.

Standards

The following is a list of all standards for this function. They are presented here for your convenience without footnotes or other explanatory text. If you have a question about a term used here, please check the Glossary.

Note: *A revised standard numbering system is being used with the reformatted standards. The revised numbering system will allow for more flexibility to add standards while maintaining the current number for each standard.*

Planning

HR.1.10   The hospital provides an adequate number and mix of staff that are consistent with the hospital's staffing plan.

HR.1.20   The hospital has a process to ensure that a person's qualifications are consistent with his or her job responsibilities.

HR.1.30   The hospital uses data on clinical/service screening indicators in combination with human resource screening indicators to assess staffing effectiveness.

Orientation, Training, and Education

HR.2.10   Orientation provides initial job training and information.

HR.2.20   Staff members, licensed independent practitioners, students, and volunteers, as appropriate, can describe or demonstrate their roles and responsibilities, based on specific job duties or responsibilities, relative to safety.

HR.2.30   Ongoing education, including in-services, training, and other activities, maintains and improves competence.

Competence Assessment

HR.3.10   Competence to perform job responsibilities is assessed, demonstrated, and maintained.

HR.3.20   The hospital periodically conducts performance evaluations.

Management of Human Resources

Understanding the Parts of This Chapter

To help you navigate this reformatted standards chapter, it may be helpful to think of its parts this way:
- The **standard** is the "goal."
- The **rationale** explains why it's important to achieve this goal.
- The **elements of performance** identify the step(s) needed to achieve this goal.

These parts are defined as follows.

Standard A statement that defines the performance expectations and/or structures or processes that must be in place in order for a hospital to provide safe, high-quality care, treatment, and services. A hospital is either "compliant" or "not compliant" with a standard.

Accreditation decisions are based on simple counts of the standards that are determined to be "not compliant."

Rationale A statement that provides background, justification, or additional information about a standard. A standard's rationale is not scored. In some instances, the rationale for a standard is self-evident. Therefore, not every standard has a written rationale.

Elements of performance (EPs) The specific performance expectations and/or structures or processes that must be in place in order for a hospital to provide safe, high-quality care, treatment, and services. The scoring of EP compliance determines a hospital's overall compliance with a standard. EPs are evaluated on the following scale:

- 0 Insufficient compliance
- 1 Partial compliance
- 2 Satisfactory compliance
- NA Not applicable

You will find a **measure of success** icon—Ⓜ—next to some EPs. Measures of success (MOS) need to be developed for certain EPs when a standard is judged to be out of compliance through either the Periodic Performance Review (PPR) or the onsite survey. An MOS is defined as a quantifiable measure, usually related to an audit, that can be used to determine whether an action has been effective and is being sustained.*

Assessing Your Compliance

Once you are familiar with the parts of this chapter, you can begin to assess your compliance with its requirements. The scoring category for each EP is noted next to the EP. If you would like to assess your hospital's performance, mark your scores for the EPs and the standards by following the simple steps described below.

---

* For more information about measures of success, *see* the "The New Joint Commission Accreditation Process" chapter in this book.

Two components are scored for each EP: (1) compliance with the requirement itself **and** (2) compliance with the track record* for that requirement. Scoring has been simplified, and track record achievements (which have always been part of the scoring) have been appropriately modified.

Note: *Some standards and EPs do not apply to a particular type of organization; these standards and EPs are marked "not applicable" and the related text is not included. Your hospital is not expected to comply with standards and EPs marked "not applicable."*

In addition, some standards and EPs that do apply to organizations may not apply to the specific care, treatment, and services that your individual hospital provides. Although these standards and EPs are included in the manual, you are not expected to comply with them. If you are unsure about the standards or EPs that apply to your hospital, please contact the Joint Commission's Standards Interpretation Group at 630/792-5900.

Step 1: Score Your Compliance with Each Element of Performance

Before you can determine your compliance with the standards, you must score your compliance with each EP. There are three scoring criterion categories: A, B, and C (described below). Please note that for each EP scoring criterion category, your hospital must meet the performance requirement itself and the track record achievements (*see* "Track Record Achievements").

Category A

These EPs relate to the presence or absence of the requirement(s) and are scored either yes (2) or no (0); however, score 1 for partial compliance is also possible based on track record achievements.

If an A EP has multiple components designated by bullets, your hospital must be compliant with all the bullets to receive a score of 2. If your hospital does not meet one or more requirements in the bullets, you will receive a score of 0.

Category B

Category B EPs are scored in two steps:
1. As with category A EPs, category B EPs relate to the presence or absence of the requirement(s). If your hospital *does not meet* the requirement(s), the EP is scored 0; there is no need to assess your compliance with the principles of good process design.
2. If your hospital *does meet* the requirement(s), but there is concern about the quality or comprehensiveness of the effort, then and only then should you assess the qualitative aspect of the EP. That is, review the applicable principles of good process design and ask how the principles were applied in the situation under discussion. Good process design has the following characteristics:

---

* **Track record** The amount of time that an organization has been in compliance with a standard, element of performance, or other requirement.

- Is consistent with your hospital's mission, values, and goals
- Meets the needs of patients
- Reflects the use of currently accepted practices (doing the right thing, using resources responsibly, using practice guidelines)
- Incorporates current safety information and knowledge such as sentinel event data and National Patient Safety Goals
- Incorporates relevant performance improvement results

This two-part evaluation applies to both simple and bulleted B EPs. First, the EPs are assessed to determine if the requirements are present. If the EP has multiple components designated by bullets, as with the category A EPs, your hospital must meet the requirements in *all* the bulleted items to get a score of 2. If your hospital meets *none* of the requirements in the bullets, it receives a score of 0. If your hospital meets *at least one, but not all*, of the bulleted requirements, it will receive a score of 1 for the EPs.

Use the following rules to determine your EP score:
- Your EP score is 0 if your hospital does not meet the requirement(s); you *do not* need to assess your compliance with the preceding applicable principles of good process design
- Your EP score is 1 if your hospital does meet the requirement(s), but considered only *some* of the preceding applicable principles of good process design
- Your EP score is 2 if your hospital does meet the requirement(s) *and* considered *all* the preceding principles of good process design

Category C

C EPs are scored 0, 1, or 2 based on the number of times your hospital does not meet the EP. These EPs are frequency based and require totaling the number of occurrences (that is, results of performance or nonperformance) related to a particular EP. Each situation discovered by a surveyor(s) will be counted as a separate occurrence.

Note: *Multiple events of the same type related to a single patient and single practitioner/staff member are counted as* one occurrence only.

Use the following rules to determine your EP score:
- Your EP score is 2 if you find one or fewer occurrences of noncompliance with the EP
- Your EP score is 1 if you find two occurrences of noncompliance with the EP
- Your EP score is 0 if you find three or more occurrences of noncompliance with the EP

If an EP in the C category has multiple requirements designated by bullets, the following scoring guidelines apply:
- If there are fewer than 2 findings in all bullets, the EP is scored 2
- If there are three or more findings in all bullets, the EP is scored 0
- In all other combinations of findings, the EP is scored 1

Track Record Achievements

In addition to meeting the requirement(s) in each EP, regardless of category, your hospital must also meet the following track record achievements:

Score	Initial Survey	Full Survey
2	4 months or more	12 months or more
1	2 to 3 months	6 to 11 months
0	Fewer than 2 months	Fewer than 6 months

Sample Sizes

If during an onsite survey, your hospital has been found to be not compliant with one or more standards, you must demonstrate Evidence of Standards Compliance (ESC) for each standard that is not compliant. The ESC must address compliance at the EP level; when an EP within a noncompliant standard requires an MOS, your hospital must demonstrate achievement with the MOS when completing the ESC.

Note: Not every EP requires an MOS. EPs that do require an MOS are clearly marked in this chapter. Organizations are required to demonstrate achievement with an MOS only for EPs within a noncompliant standard that require an MOS. Organizations do not need to demonstrate achievement with an MOS for any EP within a compliant standard.

When demonstrating achievement with the MOS during the ESC process, your hospital is **required** to use the following sample sizes, which were established because of their statistical significance, their relative simplicity in application, and their sensitivity to an organization's population size:
- For a population size of fewer than 30 cases, sample 100% of available cases
- For a population size of 30 to 100 cases, sample 30 cases
- For a population size of 101 to 500 cases, sample 50 cases
- For a population size greater than 500 cases, sample 70 cases

Note: Hospitals are encouraged, but not required, to follow this sample size when demonstrating achievement with an MOS for an EP within a noncompliant standard after conducting a full, Option 1, or Option 2 Periodic Performance Review (PPR).

When conducting PPR (optional use) or demonstrating an ESC (mandatory use), use the following percentages to determine your score: 90% through 100% of your sample size is in compliance = score 2; 80% through 89% (two instances of noncompliance) of your sample size is in compliance = score 1; less than 80% (three or more instances of noncompliance) of your sample size is in compliance = score 0.

In addition, the following information should govern your hospital's selection of samples:
- The appropriate sample size should be determined by the specific population related to the survey findings
- The sampling approach should involve either systematic random sampling (for example, your hospital selects every second or third case for review) or simple random sampling (for example, your hospital uses a series of random numbers generated by a computer to identify the cases to be reviewed)

- If your hospital chooses not to use these sample sizes while conducting PPR options 1 or 2, you should make sure that your sample size is sufficiently large enough to ensure statistical significance
- When submitting a clarifying ESC, if your hospital selects records as part of its sample, the records should be from a period of no more than three months before the last date of the survey
- Assessment of MOS compliance is conducted for a four-month period following the date of ESC approval. Your hospital should select records as a part of your sample following the date of ESC approval and use the required sample sizes. MOS percentage compliance rates are derived from the average of all four months.

Step 2: Use Your EP Scores to Gauge Your Compliance with the Standards

Now that you have evaluated and scored each EP for a particular standard, use these simple rules to determine your compliance with the standard itself:

- Your hospital is not in compliance (that is, "not compliant") with the standard if any EP is scored 0
- Otherwise, your hospital is in compliance with a standard if 65% or more of its EPs are scored 2

Standards, Rationales, Elements of Performance, and Scoring

Planning

Standard HR.1.10
The hospital provides an adequate number and mix of staff that are consistent with the hospital's staffing plan.

Element of Performance for HR.1.10
B   1. The hospital has an adequate number and mix of staff to meet the care, treatment, and service needs of the patients.

Standard HR.1.20
The hospital has a process to ensure that a person's qualifications are consistent with his or her job responsibilities.

Rationale for HR.1.20
This requirement pertains to staff and students as well as volunteers who work in the same capacity as staff when they provide care, treatment, and services.

Elements of Performance for HR.1.20
B   1. The leaders define the required competence and qualifications of staff in all program(s) or service(s).

B   2. The leaders define the required competence and qualifications of staff who make decisions about and implement and monitor restraint or seclusion use (*see* standard PC.12.30).

The hospital verifies the following (EPs 3–6):

C Ⓜ 3. Current licensure, certification, or registration

C Ⓜ 4. Education, experience, and competence appropriate for assigned responsibilities

C Ⓜ 5. Information on criminal background if required by law and regulation or hospital policy

Management of Human Resources

C Ⓜ 6. Compliance with applicable health screening requirements established by the hospital*

C Ⓜ 7. Staff supervises students when they provide patient care, treatment, and services as part of their training.

8. Through 17. Not applicable

A 18. Individuals who do not possess a license, registration, or certification do not provide or have not provided care, treatment, and services in the hospital that would, under applicable law or regulation, require such a license, registration, or certification.

A 19. Individuals who do not possess a license, registration, or certification do not provide or have not provided care, treatment, and services in the hospital that would, under applicable law or regulation, require such a license, registration, or certification and which would have placed the hospital's patients at risk for a serious adverse outcome.

Standard HR.1.30

The hospital uses data on clinical/service screening indicators† in combination with human resource screening indicators‡ to assess staffing effectiveness.§

Rationale for HR.1.30

Multiple screening indicators that relate to patient outcomes, including clinical/service and human resources screening indicators, may be indicative of staffing effectiveness.

Elements of Performance for HR.1.30

A 1. The hospital selects a minimum of four screening indicators: two clinical/service and two human resources indicators. The focus is on the relationship between human resource and clinical/service screening indicators, with the clear understanding that no one indicator, in and of itself, can directly demonstrate staffing effectiveness.

---

* The Americans with Disabilities Act (ADA) bars certain discrimination based on physical or mental impairments. To prevent such discrimination, the act prohibits or mandates various activities. Hospitals should examine their hiring and evaluation procedures for activities prohibited or mandated. For example, health care organizations need to determine whether the ADA applies to some or all applicants to their organization. If applicable, the ADA would prohibit an inquiry about the applicant's overall health status. The inquiry must be limited to dealing with the applicant's ability to perform essential job functions, perhaps defined by the privileges or position requirements sought. The Joint Commission has and will absolutely construe these standards to be consistent with the hospital's effort to meet ADA compliance efforts.

† An example of a clinical/service screening indicator is adverse drug events.

‡ Examples of human resource screening indicators are overtime and staff vacancy rate.

§ **Staffing effectiveness** The number, competency, and skill mix of staff related to the provision of needed services.

A	2.	The hospital selects at least one of the human resource and one of the clinical/service screening indicators from a list of Joint Commission-identified screening indicators. The hospital chooses additional screening indicators based on its unique characteristics, specialties, and services.
B	3.	The hospital determines the rationale for screening indicator selection.
B	4.	The hospital defines the direct and indirect caregivers included in the human resource screening indicators based on the impact, if any, the absence of such caregivers is expected to have on patient outcomes.
B	5.	The hospital uses the data collected and analyzed from the selected screening indicators to identify potential staffing effectiveness issues when performance varies from expected targets (for example, ranges of desired performance, external comparisons, or improvement goals).
B	6.	The hospital analyzes data over time per screening indicator (for example, identification of trends or patterns using a line graph, run chart, or control chart) to determine the stability of a process.
B	7.	The hospital analyzes all screening indicator data in combination (for example, a table or matrix report, multiple line graphs, spider or radar diagrams, or scatter diagrams).
A	8.	The hospital analyzes screening indicator data at the level in which staffing needs are planned in the hospital and in collaboration with other areas in the hospital, as needed.
B	9.	The hospital reports at least annually to the leaders on the aggregation and analysis of data related to staffing effectiveness (*see* standards PI.1.10 and PI.2.20) and any actions taken to improve staffing.
B	10.	The hospital can provide evidence of actions taken, as appropriate, in response to analyzed data.

List of Joint Commission Screening Indicators for Hospitals
1. Family complaints (Clinical/Service)
2. Patient complaints (Clinical/Service)
3. Patient falls (Clinical/Service)
4. Adverse drug events (Clinical/Service)
5. Injuries to patients (Clinical/Service)
6. Skin breakdown (Clinical/Service)
7. Pneumonia (Clinical/Service)
8. Postoperative infections (Clinical/Service)
9. Urinary tract infections (Clinical/Service)
10. Upper gastrointestinal bleeding (Clinical/Service)
11. Shock/cardiac arrest (Clinical/Service)
12. Length of stay (Clinical/Service)
13. Overtime (Human Resource)

Management of Human Resources

14. Staff vacancy rate (Human Resource)
15. Staff satisfaction (Human Resource)
16. Staff turnover rate (Human Resource)
17. Understaffing as compared to hospital's staffing plan (Human Resource)
18. Nursing care hours per patient day (Human Resource)
19. Staff injuries on the job (Human Resource)
20. On-call or per diem use (Human Resource)
21. Sick time (Human Resource)

Orientation, Training, and Education

Standard HR.2.10
Orientation provides initial job training and information.

Rationale for HR.2.10
Staff members, students, and volunteers are oriented to their jobs as appropriate and the work environment before providing care, treatment, and services.

Elements of Performance for HR.2.10
As appropriate, each staff member, student, and volunteer is oriented to the following:

C Ⓜ 1. The hospital's mission and goals

C Ⓜ 2. Hospitalwide policies and procedures (including safety and infection control) and relevant unit, setting, or program-specific policies and procedures

C Ⓜ 3. Specific job duties and responsibilities and service, setting, or program-specific job duties and responsibilities related to safety and infection control

4. Not applicable

C Ⓜ 5. Cultural diversity and sensitivity

C Ⓜ 6. Staff, students, and volunteers are educated about the rights of patients and ethical aspects of care, treatment, and services and the process used to address ethical issues.

7. Not applicable

C Ⓜ 8. Orientation and education for forensic staff include how to interact with patients; procedures for responding to unusual clinical events and incidents; the hospital's channels of clinical, security, and administrative communication; and distinctions between administrative and clinical seclusion and restraint.

Standard HR.2.20

Staff members, licensed independent practitioners, students, and volunteers, as appropriate, can describe or demonstrate their roles and responsibilities, based on specific job duties or responsibilities, relative to safety.

Rationale for HR.2.20

The human element is the most critical factor in any process, determining whether the right things are done correctly. The best policies and procedures for minimizing risks in the environment where care, treatment, and services are provided are meaningless if staff, licensed independent practitioners, if applicable, students, and volunteers do not know and understand them well enough to perform them properly.

It is important that everyday precautions identified by the health care hospital for minimizing various risks, including those related to patient safety and environmental safety,* are properly implemented. It is also important that the appropriate emergency procedures be instituted should an incident or failure occur in the environment.

Elements of Performance for HR.2.20

Staff members, licensed independent practitioners, students, and volunteers, as appropriate, can describe or demonstrate the following:

C Ⓜ 1. Risks within the hospital's environment

C Ⓜ 2. Actions to eliminate, minimize, or report risks

C Ⓜ 3. Procedures to follow in the event of an incident

C Ⓜ 4. Reporting processes for common problems, failures, and user errors

Standard HR.2.30

Ongoing education, including in-services, training, and other activities, maintains and improves competence.

Elements of Performance for HR.2.30

The following occurs for staff, students, and volunteers who work in the same capacity as staff providing care, treatment, and services:

B 1. Training occurs when job responsibilities or duties change

C Ⓜ 2. Participation in ongoing in-services, training, or other activities occurs to increase staff, student, or volunteer knowledge of work-related issues

C Ⓜ 3. Ongoing in-services and other education and training are appropriate to the needs of the population(s) served and comply with law and regulation

---

* The "Management of the Environment of Care" chapter of this book identifies risks associated with the following categories: safety, security, hazardous materials and waste, emergency management, laboratory/medical equipment, and utility management.

Management of Human Resources

C Ⓜ 4. Ongoing in-services, training, or other activities emphasize specific job-related aspects of safety and infection prevention and control

C Ⓜ 5. Ongoing in-services, training, or other education incorporate methods of team training, when appropriate

C Ⓜ 6. Ongoing in-services, training, or other education reinforce the need and ways to report unanticipated adverse events

C Ⓜ 7. Ongoing in-services or other education are offered in response to learning needs identified through performance improvement findings and other data analysis (that is, data from staff surveys, performance evaluations, or other needs assessments)

C Ⓜ 8. Ongoing education is documented

Competence Assessment

Standard HR.3.10
Competence to perform job responsibilities is assessed, demonstrated, and maintained.

Rationale for HR.3.10
Competence assessment is systematic and allows for a measurable assessment of the person's ability to perform required activities. Information used as part of competence assessment may include data from performance evaluations, performance improvement, and aggregate data on competence, as well as the assessment of learning needs.

Elements of Performance for HR.3.10
The competence assessment process for staff, students, and volunteers who work in the same capacity as staff providing care, treatment, and services is based on the following (EPs 1–7):

B 1. Populations served

B 2. Defined competencies to be required

B 3. Defined competencies to be assessed during orientation

B 4. Defined competencies that need to be assessed and reassessed on an ongoing basis, based on techniques, procedures, technology, equipment, or skills needed to provide care, treatment, and services

B 5. A defined time frame for how often competence assessments are performed for each person, minimally, once in the three-year accreditation cycle and in accordance with law and regulation

2005 Hospital Accreditation Standards

B   6.   Assessment methods (appropriate to determine the skill being assessed)

B   7.   The use of qualified individuals to assess competence

C Ⓜ   8.   The hospital assesses and documents each person's ability to carry out assigned responsibilities safely, competently, and in a timely manner upon completion of orientation.

C Ⓜ   9.   The hospital assesses each person according to its competence assessment process.

B   10.   When improvement activities lead to a determination that a person with performance problems is unable or unwilling to improve, the hospital modifies the person's job assignment or takes other appropriate action.

Standard HR.3.20

The hospital periodically conducts performance evaluations.

Rationale for HR.3.20

Performance is evaluated as an ongoing process for providing positive and negative feedback to staff and students as well as volunteers who work in the same capacity as staff providing care, treatment, and services. Formal performance evaluations can be conducted concurrently with competence assessments or can be completed at a separate time.

Elements of Performance for HR.3.20

C Ⓜ   1.   The hospital conducts performance evaluations periodically at time frames identified by the hospital (at a minimum, at least once in the three-year accreditation cycle).

C Ⓜ   2.   Performance is evaluated based on the performance expectations described in job descriptions.

         3.   Not applicable

C Ⓜ   4.   Performance evaluations are documented.*

---

* Effective July 1, 2004.

Management of Information

Overview

The **goal** of the information management function is to support decision making to improve patient outcomes, improve health care documentation, assure patient safety, and improve performance in patient care, treatment, and services, governance, management, and support processes. While efficiency, effectiveness, patient safety, and the quality of patient care can be improved by computerization and other technologies, the principles of good information management apply to all methods, whether paper-based or electronic. The standards in this chapter are designed to be equally compatible with paper-based systems, electronic systems, or hybrid systems.

A hospital's provision of care, treatment, and services is a complex endeavor that is highly dependent on information. This includes information about the science of care, treatment, and services; the individual patient; the care, treatment, and services provided; the results of care, treatment, and services; and the performance of the hospital itself. Furthermore, because many individuals and areas within the hospital are involved in the provision of care, treatment, and services, their work must be coordinated and integrated. As a result, hospitals must treat information as an important resource to be managed effectively and efficiently. Managing information is an active, planned activity. The hospital's leaders have overall responsibility for managing information, just as they do for managing the hospital's human, material, and financial resources.

The quality of care, treatment, and services is affected by the many transitions in information management that are currently in progress in health care, such as the transition from handwriting and traditional paper-based documentation to electronic information management, as well as the transition from free text* to structured† and interactive text.‡

To achieve the goals of this function, the following processes are performed well:
- Identifying information needs
- Designing the structure of the information management system

---

* **Free text** Free-flowing, nonstructured type of speaking, writing, or inputting of information.

† **Structured text** Process that requires authors to put specific information into specific fields with passive guidance by the information system. In paper-based systems, a form encourages a practitioner to fill in fields or boxes. Electronic systems use the same principle for templates or macros, which are guides used to create standardized information documentation. The purpose is to produce data of more consistent quality, make information more usable for decision support, make information more complete and more easily retrievable, and save documentation time.

‡ **Interactive text** A more complex version of structured text, as it interactively prompts and provides feedback to the person using it. Typically, it uses a higher level of computer intelligence that interacts with the person who records information.

- Capturing,* organizing, storing, retrieving, processing,† and analyzing‡ data and information
- Transmitting,§ reporting, displaying, integrating, and using data and information
- Safeguarding data‖ and information

The standards in this chapter focus on hospitalwide information planning and management processes to meet the hospital's internal and external information needs. They describe a vision for effectively and continuously improving information management in health care hospitals. Achieving this vision involves the following:
- Ensuring timely and easy access to complete information throughout the hospital
- Assuring data accuracy
- Balancing requirements of security# and ease of access
- Producing and using aggregate data to pursue opportunities for improvement
- Ensuring data comparability within and among organizations, where possible, by following national, state, and other recognized standards and guidelines on form and content
- Accessing and using external knowledge bases and comparative data to pursue opportunities for improvement
- Redesigning information-related processes to improve efficiency and effectiveness, as well as patient safety and quality of patient care, treatment, and services
- Increasing collaboration and information sharing to enhance patient care

---

* **Capture** The process of recording representations of human thought, perceptions, or actions, as well as device-generated data or information that is gathered and/or computed about a patient as part of a health care encounter or about other matters in an organization.

† **Processing** The process that manipulates data and information by editing and updating.

‡ **Analyzing** The process that interprets the data and transforms it into information.

§ **Transmitting** The sending of data and information from one location to another.

‖ **Data** Uninterpreted observations or facts.

Security The protection of data from intentional or unintentional destruction, modification, or disclosure.

Standards

The following is a list of all standards for this function. They are presented here for your convenience without footnotes or other explanatory text. If you have a question about a term used here, please check the Glossary.

Note: *A revised standard numbering system is being used with the reformatted standards. This revised numbering system will allow for more flexibility to add standards while maintaining the current label for each standard.*

Information Management Planning

IM.1.10 The hospital plans and designs information management processes to meet internal and external information needs.

Confidentiality and Security

IM.2.10 Information privacy and confidentiality are maintained.

IM.2.20 Information security, including data integrity, is maintained.

IM.2.30 The hospital has a process for maintaining continuity of information.

Information Management Processes

IM.3.10 The hospital has processes in place to effectively manage information, including the capturing, reporting, processing, storing, retrieving, disseminating, and displaying of clinical/service and nonclinical data and information.

Information-Based Decision Making

IM.4.10 The information management system provides information for use in decision making.

Knowledge-Based Information

IM.5.10 Knowledge-based information resources are readily available, current, and authoritative.

Patient-Specific Information

IM.6.10 The hospital has a complete and accurate medical record for every individual assessed, cared for, treated or served.

IM.6.20 Records contain patient-specific information, as appropriate, to the care, treatment, and services provided.

IM.6.30 The medical record thoroughly documents operative or other high risk procedures and the use of moderate or deep sedation or anesthesia.

IM.6.40 For patients receiving continuing ambulatory care services, the medical record contains a summary list of all significant diagnoses, procedures, drug allergies, and medications.

IM.6.50 Designated qualified personnel accept and transcribe verbal orders from authorized individuals.

IM.6.60 The hospital can provide access to all relevant information from a patient's record when needed for use in patient care, treatment, and services.

Understanding the Parts of This Chapter

To help you navigate this reformatted standards chapter, it may be helpful to think of its parts this way:
- The **standard** is the "goal."
- The **rationale** explains why it's important to achieve this goal.
- The **elements of performance** identify the step(s) needed to achieve this goal.

These parts are defined as follows.

Standard A statement that defines the performance expectations and/or structures or processes that must be in place in order for a hospital to provide safe, high-quality care, treatment, and services. A hospital is either "compliant" or "not compliant" with a standard.

Accreditation decisions are based on simple counts of the standards that are determined to be "not compliant."

Rationale A statement that provides background, justification, or additional information about a standard. A standard's rationale is not scored. In some instances, the rationale for a standard is self-evident. Therefore, not every standard has a written rationale.

Elements of performance (EPs) The specific performance expectations and/or structures or processes that must be in place in order for a hospital to provide safe, high-quality care, treatment, and services. The scoring of EP compliance determines a hospital's overall compliance with a standard. EPs are evaluated on the following scale:

- 0   Insufficient compliance
- 1   Partial compliance
- 2   Satisfactory compliance
- NA Not applicable

You will find a **measure of success** icon—Ⓜ—next to some EPs. Measures of success (MOS) need to be developed for certain EPs when a standard is judged to be out of compliance through either the Periodic Performance Review (PPR) or the onsite survey. An MOS is defined as a quantifiable measure, usually related to an audit, that can be used to determine whether an action has been effective and is being sustained.*

Assessing Your Compliance

Once you are familiar with the parts of this chapter, you can begin to assess your compliance with its requirements. The scoring category for each EP is noted next to the EP. If you would like to assess your hospital's performance, mark your scores for the EPs and the standards by following the simple steps described below.

---

* For more information about measures of success, *see* the "The New Joint Commission Accreditation Process" chapter in this book.

Two components are scored for each EP: (1) compliance with the requirement itself **and** (2) compliance with the track record* for that requirement. Scoring has been simplified, and track record achievements (which have always been part of the scoring) have been appropriately modified.

Note: *Some standards and EPs do not apply to a particular type of organization; these standards and EPs are marked "not applicable" and the related text is not included. Your hospital is not expected to comply with standards and EPs marked "not applicable."*

In addition, some standards and EPs that do apply to organizations may not apply to the specific care, treatment, and services that your individual hospital provides. Although these standards and EPs are included in the manual, you are not expected to comply with them. If you are unsure about the standards or EPs that apply to your hospital, please contact the Joint Commission's Standards Interpretation Group at 630/792-5900.

Step 1: Score Your Compliance with Each Element of Performance

Before you can determine your compliance with the standards, you must score your compliance with each EP. There are three scoring criterion categories: A, B, and C (described below). Please note that for each EP scoring criterion category, your hospital must meet the performance requirement itself and the track record achievements (*see* "Track Record Achievements").

Category A

These EPs relate to the presence or absence of the requirement(s) and are scored either yes (2) or no (0); however, score 1 for partial compliance is also possible based on track record achievements.

If an A EP has multiple components designated by bullets, your hospital must be compliant with all the bullets to receive a score of 2. If your hospital does not meet one or more requirements in the bullets, you will receive a score of 0.

Category B

Category B EPs are scored in two steps:
1. As with category A EPs, category B EPs relate to the presence or absence of the requirement(s). If your hospital *does not meet* the requirement(s), the EP is scored 0; there is no need to assess your compliance with the principles of good process design.
2. If your hospital *does meet* the requirement(s), but there is concern about the quality or comprehensiveness of the effort, then and only then should you assess the qualitative aspect of the EP. That is, review the applicable principles of good process design and ask how the principles were applied in the situation under discussion. Good process design has the following characteristics:

---

* **Track record** The amount of time that an organization has been in compliance with a standard, element of performance, or other requirement.

- Is consistent with your hospital's mission, values, and goals
- Meets the needs of patients
- Reflects the use of currently accepted practices (doing the right thing, using resources responsibly, using practice guidelines)
- Incorporates current safety information and knowledge such as sentinel event data and National Patient Safety Goals
- Incorporates relevant performance improvement results

This two-part evaluation applies to both simple and bulleted B EPs. First, the EPs are assessed to determine if the requirements are present. If the EP has multiple components designated by bullets, as with the category A EPs, your hospital must meet the requirements in *all* the bulleted items to get a score of 2. If your hospital meets *none* of the requirements in the bullets, it receives a score of 0. If your hospital meets *at least one, but not all*, of the bulleted requirements, it will receive a score of 1 for the EPs.

Use the following rules to determine your EP score:
- Your EP score is 0 if your hospital does not meet the requirement(s); you *do not* need to assess your compliance with the preceding applicable principles of good process design
- Your EP score is 1 if your hospital does meet the requirement(s), but considered only *some* of the preceding applicable principles of good process design
- Your EP score is 2 if your hospital does meet the requirement(s) *and* considered *all* the preceding principles of good process design

Category C

C EPs are scored 0, 1, or 2 based on the number of times your hospital does not meet the EP. These EPs are frequency based and require totaling the number of occurrences (that is, results of performance or nonperformance) related to a particular EP. Each situation discovered by a surveyor(s) will be counted as a separate occurrence.

Note: *Multiple events of the same type related to a single patient and single practitioner/staff member are counted as* one occurrence only.

Use the following rules to determine your EP score:
- Your EP score is 2 if you find one or fewer occurrences of noncompliance with the EP
- Your EP score is 1 if you find two occurrences of noncompliance with the EP
- Your EP score is 0 if you find three or more occurrences of noncompliance with the EP

If an EP in the C category has multiple requirements designated by bullets, the following scoring guidelines apply:
- If there are fewer than 2 findings in all bullets, the EP is scored 2
- If there are three or more findings in all bullets, the EP is scored 0
- In all other combinations of findings, the EP is scored 1

Track Record Achievements

In addition to meeting the requirement(s) in each EP, regardless of category, your hospital must also meet the following track record achievements:

Score	Initial Survey	Full Survey
2	4 months or more	12 months or more
1	2 to 3 months	6 to 11 months
0	Fewer than 2 months	Fewer than 6 months

Sample Sizes

If during an onsite survey, your hospital has been found to be not compliant with one or more standards, you must demonstrate Evidence of Standards Compliance (ESC) for each standard that is not compliant. The ESC must address compliance at the EP level; when an EP within a noncompliant standard requires an MOS, your hospital must demonstrate achievement with the MOS when completing the ESC.

Note: *Not every EP requires an MOS. EPs that do require an MOS are clearly marked in this chapter. Organizations are required to demonstrate achievement with an MOS only for EPs within a noncompliant standard that require an MOS. Organizations do not need to demonstrate achievement with an MOS for any EP within a compliant standard.*

When demonstrating achievement with the MOS during the ESC process, your hospital is **required** to use the following sample sizes, which were established because of their statistical significance, their relative simplicity in application, and their sensitivity to an organization's population size:
- For a population size of fewer than 30 cases, sample 100% of available cases
- For a population size of 30 to 100 cases, sample 30 cases
- For a population size of 101 to 500 cases, sample 50 cases
- For a population size greater than 500 cases, sample 70 cases

Note: *Hospitals are encouraged, but not required, to follow this sample size when demonstrating achievement with an MOS for an EP within a noncompliant standard after conducting a full, Option 1, or Option 2 Periodic Performance Review (PPR).*

When conducting PPR (optional use) or demonstrating an ESC (mandatory use), use the following percentages to determine your score: 90% through 100% of your sample size is in compliance = score 2; 80% through 89% (two instances of noncompliance) of your sample size is in compliance = score 1; less than 80% (three or more instances of noncompliance) of your sample size is in compliance = score 0.

In addition, the following information should govern your hospital's selection of samples:
- The appropriate sample size should be determined by the specific population related to the survey findings
- The sampling approach should involve either systematic random sampling (for example, your hospital selects every second or third case for review) or simple random sampling (for example, your hospital uses a series of random numbers generated by a computer to identify the cases to be reviewed)

- If your hospital chooses not to use these sample sizes while conducting PPR options 1 or 2, you should make sure that your sample size is sufficiently large enough to ensure statistical significance
- When submitting a clarifying ESC, if your hospital selects records as part of its sample, the records should be from a period of no more than three months before the last date of the survey
- Assessment of MOS compliance is conducted for a four-month period following the date of ESC approval. Your hospital should select records as a part of your sample following the date of ESC approval and use the required sample sizes. MOS percentage compliance rates are derived from the average of all four months.

Step 2: Use Your EP Scores to Gauge Your Compliance with the Standards

Now that you have evaluated and scored each EP for a particular standard, use these simple rules to determine your compliance with the standard itself:
- Your hospital is not in compliance (that is, "not compliant") with the standard if any EP is scored 0
- Otherwise, your hospital is in compliance with a standard if 65% or more of its EPs are scored 2

Standards, Rationales, Elements of Performance, and Scoring

Information Management Planning

Standard IM.1.10
The hospital plans and designs information management processes to meet internal and external information needs.

Rationale for IM.1.10
Hospitals vary in size, complexity, governance, structure, decision-making processes, and resources. Information management systems and processes vary accordingly. Only by first identifying the information needs can one then evaluate the extent to which they are planned for, and at what performance level the needs are being met. Planning for the management of information does not require a formal written information plan, but does require evidence of a planned approach that identifies the hospital's information needs and supports its goals and objectives.

Elements of Performance for IM.1.10

B 1. The hospital bases its information management processes on a thorough analysis of internal and external information needs.
- The analysis ascertains the flow of information in a hospital, including information storage and feedback mechanisms.
- The analysis considers what data and information are needed: within and among departments, services, or programs; within and among the staff, the administration, and governance structure; to support relationships with outside services and contractors; with licensing, accrediting, and regulatory bodies; with purchasers, payers, and employers; and to participate in national research and databases.

B 2. To guide development of processes for managing information used internally and externally, the hospital assesses its information management needs based on the following:
- Its mission
- Its goals
- Its services
- Personnel
- Patient safety considerations
- Quality of care, treatment, and services
- Mode(s) of service delivery
- Resources

- Access to affordable technology
- Identification of barriers to effective communication among caregivers

B 3. The hospital bases management, staffing, and material resource allocations for information management on the scope and complexity of care, treatment, and services provided.

B 4. Appropriate staff participates in assessment, selection, integration, and use of information management systems for clinical/service and hospital information.

B 5. The hospital has an ongoing process to assess the needs of the hospital, departments, and individuals for knowledge-based information and uses this assessment as a basis for planning.

Confidentiality and Security

Standard IM.2.10
Information privacy* and confidentiality† are maintained.

Rationale for IM.2.10
Confidentiality of data and information applies across all systems and automated, paper, and verbal communications, as well as to clinical/service, financial, and business records and employee-specific information. The capture, storage, and retrieval processes for data and information are designed to be performed on a timely‡ basis without compromising the data and information's confidentiality. Protecting privacy and confidentiality of information is the responsibility of the whole hospital. In achieving this responsibility, the hospital provides appropriate safeguards for patient privacy and the confidentiality of information. These safeguards are consistent with available technology and legitimate needs for accessibility of the information to authorized individuals for the delivery of care, treatment, and services and effective functioning of the organization, research, and education.

Elements of Performance for IM.2.10
B 1. The hospital has developed a written process (in one or more policies) based on and consistent with applicable law that addresses the privacy and confidentiality of information.

---

* **Privacy** An individual's right to limit the disclosure of personal information.

† **Confidentiality** The safekeeping of data/information so as to restrict access to individuals who have need, reason, and permission for such access.

‡ Defined by organization policy and based on the intended use of the information.

B 2. The hospital's policy, including significant changes to the policy, has been effectively communicated to applicable staff.

B 3. The hospital has a process to monitor compliance with its policy.

B 4. The hospital improves privacy and confidentiality by monitoring information and developments in technology.

C Ⓜ 5. Individuals about whom personally identifiable health data and information may be maintained or collected are made aware of what uses and disclosures of the information will be made.

B 6. For uses and disclosures of health information, the removal of personal identifiers is encouraged to the extent possible, consistent with maintaining the usefulness of the information.

C Ⓜ 7. Protected health information* is used for the purposes identified or as required by law and not further disclosed without patient authorization.

B 8. The hospital preserves the confidentiality of data and information identified as sensitive and requires extraordinary means to preserve patient privacy.

Standard IM.2.20

Information security, including data integrity,[†] is maintained.

Rationale for IM.2.20

Policies and procedures address security procedures to ensure that only authorized personnel gain access to data and information. These policies can range from access to the paper chart to the various security levels and distribution of passwords in an electronic system. The basic premise of the policies is to provide the appropriate level of security and protection for sensitive patient, employee, and other information, while facilitating access to data by those who have a legitimate need. The capture, storage, and retrieval processes for data and information are designed to provide for timely access without compromising the data and information's security and integrity.

Elements of Performance for IM.2.20

B 1. The hospital has developed a written process in one or more policies based on and consistent with applicable law that addresses information security, including data integrity.

B 2. The hospital's policy, including significant changes to the policy, has been effectively communicated to applicable staff.

---

* **Protected health information** Health information that contains information such that an individual person can be identified as the subject of that information.

[†] **Integrity** In the context of data security, data integrity means the protection of data from accidental or unauthorized intentional change.

C Ⓜ 3. The hospital has an effective process for enforcing the policy.

C Ⓜ 4. The hospital monitors compliance with its policy.

C Ⓜ 5. The hospital uses monitoring of information and developments in technology to improve information security, including data integrity.

B 6. The hospital develops controls to safeguard data and information, including the clinical record, against loss, destruction, and tampering. Controls include the following:
- Policies when the removal of records is permitted
- Data and information protection against unauthorized intrusion, corruption, or damage
- Prevention of falsification of data and information
- Guidelines to prevent the loss and destruction of records
- Guidelines for destroying copies of records
- Protection of records in a manner that minimizes the possibility of damage from fire and water

B 7. Policies and procedures, including plans for implementation, for electronic information systems address the following: data integrity, authentication,* nonrepudiation,† encryption‡ as warranted, and auditability,§ as appropriate to the system and types of information, for example, patient information and billing information.

Standard IM.2.30
The hospital has a process for maintaining continuity of information.

Rationale for IM.2.30
The overall purpose of the information continuity plan is to provide an alternative means of processing data, provide for recovery of data, and return to normal operations as soon as possible.

Elements of Performance for IM.2.30
B 1. The hospital has a business continuity/disaster recovery plan for information systems, which includes the identification of the most critical information functions for patient care, treatment, and services and business processes, and the impact on the hospital if these systems were severely interrupted, as priority areas of the continuity/disaster recovery plan.

---

* **Authentication** The validation of correctness for both the information itself and the person who is the author or user of information.

† **Nonrepudiation** The inability to dispute a document's content or authorship.

‡ **Encryption** The process of transforming plain text (readable) into cipher text that is unreadable without a special software key.

§ **Auditability** The ability to do a methodical examination and verification of all information activities such as entering and accessing.

B   2.   The plan is tested periodically to ensure that the business interruption back-up techniques are effective.

B   3.   For electronic systems, the hospital has a process for disaster recovery and business continuity, as they would impact the management of information, which includes the following:
- Plans for scheduled and unscheduled interruptions, which includes end-user training with the downtime procedures
- Contingency procedures for operations interruptions (hardware, software, or other systems failure)
- Plans for minimal interruptions as a result of scheduled downtime
- An emergency service plan
- A back-up system (electronic or manual)
- Data retrieval and what it will address, including retrieval from storage and information presently in the system, retrieval of data in the event of system interruption, and back up of data

Introduction to Managing Information for Clinical/Service and Hospital Decision Making

A hospital's ability to make the best decisions about clinical/service and hospital issues depends heavily on having ready access to reliable and accurate information. To support the decision-making process, the hospital follows certain procedures to successfully capture, process, store, and retrieve the needed information. It then supplies the information to management and others involved in the decision-making process.

Standards IM.3.10 and IM.4.10 address the procedures involved in information management in support of clinical/service and hospital decision making; as such, these procedures are critical to patient care and safety and the efficient management of the hospital. The procedures also apply in all information management environments, whether paper-based, electronic, or a hybrid of both.

The standards themselves also address all information management environments, and can be particularly helpful to hospitals transitioning from a paper-based environment to an electronic environment. The first standard addresses the tasks of collecting, processing, storing, retrieving, reporting, and disseminating data and information. The second standard addresses the use of the information.

Information Management Processes

Standard IM.3.10

The hospital has processes in place to effectively manage information, including the capturing, reporting, processing, storing, retrieving, disseminating, and displaying of clinical/service and nonclinical data and information.

Rationale for IM.3.10

Records resulting from data capture and report generation* are used for communication and continuity of the patient's care or financial and business operations over time. Records are also used for other purposes, including litigation and risk management activities, reimbursement, and statistics. Improved data capture and report generation systems enhance the value of the records. Potential benefits include improved patient care quality and safety, improved efficiency effectiveness and reduced costs in patient care, and financial and business operations. To maximize the benefits of data capture and report generation, these processes exhibit the following characteristics: unique ID, accuracy, completeness, timeliness,[†] interoperability,[‡] retrievability,[§] authentication and accountability,[‖] auditability, confidentiality, and security.

The processing, storage, and retrieval functions are integral to electronic, computerized, and paper-based information systems in hospitals. Important considerations for these functions include data elements, data accuracy, data confidentiality, data security, data integrity, permanence of storage (the time a medium can safely store information), ease of retrievability, aggregation of information, interoperability, clinical/service practice considerations, performance improvement, and decision support processing.

A goal for information storage is to be linked or centrally organized and accessible. This could include the hospital having an index identifying where the information is stored and how to access it; or, as the hospital moves to electronic systems, the hospital creates all information systems to be interoperable within the enterprise. As more hospitals automate various processes and activities, it is important to share critical data among systems. As challenges of interoperability have arisen, stan-

---

* **Report generation** The process of analyzing, organizing, and presenting recorded information for authentication and inclusion in the patient's health care record or in financial or business records.

[†] **Timeliness** The time between the occurrence of an event and the availability of data about the event. Timeliness is related to the use of the data.

[‡] **Interoperability** Enables authorized users to capture, share, and report information from any system, whether paper- or electronic-based.

[§] **Retrievability** The capability of efficiently finding relevant information.

[‖] **Accountability** All information is attributable to its source (person or device).

dards organizations have stepped in to develop industry standards. It is important that the hospital is aware of the standards development organizations and their recommendations.

Internally and externally generated data and information are accurately disseminated to users. Access to accurate information is required to deliver, improve, analyze, and advance patient care and the systems that support health care delivery. Information may be accessed and disseminated through electronic information systems or paper-based records and reports. The use of information should be considered in developing forms, screen displays, and standard or ad hoc reports.

Elements of Performance for IM.3.10

B 1. Uniform data definitions and data capture methods are used.
- Minimum data sets, terminology, definitions, classifications, vocabulary, and nomenclature are standardized as needed.
- Industry standards are used whenever possible.

C Ⓜ 2. Abbreviations, acronyms, and symbols are standardized throughout the hospital and there is a list of abbreviations, acronyms, and symbols *not* to use.

B 3. Quality control systems are used to monitor data content and collection activities.
- The method used assures timely and economical data collection with the degree of accuracy, completeness, and discrimination necessary for their intended use.
- The method used minimizes bias in the data and regularly assesses the data's reliability, validity, and accuracy.
- Those responsible for collecting and reviewing the data are accountable for information accuracy and completeness.

B 4. Storage and retrieval systems are designed to support hospital needs for clinical/service and organization-specific information.
- Storage and retrieval systems are designed to balance the ability to retrieve data and information with the intended use for the data and information.
- Storage and retrieval systems are designed to balance security and confidentiality issues with accessibility.
- Systems for paper and electronic records are designed to reduce disruption or inaccessibility during such times as diminished staffing and scheduled and unscheduled downtimes of electronic information systems.

A 5. Data and information are retained for sufficient time to comply with law and regulation.

B 6. Data and information are retained for quality of care and other hospital needs.*

---
* Effective January 1, 2005.

Management of Information

B   7. The necessary expertise and tools are available for collecting, retrieving, and analyzing data and their transformation into information.

B   8. Data are organized and transformed into information in formats useful to decision makers.

B   9. Dissemination of data and information is timely and accurate.

B   10. Data and information are disseminated in standard formats and methods to meet user needs and provide for easy retrievability and interpretation.

B   11. Industry or organization standards are used whenever possible for data display and transmission.

Information-Based Decision Making

Standard IM.4.10
The information management system provides information for use in decision making.

Rationale for IM.4.10
Information management supports timely and effective decision making at all organization levels. The information management processes support managerial and operational decisions, performance improvement activities, and patient care, treatment, and service decisions. Clinical and strategic decision making depends on information from multiple sources, including the patient record, knowledge-based information, comparative data/information, and aggregate data/information.

Elements of Performance for IM.4.10
To support clinical decision making, information found in the patient record must include the following (EPs 1–5[†]):

C Ⓜ   1. Readily accessible throughout the system

C Ⓜ   2. Accurately recorded

C Ⓜ   3. Complete

C Ⓜ   4. Organized for efficient retrieval of needed data

C Ⓜ   5. Timely

B   6. Comparative performance data and information are available for decision making, if applicable.

[†] Effective January 1, 2005

B 7. The hospital has the ability to collect and aggregate data and information to support care, treatment, and service delivery and operations, including the following:
- Individual care, treatment, and services and care, treatment, and service delivery
- Decision making
- Management and operations
- Analysis of trends over time
- Performance comparisons over time within the hospital and with other organizations
- Performance improvement
- Infection control
- Patient safety

Knowledge-Based Information

Standard IM.5.10
Knowledge-based information* resources are readily available, current, and authoritative.

Rationale for IM.5.10
Hospital practitioners and staff have access to knowledge-based information to do the following:
- Help them acquire and maintain the knowledge and skills needed to maintain and improve competence
- Help with clinical/service and management decision making
- Provide appropriate information and education to patients and families
- Support performance improvement and patient safety activities
- Support the institution's educational and research needs

Elements of Performance for IM.5.10
A 1. Library services are provided by cooperative or contractual arrangements with other institutions, if not available on site.

---

* **Knowledge-based information** A collection of stored facts, models, and information that can be used for designing and redesigning processes and for problem solving. In the context of this book, knowledge-based information is found in the clinical, scientific, and management literature.

Management of Information

B   2. The hospital provides access to information resources needed by staff in print, electronic, Internet, audio, and/or other appropriate form.*

B   3. Knowledge-based resources are available at all times to clinical/service staff, through electronic means, after-hours access to an in-house collection, or other methods.

B   4. The hospital has a plan to provide for access to information during times when electronic systems are unavailable.

Patient-Specific Information

Standard IM.6.10
The hospital has a complete and accurate medical record for every individual assessed, cared for, treated, or served.

Rationale for IM.6.10
Patient-specific data and information are contained in the medical record, both inpatient and outpatient, to facilitate patient care, treatment, and services, serve as a financial and legal record, aid in research, support decision analysis, and guide professional and organization performance improvement. This information may be maintained as a paper record or as electronic health information.†

Elements of Performance for IM.6.10

A   1. Only authorized individuals make entries in the medical record.

A   2. The hospital defines which entries made by nonindependent practitioners require countersigning consistent with law and regulation.

A   3. Standardized formats are used for documenting all care, treatment, and services provided to patients.

---

* Forms of information include current texts; periodicals; indexes; abstracts; reports; documents; databases; directories; discussion lists; successful practices; standards; protocols; practice guidelines; clinical trials; and other resources.

† **Electronic health information** A computerized format of the health care information in paper records that is used for the same range of purposes as paper records, namely to familiarize readers with the patient's status; document care, treatment, and services; plan for discharge; document the need for care, treatment, and services; assess the quality of care, treatment, and services; determine reimbursement rates; justify reimbursement claims; pursue clinical or epidemiological research; and measure outcomes of the care, treatment, and service process.

C Ⓜ 4. Every medical record entry* is dated, the author identified and, when necessary according to law or regulation and hospital policy, is authenticated.

C Ⓜ 5. At a minimum, the following are authenticated either by written signature, electronic signature, or computer key or rubber stamp:†
- The history and physical examination
- Operative report
- Consultations
- Discharge summary

C Ⓜ 6. The medical record contains sufficient information to identify the patient; support the diagnosis/condition; justify the care, treatment, and services; document the course and results of care, treatment, and services; and promote continuity of care among providers.

C Ⓜ 7. A concise discharge summary‡ providing information to other caregivers and facilitating continuity of care includes the following:
- The reason for hospitalization
- Significant findings
- Procedures performed and care, treatment, and services provided
- The patient's condition at discharge
- Information to the patient and family, as appropriate

B 8. The hospital has a policy and procedures on the timely entry of all significant information into the patient's medical record.

A 9. The hospital defines a complete record and the time frame within which the record must be completed.

B 10. The hospital measures medical record delinquency at regular intervals, no less frequently than every three months.

---

* Signatures do not have to be dated if they occur in real time of the entry. For paper-based records, counter-signatures entered for purposes of authentication after transcription or for verbal orders are dated when required by state or federal law and regulations and organization policy. For electronic records, electronic signatures will be date-stamped.

† Authentication can be shown by written signatures or initials, rubber-stamp signatures, or computer key. Authorized users of signature stamps or computer keys sign a statement assuring that they alone will use the stamp or key.

§ Exceptions to the discharge summary: When individuals are seen for minor problems or interventions (as defined by the medical staff), a final progress note may be substituted for the discharge summary. When individuals are transferred to a different level of care within the organization, and the caregivers change, a transfer summary may be substituted for the discharge summary. When the caregivers are the same, a progress note may be used.

Management of Information

B   11. The medical record delinquency rate averaged from the last four quarterly measurements is not greater than 50% of the average monthly discharge (AMD) rate and no quarterly measurement is greater than 50% of the AMD rate.*

Note: The score for this EP will result from the following described conditions:

The medical record delinquency rate averaged from the last four quarterly measurements is the following:
- *Not greater than 50% of the AMD rate and no single quarterly measurement is greater than 50% of the AMD rate the score is **2–Compliance**.*
- *Not greater than 50% of the AMD rate but one or more quarterly measurements are greater than 50% of the AMD rate the score is **1–Partial Compliance**.*
- *Greater than 50% of the AMD rate but less than twice (that is, 200%) of the AMD rate the score is **0–Insufficient Compliance**.*
- *Equal to or greater than twice (that is, 200%) of the AMD rate the score is **0–Insufficient Compliance and a decision of Conditional Accreditation**.*

B   12. Medical records are reviewed on an ongoing basis at the point of care.*

B   13. The review of medical records is based on hospital-defined indicators that address the presence, timeliness, readability (whether handwritten or printed), quality, consistency, clarity, accuracy, completeness, and authentication of data and information contained within the record.*

B   14. The retention time of medical record information is determined by the hospital based on law and regulation, and on its use for patient care, treatment, and services, legal, research, and operational purposes, as well as educational activities.

15. Not applicable

16. Not applicable

A   17. Original medical records are not released unless the hospital is responding appropriately to federal or state laws, court orders, or subpoenas.

C Ⓜ   18. Records of patients who have received emergency care, treatment, and services contain the following information:
- Times and means of arrival
- Whether the patient left against medical advice

---

* Effective January 1, 2005.

† *See* the "Provision of Care, Treatment, and Services" chapter in this book.

- The conclusions at termination of treatment, including final disposition, condition, and instructions for follow-up care, treatment, and services
- A copy of the record that is available to the practitioner or medical organization providing follow-up care, treatment, and services

Standard IM.6.20

Records contain patient-specific information, as appropriate, to the care, treatment, and services provided.

Elements of Performance for IM.6.20

C Ⓜ 1. Each medical record contains, as applicable, the following clinical/case information:
- Emergency care, treatment, and services provided to the patient before his or her arrival, if any
- Documentation and findings of assessments*
- Conclusions or impressions drawn from medical history and physical examination
- The diagnosis, diagnostic impression, or conditions
- The reason(s) for admission or care, treatment, and services
- The goals of the treatment and treatment plan
- Diagnostic and therapeutic orders
- All diagnostic and therapeutic procedures, tests, and results
- Progress notes made by authorized individuals
- All reassessments and plan of care revisions, when indicated
- Relevant observations
- The response to care, treatment, and services provided
- Consultation reports
- Allergies to foods and medicines
- Every medication ordered or prescribed
- Every dose of medication administered, including the strength, dose, or rate of administration, administration devices used, access site or route, known drug allergies, and any adverse drug reaction
- Every medication dispensed or prescribed on discharge
- All relevant diagnoses/conditions established during the course of care, treatment, and services

C Ⓜ 2. Each medical record contains, as applicable, the following demographic information:
- The patient's name, sex, address, date of birth, and authorized representative, if any
- Legal status of patients receiving behavioral health care services

---

* *See* the "Provision of Care, Treatment, and Services" chapter in this book.

Management of Information

C Ⓜ 3. Each medical record contains, as applicable, the following information:
- Evidence of known advance directives
- Evidence of informed consent patient care
- Records of communication with the patient regarding care, treatment, and services, for example, telephone calls or e-mail, if applicable
- Patient-generated information (for example, information entered into the record over the Web or in previsit computer systems), if applicable

Standard IM.6.30*
The medical record thoroughly documents operative or other high risk procedures† and the use of moderate or deep sedation or anesthesia.

Elements of Performance for IM.6.30

C Ⓜ 1. The history and physical examination, the results of any indicated diagnostic tests, as well as a provisional diagnosis are recorded before the operative or other procedures by the licensed independent practitioner responsible for the patient.

C Ⓜ 2. Operative or other high risk procedure reports dictated or written immediately‡ after an operative or other high risk procedure record appropriate information as defined by the medical staff.

C Ⓜ 3. An operative or other high risk procedure progress note is entered in the medical record immediately after the procedure, when the full operative or other high risk procedure report cannot be entered into the record immediately after the operation or procedure.

C Ⓜ 4. The completed operative or other high risk procedure report is authenticated by the surgeon and made available in the medical record as soon as possible after the procedure.

C Ⓜ 5. Postoperative documentation records the patient's vital signs and level of consciousness; medications (including intravenous fluids) and blood and blood components administered, if applicable; and any unusual events or complications, including blood transfusion reactions and the management of those events.

---

* **Note:** Also see *the "Provision of Care, Treatment, and Services" chapter, standards PC.13.30 and PC.13.40.*

† **Operative and other high risk procedures** Procedures including operative, other invasive, and noninvasive procedures that place the patient at risk. The focus is on procedures and therefore is not meant to include use of medications that place patients at risk.

‡ "Immediately after a procedure" is defined as "upon completion of the operation or procedure, before the patient is transferred to the next level of care." This is to ensure that pertinent information is available to the next caregiver. In addition, if the surgeon accompanies the patient from the operating room to the next unit or area of care, the operative note or progress note can be written in that unit or area of care.

C Ⓜ 6. Postoperative documentation records the patient's discharge from the postsedation or postanesthesia care area by the responsible licensed independent practitioner or according to discharge criteria.

C Ⓜ 7. The use of approved discharge criteria to determine the patient's readiness for discharge is documented in the medical record.

C Ⓜ 8. Postoperative documentation records the name of the licensed independent practitioner responsible for discharge.

Standard IM.6.40

For patients receiving continuing ambulatory care services, the medical record contains a summary list of all significant diagnoses, procedures, drug allergies, and medications.

Rationale for IM.6.40

Summary lists facilitate continuity of care over time for a single provider or among several providers.

Elements of Performance for IM.6.40

Ⓜ 1. The list is initiated for each patient by the third visit and maintained thereafter.

Ⓜ 2. The list is always stored in the same location to help practitioners access needed information quickly and easily.

Ⓜ 3. The list contains the following information:
- Known* significant medical diagnoses and conditions
- Known significant operative and invasive procedures
- Known adverse and allergic drug reactions
- Known long-term medications, including current prescriptions, over-the-counter drugs, and herbal preparations

Standard IM.6.50

Designated qualified personnel accept and transcribe verbal orders from authorized individuals.

Rationale for IM.6.50

Processes for receiving, transcribing, and authenticating verbal orders are established to protect the quality of patient care, treatment and services.

---

* "Known" refers to information gathered during ambulatory care assessment and treatment.

Management of Information

Elements of Performance for IM.6.50

A 1. Qualified personnel are identified, as defined by hospital policy and, as appropriate, in accordance with state and federal law, and authorized to receive and record verbal orders.

C Ⓜ 2. Each verbal order is dated and identifies the names of the individuals who gave and received it, and the record indicates who implemented it.

A 3. When required by state or federal law and regulation, verbal orders are authenticated within the specified time frame.

A 4. Implement a process for taking verbal or telephone orders or receiving critical test results that require a verification "read-back" of the complete order or test result by the person receiving the order or test result.

Standard IM.6.60

The hospital can provide access to all relevant information from a patient's record when needed for use in patient care, treatment, and services.

Rationale for IM.6.60

To facilitate continuity of care, providers have access to information about all previous care, treatment, and services provided to a patient by the hospital.

Elements of Performance for IM.6.60

B 1. There is a manual or automated mechanism to track the location of all components of the medical record.

B 2. The hospital uses a system to assemble required information or make available a summary of information relative for patient care, treatment, and services when the patient is seen.

Medical Staff

Overview

The organized medical staff has a critical role in the process of providing oversight of quality of care, treatment, and services. The organized medical staff is a self-governing body that is charged with overseeing the quality of care, treatment, and services delivered by practitioners who are credentialed and privileged through the medical staff process. The organized medical staff must credential and privilege all licensed independent practitioners. Physician assistants (PAs) and advanced practiced registered nurses (APRNs) who are not licensed independent practitioners may be privileged through the medical staff process or a process that has been developed and approved by the hospital that is equivalent to the process and criteria set forth in the credentialing and privileging standards contained in this chapter. When medical staff processes are not used, there are mechanisms to assure communication with and input from the Medical Staff Executive Committee regarding those privileges.

The self-governing, organized medical staff must create and maintain a set of bylaws that defines its role within the context of a hospital setting and clearly delineates its responsibilities in the oversight of care, treatment, and services. The medical staff bylaws, rules, and regulations create a framework within which medical staff members can act with a reasonable degree of freedom and confidence. The organized medical staff also provides leadership in performance improvement activities within the organization. The tasks of the medical staff are numerous and require a dedicated and organized leadership to adequately perform their duties. Evaluating the competency of privileged practitioners and delineating the scope of privileges of privileged practitioners are key areas of responsibility for the organized medical staff.

The hospital's governing body has the ultimate authority and responsibility for the oversight and delivery of health care rendered by licensed independent practitioners, and other practitioners credentialed and privileged through the medical staff process or any equivalent process. The governing body and the medical staff define medical staff membership criteria that must include licensed independent practitioners but may include other practitioners as deemed necessary by the governing body and the medical staff. The Joint Commission does not dictate who is eligible for medical staff membership at accredited hospitals. Membership on the medical staff is not synonymous with privileges. The medical staff may create categories of membership, as in active member, courtesy member, and so forth. These categories may be helpful in defining the roles and expectations for the various members of the medical staff.

The Joint Commission does not determine if a practitioner is a licensed independent practitioner. State law and hospital policy determine whether a practitioner can practice independently. The Joint Commission defines a licensed independent practitioner as "any individual permitted by law and by the organization to provide care, treatment, and services, without direction or supervision."

Practitioners who are responsible for the oversight of health care delivered by all medical staff practitioners must be licensed independent practitioners. The organized medical staff develops and uses criteria to determine which licensed independent practitioners are eligible to participate in the oversight process.

Standards

The following is a list of all standards for this function. They are presented here for your convenience without footnotes or other explanatory text. If you have a question about a term used here, please check the Glossary.

Note: *A revised standard numbering system is being used with the reformatted standards. This revised numbering system will allow for more flexibility to add standards while maintaining the current number for each standard.*

The Organized Medical Staff
Organized Medical Staff Structure

MS.1.10 The hospital has an organized, self-governing medical staff that provides oversight of care, treatment, and services provided by practitioners with privileges, provides for a uniform quality of patient care, treatment, and services, and reports to and is accountable to the governing body.

MS.1.20 Medical staff bylaws address self governance and accountability to the governing body.

MS.1.30 Neither the organized medical staff nor the governing body may unilaterally amend the medical staff bylaws or rules and regulations.

MS.1.40 There is a medical staff executive committee.

Management of Patient Care, Treatment, and Services

MS.2.10 The organized medical staff oversees the quality of patient care, treatment, and services provided by practitioners privileged through the medical staff process.

MS.2.20 The management and coordination of each patient's care, treatment, and services is the responsibility of a practitioner with appropriate privileges.

MS.2.30 In hospitals participating in a professional graduate education program(s), the organized medical staff has a defined process for supervision by a licensed independent practitioner with appropriate clinical privileges of each member in the program in carrying out his or her patient care responsibilities.

Performance Improvement

MS.3.10 The organized medical staff has a leadership role in hospital performance improvement activities to improve quality of care, treatment, and services and patient safety.

MS.3.20 The organized medical staff participates in the measurement, assessment, and improvement of other processes.

Credentialing, Privileging, and Appointment

MS.4.10 The organized medical staff has a credentialing process that is defined in the medical staff bylaws.

MS.4.20 There is a process for granting, renewing, or revising setting-specific clinical privileges.

MS.4.30 An organized medical staff may use an expedited process for appointing to the medical staff and when granting privileges when criteria for that process are met.

MS.4.40 At the time of renewal of privileges, the organized medical staff evaluates individuals for their continued ability to provide quality care, treatment, and services for the privileges requested as defined in the medical staff bylaws.

MS.4.50 There are mechanisms including a fair hearing and appeal process for addressing adverse decisions regarding reappointment, denial, reduction, suspension, or revocation of privileges that may relate to quality of care, treatment, and services issues.

MS.4.60 The organized medical staff provides oversight for the quality of care, treatment, and services by recommending members for appointment to the medical staff.

MS.4.70 Peer recommendations from peers in the same professional discipline as the applicant are used as part of the basis for the initial granting of privileges. Peer recommendations are used to recommend individuals for the renewal of clinical privileges when insufficient practitioner-specific data are available.

MS.4.80 The medical staff implements a process to identify and manage matters of individual health for licensed independent practitioners. This identification process is separate from actions taken for disciplinary purposes.

MS.4.90 There is a process that defines circumstances requiring a focused review of a practitioner's performance and evaluation of a practitioner's performance by peers.

Medical Staff

MS.4.100 Under certain circumstances, temporary clinical privileges may be granted for a limited period of time.

MS.4.110 Disaster privileges may be granted when the emergency management plan has been activated and the hospital is unable to handle the immediate patient needs (*see* standard EC.4.10).

MS.4.120 Licensed independent practitioners who are responsible for the care, treatment, and services of the patient via telemedicine link are subject to the credentialing and privileging processes of the originating site.

MS.4.130 The medical staffs at both the originating and distant sites recommend the clinical services to be provided by licensed independent practitioners through a telemedical link at their respective sites.

Continuing Education

MS.5.10 All licensed independent practitioners and other practitioners privileged through the medical staff process participate in continuing education.

Understanding the Parts of This Chapter

To help you navigate this reformatted standards chapter, it may be helpful to think of its parts this way:
- The **standard** is the "goal."
- The **rationale** explains why it's important to achieve this goal.
- The **elements of performance** identify the step(s) needed to achieve this goal.

These parts are defined as follows.

Standard A statement that defines the performance expectations and/or structures or processes that must be in place in order for a hospital to provide safe, high-quality care, treatment, and services. A hospital is either "compliant" or "not compliant" with a standard.

Accreditation decisions are based on simple counts of the standards that are determined to be "not compliant."

Rationale A statement that provides background, justification, or additional information about a standard. A standard's rationale is not scored. In some instances, the rationale for a standard is self-evident. Therefore, not every standard has a written rationale.

Elements of performance (EPs) The specific performance expectations and/or structures or processes that must be in place in order for a hospital to provide safe, high-quality care, treatment, and services. The scoring of EP compliance determines a hospital's overall compliance with a standard. EPs are evaluated on the following scale:

> 0 Insufficient compliance
> 1 Partial compliance
> 2 Satisfactory compliance
> NA Not applicable

You will find a **measure of success** icon—Ⓜ—next to some EPs. Measures of success (MOS) need to be developed for certain EPs when a standard is judged to be out of compliance through either the Periodic Performance Review (PPR) or the onsite survey. An MOS is defined as a quantifiable measure, usually related to an audit, that can be used to determine whether an action has been effective and is being sustained.*

Assessing Your Compliance

Once you are familiar with the parts of this chapter, you can begin to assess your compliance with its requirements. The scoring category for each EP is noted next to the EP. If you would like to assess your hospital's performance, mark your scores for the EPs and the standards by following the simple steps described below.

---

* For more information about measures of success, *see* the "The New Joint Commission Accreditation Process" chapter in this book.

Medical Staff

Two components are scored for each EP: (1) compliance with the requirement itself **and** (2) compliance with the track record* for that requirement. Scoring has been simplified, and track record achievements (which have always been part of the scoring) have been appropriately modified.

Note: *Some standards and EPs do not apply to a particular type of organization; these standards and EPs are marked "not applicable" and the related text is not included. Your hospital is not expected to comply with standards and EPs marked "not applicable."*

In addition, some standards and EPs that do apply to organizations may not apply to the specific care, treatment, and services that your individual hospital provides. Although these standards and EPs are included in the manual, you are not expected to comply with them. If you are unsure about the standards or EPs that apply to your hospital, please contact the Joint Commission's Standards Interpretation Group at 630/792-5900.

Step 1: Score Your Compliance with Each Element of Performance

Before you can determine your compliance with the standards, you must score your compliance with each EP. There are three scoring criterion categories: A, B, and C (described below). Please note that for each EP scoring criterion category, your hospital must meet the performance requirement itself and the track record achievements (*see* "Track Record Achievements").

Category A

These EPs relate to the presence or absence of the requirement(s) and are scored either yes (2) or no (0); however, score 1 for partial compliance is also possible based on track record achievements.

If an A EP has multiple components designated by bullets, your hospital must be compliant with all the bullets to receive a score of 2. If your hospital does not meet one or more requirements in the bullets, you will receive a score of 0.

Category B

Category B EPs are scored in two steps:
1. As with category A EPs, category B EPs relate to the presence or absence of the requirement(s). If your hospital *does not meet* the requirement(s), the EP is scored 0; there is no need to assess your compliance with the principles of good process design.
2. If your hospital *does meet* the requirement(s), but there is concern about the quality or comprehensiveness of the effort, then and only then should you assess the qualitative aspect of the EP. That is, review the applicable principles of good process design and ask how the principles were applied in the situation under discussion. Good process design has the following characteristics:

---

* **Track record** The amount of time that an organization has been in compliance with a standard, element of performance, or other requirement.

MS – 7

- Is consistent with your hospital's mission, values, and goals
- Meets the needs of patients
- Reflects the use of currently accepted practices (doing the right thing, using resources responsibly, using practice guidelines)
- Incorporates current safety information and knowledge such as sentinel event data and National Patient Safety Goals
- Incorporates relevant performance improvement results

This two-part evaluation applies to both simple and bulleted B EPs. First, the EPs are assessed to determine if the requirements are present. If the EP has multiple components designated by bullets, as with the category A EPs, your hospital must meet the requirements in *all* the bulleted items to get a score of 2. If your hospital meets *none* of the requirements in the bullets, it receives a score of 0. If your hospital meets *at least one, but not all*, of the bulleted requirements, it will receive a score of 1 for the EPs.

Use the following rules to determine your EP score:
- Your EP score is 0 if your hospital does not meet the requirement(s); you *do not* need to assess your compliance with the preceding applicable principles of good process design
- Your EP score is 1 if your hospital does meet the requirement(s), but considered only *some* of the preceding applicable principles of good process design
- Your EP score is 2 if your hospital does meet the requirement(s) *and* considered *all* the preceding principles of good process design

Category C

C EPs are scored 0, 1, or 2 based on the number of times your hospital does not meet the EP. These EPs are frequency based and require totaling the number of occurrences (that is, results of performance or nonperformance) related to a particular EP. Each situation discovered by a surveyor(s) will be counted as a separate occurrence.

Note: *Multiple events of the same type related to a single patient and single practitioner/staff member are counted as* one occurrence only.

Use the following rules to determine your EP score:
- Your EP score is 2 if you find one or fewer occurrences of noncompliance with the EP
- Your EP score is 1 if you find two occurrences of noncompliance with the EP
- Your EP score is 0 if you find three or more occurrences of noncompliance with the EP

If an EP in the C category has multiple requirements designated by bullets, the following scoring guidelines apply:
- If there are fewer than 2 findings in all bullets, the EP is scored 2
- If there are three or more findings in all bullets, the EP is scored 0
- In all other combinations of findings, the EP is scored 1

Track Record Achievements

In addition to meeting the requirement(s) in each EP, regardless of category, your hospital must also meet the following track record achievements:

Score	Initial Survey	Full Survey
2	4 months or more	12 months or more
1	2 to 3 months	6 to 11 months
0	Fewer than 2 months	Fewer than 6 months

Sample Sizes

If during an onsite survey, your hospital has been found to be not compliant with one or more standards, you must demonstrate Evidence of Standards Compliance (ESC) for each standard that is not compliant. The ESC must address compliance at the EP level; when an EP within a noncompliant standard requires an MOS, your hospital must demonstrate achievement with the MOS when completing the ESC.

Note: *Not every EP requires an MOS. EPs that do require an MOS are clearly marked in this chapter. Organizations are required to demonstrate achievement with an MOS only for EPs within a noncompliant standard that require an MOS. Organizations do not need to demonstrate achievement with an MOS for any EP within a compliant standard.*

When demonstrating achievement with the MOS during the ESC process, your hospital is **required** to use the following sample sizes, which were established because of their statistical significance, their relative simplicity in application, and their sensitivity to an organization's population size:
- For a population size of fewer than 30 cases, sample 100% of available cases
- For a population size of 30 to 100 cases, sample 30 cases
- For a population size of 101 to 500 cases, sample 50 cases
- For a population size greater than 500 cases, sample 70 cases

Note: *Hospitals are encouraged, but not required, to follow this sample size when demonstrating achievement with an MOS for an EP within a noncompliant standard after conducting a full, Option 1, or Option 2 Periodic Performance Review (PPR).*

When conducting PPR (optional use) or demonstrating an ESC (mandatory use), use the following percentages to determine your score: 90% through 100% of your sample size is in compliance = score 2; 80% through 89% (two instances of noncompliance) of your sample size is in compliance = score 1; less than 80% (three or more instances of noncompliance) of your sample size is in compliance = score 0.

In addition, the following information should govern your hospital's selection of samples:
- The appropriate sample size should be determined by the specific population related to the survey findings
- The sampling approach should involve either systematic random sampling (for example, your hospital selects every second or third case for review) or simple random sampling (for example, your hospital uses a series of random numbers generated by a computer to identify the cases to be reviewed)

- If your hospital chooses not to use these sample sizes while conducting PPR options 1 or 2, you should make sure that your sample size is sufficiently large enough to ensure statistical significance
- When submitting a clarifying ESC, if your hospital selects records as part of its sample, the records should be from a period of no more than three months before the last date of the survey
- Assessment of MOS compliance is conducted for a four-month period following the date of ESC approval. Your hospital should select records as a part of your sample following the date of ESC approval and use the required sample sizes. MOS percentage compliance rates are derived from the average of all four months.

Step 2: Use Your EP Scores to Gauge Your Compliance with the Standards

Now that you have evaluated and scored each EP for a particular standard, use these simple rules to determine your compliance with the standard itself:
- Your hospital is not in compliance (that is, "not compliant") with the standard if any EP is scored 0
- Otherwise, your hospital is in compliance with a standard if 65% or more of its EPs are scored 2

Standards, Rationales, Elements of Performance, and Scoring

Organized Medical Staff* Structure

The organized medical staff is structured such that it has the ability to function in guiding and governing its members. The primary function of the organized medical staff is to provide oversight for the quality of care, treatment, and services provided by practitioners with privileges.

The organized medical staff must be structured using the following guiding principles:
- Designated members of the organized medical staff who have independent privileges provide oversight of care, treatment, and services provided by practitioners with privileges
- The organized medical staff is responsible for structuring itself to provide a uniform standard of quality patient care, treatment, and services
- The organized medical staff is accountable to the governing body

Self governance of the organized medical staff includes the following and is located in the medical staff's bylaws:
- Initiating, developing, and approving medical staff bylaws and rules and regulations
- Approving or disapproving amendments to the medical staff bylaws and rules and regulations
- Selecting and removing medical staff officers
- Determining the mechanism for establishing and enforcing criteria and standards for medical staff membership
- Determining the mechanism for establishing and enforcing criteria for delegating oversight responsibilities to practitioners with independent privileges
- Determining the mechanism for establishing and maintaining patient care standards and credentialing and delineation of clinical privileges
- Engaging in performance improvement activities

An organized medical staff is self governing and has the responsibility to oversee care, treatment, and services provided by practitioners with privileges. Oversight of care, treatment, and services is provided by a variety of mechanisms, one of which is the development of bylaws that govern the actions of the medical staff. The governing body must approve the medical staff bylaws.

Under most circumstances, the organized medical staff should be a single, organized medical staff. There may be exceptions to the general requirement for a single medical staff (*see* note below regarding requirements for exception.) When

---

* The term *medical staff* takes on various meanings within different organizations. The standards and elements of performance in this chapter are intended to apply to all practitioners privileged through the medical staff process.

more than one organized medical staff exists, it is incumbent upon the medical staffs to have a mechanism to ensure that the same principles that guide a single medical staff are fully integrated into any multiple medical staff structure.

Note: *The following bases are used in determining whether a hospital may have more than one organized medical staff:**
- *A hospital with a single governing body that has multiple inpatient care sites, each of which serves two or more geographically distinct patient populations, may have a separate organized medical staff at each site.*
- *The patient population consists of those individuals who chose the hospital as their primary source of inpatient care, treatment, and services and for whom the hospital designs and delivers services consistent with its mission.*

Standard MS.1.10

The hospital has an organized, self-governing medical staff that provides oversight of care, treatment, and services provided by practitioners with privileges, provides for a uniform quality of patient care, treatment, and services, and reports to and is accountable to the governing body.

Elements of Performance for MS.1.10

A   1. The organized medical staff is self governing, as referenced in the bullets defining self-governance on page MS-11.

A   2. There is a single, organized medical staff, unless the requirements for an exception to the single medical staff rule exist.

A   3. When more than one medical staff exists, the guiding principles for medical staffs are addressed by the structure of the multiple medical staffs.

B   4. The organized medical staff provides a mechanism to ensure a uniform standard of quality patient care, treatment, and services.

A   5. The organized medical staff is accountable to the governing body for the quality of the medical care, treatment, and services provided to patients.

A   6. The medical staff is organized in a manner approved by the governing body.

Standard MS.1.20

Medical staff bylaws address self governance and accountability to the governing body.

---

* Please note that the Medicare Conditions of Participation address requirements related to a single medical staff.

Medical Staff

Rationale for MS.1.20
The organized medical staff and governing body must work collaboratively, reflecting clearly recognized roles, responsibilities, and accountabilities, to enhance the quality and safety of care, treatment, and services provided to patients. The organized medical staff creates a written set of documents that describes the organizational structure of the medical staff and the rules for self governance. These documents are called medical staff bylaws. The medical staff bylaws create a system of rights and responsibilities between the organized medical staff and the governing body, and between the organized medical staff and its members. As required by and pursuant to the medical staff bylaws, the organized medical staff may create additional governance documents such as policies, procedures, protocols, rules, and regulations, but the requirements listed below must be retained in the medical staff bylaws.

Elements of Performance for MS.1.20

A 1. The medical staff develops medical staff bylaws.

A 2. The medical staff bylaws define the medical staff structure.

A 3. The medical staff bylaws define the criteria and qualifications for appointment to the medical staff.

A 4. The medical staff bylaws are adopted and amended by the medical staff.

A 5. The governing body approves and complies with the medical staff bylaws.

B 6. The organized medical staff enforces and complies with the medical staff bylaws.

A 7. The medical staff bylaws, rules and regulations, and policies and the governing body bylaws do not conflict.

B 8. When medical departments exist, the qualifications and roles and responsibilities of the medical department chair are defined in the medical staff bylaws and include the following:

   Qualifications
   - Certification by an appropriate specialty board or affirmatively established comparable competence through the credentialing process

   Roles and Responsibilities
   - Clinically related activities of the department
   - Administratively related activities of the department, unless otherwise provided by the hospital
   - Continuing surveillance of the professional performance of all individuals in the department who have delineated clinical privileges
   - Recommending to the medical staff the criteria for clinical privileges that are relevant to the care provided in the department

- Recommending clinical privileges for each member of the department
- Assessing and recommending to the relevant hospital authority off-site sources for needed patient care, treatment, and services not provided by the department or the organization
- The integration of the department or service into the primary functions of the organization
- The coordination and integration of interdepartmental and intradepartmental services
- The development and implementation of policies and procedures that guide and support the provision of care, treatment, and services
- The recommendations for a sufficient number of qualified and competent persons to provide care, treatment, and service
- The determination of the qualifications and competence of department or service personnel who are not licensed independent practitioners and who provide patient care, treatment, and services
- The continuous assessment and improvement of the quality of care, treatment, and services
- The maintenance of quality control programs, as appropriate
- The orientation and continuing education of all persons in the department or service
- Recommendations for space and other resources needed by the department or service

The medical staff bylaws must also include the following:

Medical Staff Executive Committee

A   9. The medical staff executive committee includes physicians and may include other licensed independent practitioners

B   10. The medical staff bylaws include a description of the executive committee's function, size, composition, and method of selecting and removing officers

B   11. The medical staff bylaws empower the medical staff executive committee to act for the organized medical staff between meetings of the organized medical staff

Corrective Actions

B   12. A description of indications and procedures for automatic suspension of a practitioner's medical staff membership or clinical privileges

B   13. A description of indications and procedures for summary suspension of a practitioner's medical staff membership or clinical privileges

B   14. A description of when automatic suspension procedures are indicated and implemented

B   15. A description of when summary suspension procedures are indicated and implemented

B 16. A description of the mechanism to recommend medical staff membership and/or terminations, suspensions, or reduction in privileges

Fair Hearing
B 17. A mechanism for a fair hearing and appeal procedure is defined in the medical staff bylaws

Credentialing, Privileging, and Appointment
B 18. A description of the credentialing process

B 19. A description of the privileging process (including temporary and disaster privileging)

B 20. A description of the process of appointment to membership of the medical staff

Standard MS.1.30
Neither the organized medical staff nor the governing body may unilaterally amend the medical staff bylaws or rules and regulations.

Rationale for MS.1.30
A hospital with an organized medical staff and governing body that cannot agree on amendments to critical documents has evidenced a breakdown in the required collaborative relationship.

Element of Performance for MS.1.30
A 1. The medical staff bylaws, rules, and regulations are not unilaterally amended.

Medical Staff Executive Committee

Standard MS.1.40
There is a medical staff executive committee.*

Rationale for MS.1.40
The organized medical staff delegates authority to the medical staff executive committee to carry out medical staff responsibilities. The medical staff executive committee carries out its work within the context of the hospital functions of governance, leadership, and performance improvement. The medical staff executive committee has the primary authority for activities related to self governance of the medical staff and for

---

* The medical staff as a whole may serve as the executive committee. In smaller, less complex hospitals where the entire medical staff functions as the executive committee, it is often designated as a committee of the whole.

performance improvement of the professional services provided by licensed independent practitioners and other practitioners privileged through the medical staff process.

Elements of Performance for MS.1.40

A   1. The structure and function of the medical staff executive committee conforms to the medical staff bylaws.

A   2. The chief executive officer (CEO) of the hospital or his or her designee attends each executive committee meeting on an ex-officio basis, with or without a vote.

A   3. All members of the organized medical staff, of any discipline or specialty, are eligible for membership on the executive committee.

A   4. The majority of voting medical staff executive committee members are fully licensed physicians actively practicing in the hospital.

C Ⓜ   5. The medical staff executive committee acts on behalf of the organized medical staff between medical staff meetings.

B   6. The medical staff executive committee has a mechanism to recommend medical staff membership termination.

B   7. The medical staff executive committee requests evaluations of practitioners privileged through the medical staff process in instances where there is doubt about an applicant's ability to perform the privileges requested.

The medical staff executive committee makes recommendations, as defined in the medical staff bylaws, directly to the governing body on at least the following:

A   8. The organized medical staff's structure

B   9. The process used to review credentials and delineate privileges

A   10. The delineation of privileges for each practitioner privileged through the medical staff process

A   11. Medical staff membership

B   12. The executive committee reviews and acts on reports of medical staff committees, departments, and other assigned activity groups

Management of Patient Care, Treatment, and Services

Caring for patients is the nucleus of activity around which all health care organization functions revolve. The organized medical staff is intricately involved in carrying out, and in providing leadership in, all patient care functions conducted by practitioners privileged through the medical staff process.

Medical Staff

Standard MS.2.10
The organized medical staff oversees the quality of patient care, treatment, and services provided by practitioners privileged through the medical staff process.

Rationale for MS.2.10
The organized medical staff is responsible for establishing and maintaining patient care standards and oversight of the quality of care, treatment, and services rendered by practitioners privileged through the medical staff process. The organized medical staff designates member licensed independent practitioners to provide oversight of care, treatment, and services rendered by practitioners privileged through the medical staff process. The organized medical staff recommends practitioners for privileges to perform medical histories and physical examinations; the governing body approves such privileges. Licensed independent practitioners (that is, physicians, oral and maxillofacial surgeons, dentists, podiatrists and some APRNs), physician assistants, and some APRNs may perform medical histories and physical examinations if permitted by law, the medical staff bylaws, and the hospital to do so.

Elements of Performance for MS.2.10
Oversight Domains

B   1. Licensed independent practitioner members of the organized medical staff are designated to perform the oversight activities of the organized medical staff.

B   2. The organized medical staff has a mechanism to ensure that patients receive appropriate care, treatment, and services from a licensed independent practitioner who has been credentialed through the medical staff process during the entire length of stay with the organization.

B   3. Licensed independent practitioners are responsible for the oversight activities of the organized medical staff.

B   4. The organized medical staff, through its designated mechanisms, provides leadership in activities related to patient safety.

B   5. The organized medical staff provides oversight in the process of analyzing and improving patient satisfaction.

Medical History and Physical Examinations

A   6. The organized medical staff specifies the minimal content of medical histories and physical examinations, which may vary by setting or level of care, treatment, and services.

B   7. The organized medical staff monitors the quality of medical histories and physical examinations.

A   8. The organized medical staff requires that a practitioner who has been granted privileges by the hospital to do so performs a patient's medical history and physical examination.

A 9. As permitted by state law and policy, the organized medical staff may choose to allow individuals who are not licensed independent practitioners to perform part or all of a patient's medical history and physical examination under the supervision of, or through appropriate delegation by, a specific qualified physician who is accountable for the patient's medical history and physical examination.

A 10. The organized medical staff defines when a medical history and physical examination must be validated and countersigned by a licensed independent practitioner with appropriate privileges.

A 11. The organized medical staff defines the scope of the medical history and physical examination when required for non-inpatient services.

Standard MS.2.20

The management and coordination of each patient's care, treatment, and services is the responsibility of a practitioner with appropriate privileges.

Rationale for MS.2.20

Quality of care, treatment, and services is dependent upon coordination and communication of the plan of care and is given to all relevant health care providers to optimize resources and provide for patient safety. Practitioners have privileges that correspond to the care, treatment, and services needed by individual patients. Such privileges are specific to each patient's needs and therefore are "appropriate" for that particular patient. Communication and coordination is key to the safe management of patient care, treatment, and services. Communication among all practitioners and staff involved in a patient's care, treatment, and services is vital to ensuring coordinated, high-quality care.

Elements of Performance for MS.2.20

A 1. A patient's general medical condition is managed and coordinated by a physician.

C 2. There is communication among all practitioners involved in a patient's care, treatment, and services.

B 3. Licensed independent practitioners with appropriate privileges manage and coordinate a patient's care, treatment, and services.

A 4. The organized medical staff, through its designated mechanism, determines the circumstances under which consultation or management by a physician or other licensed independent practitioner is required and consultation is obtained as required.

Medical Staff

Graduate Education Programs

Standard MS.2.30
In hospitals participating in a professional graduate education program(s), the organized medical staff has a defined process for supervision by a licensed independent practitioner with appropriate clinical privileges of each member in the program in carrying out his or her patient care responsibilities.

Rationale for MS.2.30
This standard applies to participants registered in a professional graduate education program when the graduate practitioner will be a licensed independent practitioner. The management of each patient's care, treatment, and services (including patients under the care of participants in professional graduate education programs) is the responsibility of a licensed independent practitioner with appropriate clinical privileges.

Elements of Performance for MS.2.30

B 1. The organized medical staff has a defined process for supervision by a licensed independent practitioner with appropriate clinical privileges of each participant in the program in carrying out patient care responsibilities.

A 2. Written descriptions of the roles, responsibilities, and patient care activities of the participants of graduate educational programs are provided to the organized medical staff and hospital staff.

A 3. The descriptions include identification of mechanisms by which the supervisor(s) and graduate education program director make decisions about each participant's progressive involvement and independence in specific patient care activities.

B 4. Organized medical staff rules and regulations and policies delineate participants in professional education programs who may write patient care orders, the circumstances under which they may do so (without prohibiting licensed independent practitioners from writing orders), and what entries, if any, must be countersigned by a supervising licensed independent practitioner.

B 5. There is a mechanism for effective communication between the committee(s) responsible for professional graduate education and the organized medical staff and the governing body.

B 6. There is responsibility for effective communication (whether training occurs at the organization that is responsible for the professional graduate education program or in a participating local or community organization or hospital).
   - The professional graduate medical education committee(s) (GMEC)* must communicate with the medical staff and governing

2005 Hospital Accreditation Standards

body about the safety and quality of patient care, treatment, and services provided by, and the related educational and supervisory needs of, the participants in professional graduate education programs.
- If the graduate medical education program uses a community or local participating hospital or organization, the person(s) responsible for overseeing the participants from the program communicates to the organized medical staff and its governing body about the patient care, treatment, and services provided by, and the related educational and supervisory needs of, its participants in the professional graduate education programs.

B   7. There is a mechanism for an appropriate person from the community or local hospital or organization to communicate information to the GMEC about the quality of care, treatment, and services and educational needs of the participants.

A   8. Information about the quality of care, treatment, and services and educational needs is included in the communication that the GMEC has with the governing board of the sponsoring organization.

C Ⓜ   9. Medical staff demonstrates compliance with residency review committee citations.

Note: *Graduate medical education programs accredited by the Accreditation Counsel on Graduate Medical Education (ACGME), the American Osteopathic Association (AOA), or the American Dental Association's Commission on Dental Accreditation are expected to be in compliance with the above requirements; the hospital should be able to demonstrate compliance with any residency review committee citations related to this standard.*

Performance Improvement

Standard MS.3.10
The organized medical staff has a leadership role in hospital performance improvement activities to improve quality of care, treatment, and services and patient safety.

Rationale for MS.3.10
Relevant information developed from the following processes is integrated into performance improvement initiatives and consistent with hospital preservation of confidentiality and privilege of information.

Medical Staff

Elements of Performance for MS.3.10

B 1. The organized medical staff provides leadership for measuring, assessing, and improving processes that primarily depend on the activities of one or more licensed independent practitioners, and other practitioners credentialed and privileged through the medical staff process.

The medical staff is actually involved in the following processes:

B 2. Medical assessment and treatment of patients

B 3. Use of information about adverse privileging decisions for any practitioner privileged through the medical staff process

B 4. Use of medications (standard PI.1.10)

B 5. Use of blood and blood components (standard PI.1.10)

B 6. Operative and other procedure(s) (standard PI.1.10)

B 7. Appropriateness of clinical practice patterns

B 8. Significant departures from established patterns of clinical practice

B 9. The use of developed criteria for autopsies (standard PI.1.10)

Information used as part of the performance improvement mechanisms, measurement, or assessment includes the following:

B 10. Sentinel event data

B 11. Patient safety data (standard LD.4.40)

Standard MS.3.20

The organized medical staff participates in the measurement, assessment, and improvement of other processes.

Elements of Performance for MS.3.20

The organized medical staff participates in the following activities when the hospital is engaged in any of these activities:

B 1. Education of patients and families

B 2. Coordination of care, treatment, and services with other practitioners and hospital personnel, as relevant to the care, treatment, and services of an individual patient

B 3. Accurate, timely, and legible completion of patient's medical records (standard IM.6.10)

B 4. Findings of the assessment process that are relevant to an individual's performance. The organized medical staff is responsible for determining the use of this information in the ongoing evaluations of a practitioner's competence.

B   5. Communication of findings, conclusions, recommendations, and actions to improve performance to appropriate staff members and the governing body

Credentialing, Privileging, and Appointment

The credentialing process includes a series of activities designed to collect relevant data that serve as the basis for decisions regarding appointment to membership on the medical staff, as well as privileges recommended and delineation of privileges recommended by the organized medical staff. Credentialing is the first step in the process that leads to privileging and that may lead to appointment to membership on the medical staff, if requested by the applicant.

The typical credentialing process includes processing applications, verifying credentials, evaluating applicant-specific information, and making recommendations to the governing body for appointment and privileges. The required information should include data on qualifications, such as licensure and training or experience.

Although much of the specific information used to make decisions about privileges and appointment to membership is at the discretion of the organized medical staff, the range of information used should be explicit. The governance documents specify professional criteria for medical staff membership and clinical privileges. These criteria are designed to help establish an applicant's background, current competence, and physical and mental ability to discharge patient care responsibilities. Moreover, they are designed to help assure the medical staff and governing body that patients will receive quality care, treatment, and services.

The organized medical staff is also responsible for planning and implementing a privileging process. At the organization's discretion, the criteria for granting initial privileges and renewing privileges may differ. The privileging process typically entails developing and approving a procedures list, processing the application, evaluating applicant-specific information and making recommendations to the governing body for applicant-specific delineated privileges, notifying the applicant and relevant personnel, and monitoring the use of privileges and quality of care issues. The required information should include data on the individual practitioner's performance that are collected and assessed on an ongoing basis.

Appointment refers to the process whereby an individual is selected as a member of the organized medical staff. The processes for credentialing for appointment to membership of the medical staff and delineating privileges are essentially identical. The organized medical staff defines the criteria for categories of medical staff membership. The categories and criteria include a category of membership that is responsible for the oversight of care, treatment, and services and requires the members in that category to have the requisite skills for oversight. Applicants for membership may receive appointment to membership without receiving privileges; applicants for privileges need not necessarily be members of the medical staff.

Credentialing Applications

Standard MS.4.10
The organized medical staff has a credentialing process that is defined in the medical staff bylaws.

Rationale for MS.4.10
Credentials review is the process of obtaining, verifying, and assessing the qualifications of an applicant to provide patient care, treatment, and services in or for a health care organization. The credentials review process is the basis for making appointments to membership of the medical staff; it also provides information for granting clinical privileges to licensed independent practitioners and other practitioners credentialed and privileged through the hospital's medical staff process. The purpose of verifying credentials data is to ensure the following:
- The individual requesting privileges is in fact the same individual that is identified in the credentialing documents
- The applicant has attained the credentials as stated
- The credentials are current
- There are no challenges to any of the credentials

Note: *Acceptable documentation for credentialing criteria includes the following:*
- ***Current licensure.*** *The medical staff verifies and documents current licensure for all practitioners. Licensure is verified with the primary source at the time of appointment to membership and initial granting of clinical privileges, reappointment, and at renewal of clinical privileges by a letter or secure electronic communication obtained from the appropriate state licensing board or from any state licensing board if in a federal service. Verification of current licensure through the primary source via a secure electronic communication or by telephone is acceptable, if this verification is documented. Physician assistants in federal service use criteria established by federal standards.*
- ***Relevant training or experience.*** *At the time of appointment to membership and initial granting of clinical privileges, the hospital obtains verification of relevant training or experience from the primary source(s), whenever feasible. The primary source is the original source of the specific credential that can be used to verify the accuracy of a credential reported by the practitioner. Primary sources include, for example, the specialty certifying boards approved by the American Dental Association for a dentist's board certification, and letters from professional schools (for example, medical, dental and podiatric) and from residency or postdoctoral programs for completion of training. Information from credentials verification organizations (CVOs) may be used. Verification of relevant training and experience may be obtained by contacting the primary source via a secure electronic communication or telephone, if this verification is documented. Relevant training or experience is defined by the specific circumstances of the applicant, requiring that the hospital believes there is sufficient information on which to base a reasoned decision. Relevant training and experience may vary among specialties.*

- **Current competence.** Current competence at the time of appointment to membership and initial granting of clinical privileges is verified in writing by peers knowledgeable about the applicant's professional performance. The hospital has obtained information directly from the primary source(s) in the form of written documentation from authoritative sources, which contain informed opinions on each applicant's scope and level of performance. Such primary source verification may be obtained through a secure electronic communication or by phone contact with the primary source. Written documentation that describes the applicant's actual clinical performance in general terms, the satisfactory discharge of his or her professional obligations as a medical staff member, and his or her ethical performance are acceptable. However, ideally the documentation also addresses at least the following two specific aspects of current competence:
    1. For applicants in fields performing operative and other procedure(s), the types of operative procedures performed as the surgeon of record; the handling of complicated deliveries; or the skill demonstrated in performing invasive procedures, including information on appropriateness and outcomes. In the case of applicants in nonsurgical fields, the types and outcomes of medical conditions managed by the applicant as the responsible physician should be addressed.
    2. The applicant's clinical judgment and technical skills.

It may not always be feasible to obtain information from the primary source. In rare or occasional instances, a primary source, such as an educational institution or a hospital, no longer exists, or the applicant's records have been lost or destroyed. Applicants may have received education, training, and experience partially or wholly in a foreign country, and for political or other reasons, information regarding their professional background is not accessible. However, when undue delay occurs in deriving information from a primary source, medical staff appointment is withheld pending receipt of this information. Under these circumstances, the applicant may be given temporary privileges for a limited time in accordance with applicable medical staff bylaws, rules and regulations, and policies, as well as state and federal regulations. Reliable secondary sources may also be used if there has been a documented attempt to contact the primary source.

Designated equivalent sources are selected agencies that have been determined to maintain a specific item(s) of credential information that is identical to the information at the primary source. These sources may be used to verify the specific issues of credential information in lieu of using the primary source. These designated equivalent sources are the following:
- The American Medical Association (AMA) Physician Masterfile for verification of a physician's medical school graduation and residency completion
- The American Board of Medical Specialties (ABMS) for verification of a physician's board certification
- The Educational Commission for Foreign Medical Graduates (ECFMG) for verification of a physician's graduation from a foreign medical school
- The American Osteopathic Association (AOA) Physician Database for predoctoral education accredited by the AOA Bureau of Professional Education; postdoctoral education approved by the AOA Council on Postdoctoral Training; and Osteopathic Specialty Board Certification

- The Federation of State Medical Boards (FSMB) for all actions against a physician's medical license

These designated equivalent sources may be used by a hospital, a network, the network's components, or a CVO that is used by the hospital, network, or its components. Other designated equivalent sources may exist for certain applicants, such as for licensure verification of an applicant in the federal service. The physician profiles from the AMA Physician Masterfile also include other primary source-reported information that is similar to primary source-verified information provided by a CVO. Use of this additional information is subject to the guidelines set forth below.

Verification of data from the primary source: Any hospital that bases its decisions in part on information from a CVO should have confidence in the completeness, accuracy, and timeliness of that information. To achieve this level of confidence in the information, the hospital should evaluate the agency providing the information initially and then periodically as appropriate. The principles that guide such an evaluation include the following:

- The agency makes known to the user what data and information it can provide.
- The agency provides documentation to the user describing how its data collection, information and development, and verification process(es) are performed.
- The user is provided with sufficient, clear information on database functions. This information includes any limitations on information available from the agency (for example, practitioners not included in the database); the time frame for agency responses to requests for information; and a summary overview of quality control processes relating to data integrity, security, transmission accuracy, and technical specifications.
- The user and agency agree on the format for transmission of an individual's credentials information from the agency.
- The user can easily discern which information, transmitted by the agency, is from a primary source and which is not.
- When the agency transmits information that can become out of date, it provides the date on which the information was last updated from the primary source.
- The agency certifies that the information transmitted to the user accurately presents the information obtained by it.
- The user can discern whether the information transmitted by the agency from a primary source is all the primary source information in the agency's possession pertinent to a given item and, if not, where additional information can be obtained.
- When necessary, the user can engage the agency's quality control processes to resolve concerns about transmission errors, inconsistencies, or other data issues that may be identified from time to time.
- The user has a formal arrangement with the CVO for communication of any changes in credentialing information.

There may be circumstances when it is impossible to obtain data from the primary source. In these circumstances the hospital may rely on a secondary source if the secondary source obtained the information from the primary source and the hospital believes the information to be credible and accurate.

A primary source of verified information may designate to an agency the role of communicating credentials information. The delegated agency then becomes acceptable to be used as a primary source.

Elements of Performance for MS.4.10

B   1. There are credentialing processes (*see* standard MS.1.20) that are designed to ensure that patients receive care, treatment, and services from qualified providers.

B   2. The credentialing process follows the steps outlined in the medical staff bylaws or other documents as previously approved by the governing body.

A   3. The credentialing process includes a mechanism to ensure that the individual requesting approval is the same individual identified in the credentialing documents.

A   4. The credentialing process requires that the hospital verifies in writing and from the primary source whenever feasible or from a CVO (*see* note in standard MS.4.10, pages MS-23–MS-26) the following information:
- The applicant's current licensure, at time of granting and renewal of privileges
- The applicant's specific relevant training
- The applicant's current competence

Initial Granting, Renewal, and Revision of Privileges

Standard MS.4.20
There is a process for granting, renewing, or revising setting-specific clinical privileges.

Rationale for MS.4.20
Essential information needs to be gathered in the process of granting, renewing, or revising clinical privileges. The information will dictate the type(s) of care, treatment, and services or procedures that a practitioner will be authorized to perform. Privileges are setting-specific because they require consideration of setting characteristics, such as adequate facilities, equipment, number, and type of qualified support personnel and resources. Setting-specific decisions mean that privileges granted to an applicant are based not only on the applicant's qualifications, but also on consideration of the procedures and types of care, treatment, and services that can be performed or provided within the proposed setting. All licensed independent practitioners are privileged through the medical staff process.

Elements of Performance for MS.4.20
A   1. There is a mechanism for granting and renewing clinical privileges.

A   2. There is a mechanism for revising clinical privileges.

B   3. Criteria are developed that determine an applicant's ability to provide patient care, treatment, and services within the scope of privileges requested.
- The criteria include evidence of current competence.
- The criteria include peer recommendations when required.

A   4. Setting-specific privileges are granted, renewed, or revised and do not exceed a period of two years.

A   5. The governing body or delegated committee has final authority for granting, renewing, revising, or denying privileges.

B   6. Before granting privileges, the organized medical staff evaluates the following:
- Challenges to any licensure or registration
- Voluntary and involuntary relinquishment of any license or registration
- Voluntary and involuntary termination of medical staff membership
- Voluntary and involuntary limitation, reduction, or loss of clinical privileges
- Any evidence of an unusual pattern or an excessive number of professional liability actions resulting in a final judgment against the applicant
- Documentation as to the applicant's health status
- Relevant practitioner-specific data are compared to aggregate data, when available
- Morbidity and mortality data, when available

C Ⓜ   7. Each reappraisal includes information concerning professional performance, including clinical and technical skills and information from hospital performance improvement activities, when such data are available.

C Ⓜ   8. When department chairpersons exist, the chairperson participates in the evaluation of practitioners practicing within the department.

The process for privileges includes the following:

A   9. A clearly defined mechanism for the processing of applications for initial, renewal, or revisions of clinical privileges.

A   10. An applicant submits a statement that no health problems exist that could affect his or her ability to perform the privileges requested.

A   11. If the hospital uses a provisional period of initial appointment to membership, a description is included.

C Ⓜ   12. Completed applications for privileges are acted on within the time period specified in the bylaws.

C Ⓜ 13. Information regarding each practitioner's scope of privileges is updated as changes in clinical privileges for each practitioner are made.

C Ⓜ 14. Decisions on membership and granting of privileges must consider criteria that are directly related to the quality of health care, treatment, and services. If privileging criteria are used that are unrelated to quality of care, treatment, and services or professional competence, evidence exists that the impact of resulting decisions on the quality of care, treatment, and services is evaluated.

A 15. The hospital queries the National Practitioner Data Bank (NPDB) at the time of initial medical staff appointments to membership and initial granting of clinical privileges, and at the time of expanding privileges or requesting to add new privileges, as well as at least every two years thereafter for information on physicians, dentists, and other health care practitioners granted clinical privileges.

Note 1: *Ability to perform privileges requested. The applicant's ability to perform privileges requested must be evaluated. This evaluation is documented in the individual's credentials file. Such documentation may include the applicant's statement that no health problems exist that could affect his or her practice. Documentation regarding an applicant's health status and their ability to practice should be confirmed. Initial applicants may have his or her health status confirmed by the director of a training program, the chief of services or chief of staff at another hospital at which the applicant holds privileges, or a currently licensed physician approved by the organized medical staff.*

In instances where there is doubt about an applicant's ability to perform privileges requested, an evaluation by an external and internal source may be required. The request for an evaluation rests with the organized medical staff.

Note 2: *The Americans with Disabilities Act (ADA) bars certain discrimination based on physical or mental impairment. Toward preventing such discrimination, the act prohibits or mandates various activities.*

Hospitals need to determine the applicability of the ADA to their medical staff. If applicable, the hospital should examine its privileging or credentialing procedures as to how and when it ascertains and confirm an applicant's ability to perform the privileges requested.

The Joint Commission cannot provide legal advice to hospitals. However, the Joint Commission has and will absolutely construe standard MS.4.20 in such a manner as not to be inconsistent with hospital efforts to comply with the ADA.

Expedited Credentialing and Privileging Process

Standard MS.4.30
An organized medical staff may use an expedited process for appointing to the medical staff and when granting privileges when criteria for that process are met.*

Elements of Performance for MS.4.30

B   1. The organized medical staff develops criteria for an expedited process for granting privileges.

C   2. The criteria provide that an applicant for privileges is ineligible for the expedited process if any of the following has occurred:
- The applicant submits an incomplete application
- The medical staff executive committee makes a final recommendation that is adverse or has limitations

C Ⓜ   3. The organized medical staff uses the criteria developed for the expedited process when recommending privileges.

The following situations are evaluated on a case-by-case basis and usually result in ineligibility for the expedited process:

C Ⓜ   4. There is a current challenge or a previously successful challenge to licensure or registration

C Ⓜ   5. The applicant has received an involuntary termination of medical staff membership at another organization

C Ⓜ   6. The applicant has received involuntary limitation, reduction, denial, or loss of clinical privileges

        or

C Ⓜ   7. The hospital determines that there has been either an unusual pattern of, or an excessive number of, professional liability actions resulting in a final judgment against the applicant

Renewal or Reappraisal Process for Privileging

Standard MS.4.40
At the time of renewal of privileges, the organized medical staff evaluates individuals for their continued ability to provide quality care, treatment, and services for the privileges requested as defined in the medical staff bylaws.

---

* To expedite initial appointments to membership and granting of privileges, reappointment to membership, or renewal or modification of privileges, the governing body may delegate the authority to render those decisions to a committee of at least two voting members of the governing body.

Rationale for MS.4.40

The process for renewal of privileges involves the same steps as those outlined under standard MS.4.20 for granting initial privileges and additionally requires the medical staff to evaluate a practitioner's ability to perform the privileges requested based upon his or her performance during the period of time he or she has been practicing at the organization. A hospital reviews the performance of each practitioner for every setting, under the control of the hospital, where the individual practices. Current competence is determined by the results of performance improvement activities and peer recommendations.

Evidence of current ability to perform privileges requested is required of all applicants for renewal of clinical privileges. The process should emphasize the organization's performance improvement philosophy. The process should identify quality of care, treatment, and services issues for groups of individuals as well as individual practitioners (*see also* the "Improving Organization Performance" chapter in this book).

In evaluating the ability to perform requested privileges and when renewing or revising privileges, criteria could include procedures performed and their outcomes and could be based on pertinent results of review of operative procedures and other procedure(s),* medication usage, blood usage, medical records, and other performance improvement activities, as appropriate. Additional criteria may be based on mortality rates, utilization management, meeting and committee attendance, and risk management data. Relevant information developed from these activities is integrated into performance improvement initiatives consistent with any of the organization's policies or procedures intended to preserve any confidentiality or privilege of information established by applicable law. The hospital may wish to add other reasonable criteria, such as patient care, treatment, and service needs for additional staff members with the applicant's skill and training.

In instances where there is doubt about an applicant's ability to perform privileges requested, an evaluation by someone other than the applicant's chairperson or chief of service may be necessary to resolve the issue. The executive committee of the organized medical staff is responsible for requesting such an evaluation.

One indicator of the effectiveness of the reappraisal process may be objective documentation in an individual's file that, within the past few years, an individual's privileges were increased, reduced, or terminated because of the following:
- Assessments of his or her documented performance
- Nonuse of privileges for a procedures or treatments
- Emergence of new technologies

Elements of Performance for MS.4.40

In addition to meeting the requirements of standard MS.4.20, upon renewal or revision of privileges an individual must also meet the following additional requirements:

---

* **Operative and other high-risk procedures** Includes operative, other invasive, and noninvasive procedures such as radiotherapy, hyperbaric treatment, CAT scan, and MRI that place the patient at risk. The focus is on procedures and is not meant to include medications that place the patient at risk.

Medical Staff

A   1. Each renewal or revision of privileges is based on a reappraisal*

A   2. There are criteria that pertain to evidence of current competence and ability to perform the privileges requested

B   3. Upon renewing or revising privileges, the organized medical staff evaluates the following:
- Challenges to any licensure or registration
- Voluntary and involuntary relinquishment of any license or registration
- Voluntary and involuntary termination of medical staff membership
- Voluntary and involuntary limitation, reduction, or loss of clinical privileges
- Involvement in a professional liability action, as defined in the medical staff bylaws, including final judgments and settlements involving a practitioner
- Documentation as to applicant's health status
- Relevant practitioner-specific data are compared to aggregate data if such data are available for that practitioner
- Morbidity and mortality data if such data are available for that practitioner
- Peer recommendations

C (M)   4. Each reappraisal includes information concerning professional performance, including clinical and technical skills and information from hospital performance improvement activities, when such data are available.

A   5. Practitioners do not practice outside the scope of their privileges.

Fair Hearing and Appeal Process for Adverse Privileging Decisions

Standard MS.4.50
There are mechanisms including a fair hearing and appeal process for addressing adverse decisions regarding reappointment, denial, reduction, suspension, or revocation of privileges that may relate to quality of care, treatment, and services issues.

Rationale MS.4.50
Mechanisms for fair hearing and appeals processes are designed to allow the affected individual a fair opportunity to defend herself or himself regarding the adverse decision to an unbiased hearing body of the medical staff, and an opportunity to appeal the decision of the hearing body to the governing body. The purpose

---

* Renewal of privileges may not exceed a period of two years.

of a fair hearing and appeal is to assure full consideration and reconsideration of quality and safety issues and, under the current structure of reporting to the NPDB, allow practitioners an opportunity to defend themselves.

Elements of Performance for MS.4.50
The organized medical staff has developed a fair hearing and appeal process addressing quality of care issues that has the following characteristics:

B   1. Is designed to provide a fair process that may differ for members and non-members of the medical staff

A   2. Has a mechanism to schedule a hearing of such requests

A   3. Has identified the procedures for the hearing to follow

A   4. Identifies the composition of the hearing committee as a committee of impartial peers

A   5. With the governing body provides a mechanism to appeal adverse decisions as provided in the medical staff bylaws

Appointment to Membership on the Medical Staff

Standard MS.4.60
The organized medical staff provides oversight for the quality of care, treatment, and services by recommending members for appointment to the medical staff.

Elements of Performance for MS.4.60

A   1. The organized medical staff develops criteria for medical staff membership.

C Ⓜ   2. The professional criteria are designed to assure the medical staff and governing body that patients will receive quality care, treatment, and services.

C Ⓜ   3. The organized medical staff uses the criteria in appointing members to the medical staff and appointment does not exceed a period of two years.

C Ⓜ   4. The members of the organized medical staff who are responsible for the oversight of quality of care, treatment, and services are licensed independent practitioners.

C Ⓜ   5. Membership is recommended by the medical staff and granted by the governing body.

Peer Recommendation

Standard MS.4.70
Peer recommendations from peers in the same professional discipline as the applicant are used as part of the basis for the initial granting of privileges. Peer recommendations are used to recommend individuals for the renewal of clinical privileges when insufficient practitioner-specific data are available.

Rationale for MS.4.70
In circumstances where there are insufficient peer review data available when evaluating an applicant for privileges, the organized medical staff uses peer recommendations.

A recommendation(s) from peers (appropriate practitioners in the same professional discipline as the applicant who have personal knowledge of the applicant) reflects a basis for recommending the granting of privileges.

Sources for peer recommendations may include the following:
- A hospital performance improvement committee, the majority of whose members are the applicant's peers
- A reference letter(s), written documentation, or documented telephone conversation(s) about the applicant from a peer(s) who is knowledgeable about the applicant's professional performance and competence
- A department or major clinical service chairperson who is a peer
- The medical staff executive committee

Elements of Performance for MS.4.70

C Ⓜ 1. Peer recommendations are obtained and evaluated for all new applicants for privileges.

C Ⓜ 2. Upon renewal of privileges, when insufficient practitioner-specific data are available, the medical staff obtains and evaluates peer recommendations.

C Ⓜ 3. Peer recommendations include the following information:
- Relevant training and experience
- Current competence
- Any effects of health status on privileges being requested

C Ⓜ 4. Peer recommendations are obtained from a practitioner in the same professional discipline as the applicant with personal knowledge of the applicant's ability to practice.

Licensed Independent Practitioner Health

Standard MS.4.80
The medical staff implements a process to identify and manage matters of individual health for licensed independent practitioners. This identification process is separate from actions taken for disciplinary purposes.

Rationale for MS.4.80
The organized medical staff and hospital leaders have an obligation to protect patients, its members, and other persons present in the hospital from harm. Therefore, the organized medical staff designs a process that provides education about licensed independent practitioner health, addresses prevention of physical, psychiatric, or emotional illness, and facilitates confidential diagnosis, treatment, and rehabilitation of licensed independent practitioners who suffer from a potentially impairing condition.

The purpose of the process is to help with the rehabilitation, rather than discipline, to aid a practitioner in retaining and regaining optimal professional functioning that is consistent with protection of patients. If at any time during the diagnosis, treatment, or rehabilitation phase of the process it is determined that a practitioner is unable to safely perform the privileges he or she has been granted, the matter is forwarded for appropriate corrective action that includes strict adherence to any state or federally mandated reporting requirements.

Elements of Performance for MS.4.80
Process design addresses the following issues:

B 1. Education of licensed independent practitioners and other hospital staff about illness and impairment recognition issues specific to licensed independent practitioners (at-risk criteria)

A 2. Self referral by a licensed independent practitioner

A 3. Referral by others and creation of confidentiality of informants

A 4. Referral of the affected licensed independent practitioner to appropriate professional internal or external resources for evaluation, diagnosis, and treatment of the condition or concern

A 5. Maintenance of confidentiality of the licensed independent practitioner seeking referral or referred for assistance, except as limited by law, ethical obligation, or when the health and safety of a patient is threatened

A 6. Evaluation of the credibility of a complaint, allegation, or concern

A 7. Monitoring the affected licensed independent practitioner and the safety of patients until the rehabilitation or any disciplinary process is complete and periodically thereafter, if required

A   8. Reporting to the organized medical staff leadership instances in which a licensed independent practitioner is providing unsafe treatment

Note: *The Americans with Disabilities Act (ADA) bars certain discrimination based on physical or mental impairment. Toward preventing such discrimination, the act prohibits or mandates various activities.*

Hospitals need to determine the applicability of the ADA to their medical staff. If applicable, the hospital should examine its privileging or credentialing procedures as to how and when it ascertains and confirms the ability of an applicant to perform the privileges requested.

The Joint Commission cannot provide legal advice to hospitals. However, the Joint Commission has and will absolutely construe standard MS.4.80 in such a manner as not to be inconsistent with hospital efforts to comply with the ADA.

Focused Review of Practitioner's Performance

Standard MS.4.90
There is a process that defines circumstances requiring a focused review of a practitioner's performance and evaluation of a practitioner's performance by peers.

Rationale for MS.4.90
The purpose of this standard is to require a hospital to identify a minimum set of circumstances that will require further intensive review to determine whether a practitioner's performance may require further action to improve that practitioner's performance. This process allows a hospital to define its own circumstances for review of a practitioner's performance and also to define when external reviewers are necessary. Additionally, the goal of this process is not necessarily disciplinary but primarily to improve a practitioner's performance.

The practitioner's peers conduct the focused review of a practitioner's performance. Members of the organized medical staff are involved in activities to measure, assess, and improve performance on an organizationwide basis, including a focused practitioner review process. The focused review process involves monitoring, analyzing, and understanding those special circumstances of practitioner performance, as defined by the organized medical staff, which requires further evaluation. When the findings of the assessment process are relevant to an individual's performance, the organized medical staff is responsible for determining their use in ongoing evaluations of a licensed independent practitioner's competence, in accordance with the standards on renewing or revising clinical privileges identified in this chapter.

Relevant information developed from the following processes is integrated into performance improvement initiatives and consistent with hospital preservation of confidentiality and privilege of information.

Elements of Performance for MS.4.90
The focused review process includes the following:

- **A** 1. Definition of the special circumstances requiring focused review
- **A** 2. Method for selecting focused review panels for specific circumstances
- **A** 3. Time frames in which focused review activities are reasonably adhered to
- **A** 4. Circumstances under which external peer review is required
- **A** 5. Provision of participation in the review process by the individual whose performance is being reviewed
- **C Ⓜ** 6. The focused review is conducted in accordance with circumstances requiring a focused review, as defined by the organization

The organized medical staff is involved in the following:

- **C Ⓜ** 7. Evaluation of individuals with clinical privileges whose performance is questioned as a result of the measurement and assessment activities
- **C Ⓜ** 8. Communication to the appropriate parties of the findings, conclusions, recommendations, and actions taken to improve practitioner performance
- **C Ⓜ** 9. Implementation of changes to improve performance

Temporary Privileges

Standard MS.4.100
Under certain circumstances, temporary clinical privileges may be granted for a limited period of time.

Rationale for MS.4.100
There are two circumstances in which temporary privileges may be granted. Each circumstance has different criteria for granting privileges.

The circumstances for which the granting of temporary privileges are acceptable include the following:
- To fulfill an important patient care, treatment, and service need
- When a new applicant with a complete application that raises no concerns is awaiting review and approval of the medical staff executive committee and the governing body

Temporary privileges for the fulfillment of important patient care, treatment, and service needs are time limited as determined in the medical staff bylaws or other documents. Temporary privileges for new applicants are not to exceed 120 days.

Medical staff bylaws or other documents may stipulate that in an emergency, any medical staff member with clinical privileges is permitted to provide any type of patient care, treatment, and services necessary as a life-saving measure or to prevent serious harm—regardless of his or her medical staff status or clinical privileges—provided that the care, treatment, and services provided are within the scope of the individual's license.

Elements of Performance for MS.4.100

Temporary privileges granted for an important patient care need:

C Ⓜ 1. Temporary privileges are granted to meet an important patient care need.

A 2. When temporary privileges are granted to meet an important care need, the organized medical staff verifies current licensure and current competence.

Temporary privileges for new applicants:

A 3. Temporary privileges for new applicants may be granted while awaiting review and approval by the organized medical staff upon verification of the following:
- Current licensure
- Relevant training or experience
- Current competence
- Ability to perform the privileges requested
- Other criteria required by the organized medical staff bylaws
- A query and evaluation of the NPDB information
- A complete application
- No current or previously successful challenge to licensure or registration
- No subjection to involuntary termination of medical staff membership at another organization
- No subjection to involuntary limitation, reduction, denial, or loss of clinical privileges

A 4. All temporary privileges are granted by the CEO or authorized designee.

A 5. All temporary privileges are granted on the recommendation of the medical staff president or authorized designee.

A 6. Temporary privileges for new applicants are granted for no more than 120 days.

Disaster Privileges

Standard MS.4.110
Disaster privileges may be granted when the emergency management plan has been activated and the hospital is unable to handle the immediate patient needs (*see* standard EC.4.10).

Rationale for MS.4.110
During disaster(s) in which the emergency management plan has been activated, the CEO or medical staff president or their designee(s) has the option to grant disaster privileges.

Elements of Performance for MS.4.110

A 1. The medical staff identifies in writing the individual(s) responsible for granting disaster privileges.

A 2. The medical staff describes in writing the responsibilities of the individual(s) granting disaster privileges. (The responsible individual is not required to grant privileges to any individual and is expected to make such decisions on a case-by-case basis at his or her discretion.)

B 3. The medical staff describes in writing a mechanism to manage individuals who receive disaster privileges.

A 4. The medical staff includes a mechanism to allow staff to readily identify these individuals.

A 5. The medical staff addresses the verification process as a high priority.

A 6. The medical staff begins the verification process of the credentials and privileges of individuals who receive disaster privileges as soon as the immediate situation is under control.

A 7. This verification process is identical to the process established under the medical staff bylaws or other documents for granting temporary privileges to meet an important patient care need (*see* standard MS.4.100).

B 8. The CEO or president of the medical staff or their designee(s) *may* grant disaster privileges upon presentation of any of the following:
- A current picture hospital ID card
- A current license to practice and a valid picture ID issued by a state, federal, or regulatory agency
- Identification indicating that the individual is a member of a Disaster Medical Assistance Team (DMAT)
- Identification indicating that the individual has been granted authority to render patient care, treatment, and services in disaster circumstances (such authority having been granted by a federal, state, or municipal entity)

- Presentation by current hospital or medical staff member(s) with personal knowledge regarding practitioner's identity

Telemedicine

Introduction
The services covered under these standards are narrowly defined, focusing solely on licensed independent practitioners who have either total or shared responsibility for patient care, treatment, and services (as evidenced by having the authority to write orders and direct care, treatment, and services) through a telemedicine* link. Licensed independent practitioners who provide official readings of images, tracings, or specimens through a telemedicine link are credentialed and privileged under the contracted services standard LD.3.50.

If the hospital has a pressing clinical need and a practitioner can supply that service through a telemedicine link, the hospital can evaluate the use of temporary privileges (standard MS.4.100) for this clinical situation.

These standards introduce the concept of credentialing and privileging by proxy. Under special circumstances, the originating site (the site where the patient is located at the time the service is provided) is allowed to accept the credentialing and privileging decisions of the distant site (the site where the practitioner providing the professional service is located). As in all other standards, these standards assume that the hospital is following applicable law and regulation such as appropriate licensure to practice medicine or telemedicine in the states where the originating sites and distant sites are located. This approach involves the following:
- Reduces the credentialing and privileging burden for the originating site, especially where there are large numbers of licensed independent practitioners who might provide telemedicine services
- Recognizes that the distant site has more relevant information upon which to base its privileging decisions
- Acknowledges that the originating site may have little experience in privileging in certain specialties

Other Standards Related to the Delivery of Telemedicine
Clinical privileging decisions encompass consideration of the appropriate use of telemedicine equipment by the telemedicine practitioner. *See* the "Management of the Environment of Care" chapter, standards EC.6.10 and EC.6.20, for additional standards related to maintaining telemedical equipment.

---

* **Telemedicine** The use of medical information exchanged from one site to another via electronic communications for the health and education of the patient or health care provider and for the purpose of improving patient care, treatment, and services. **Source:** *American Telemedicine Association.*

For Originating Sites Only
Standard MS.4.120
Licensed independent practitioners who are responsible for the care, treatment, and services of the patient via telemedicine link are subject to the credentialing and privileging processes of the originating site.

Rationale for MS.4.120
The originating site retains responsibility for overseeing the safety and quality of services offered to its patients.

Elements of Performance for MS.4.120
A   1. All licensed independent practitioners who are responsible for the patient's care, treatment, and services via telemedicine link are credentialed and privileged to do so at the originating site through one of the following mechanisms:
a. The originating site may fully privilege and credential the practitioner according to standards MS.4.10 through MS.4.110
b. The practitioner may be privileged at the originating site using credentialing information from the distant site if the distant site is a Joint Commission-accredited organization
or
c. The originating site may use the credentialing and privileging information from the distant site if all the following requirements are met:
   1. The distant site is Joint Commission-accredited
   2. The practitioner is privileged at the distant site for those services to be provided at the originating site
   3. The originating site has evidence of an internal review of the practitioner's performance of these privileges and sends to the distant site information that is useful to assess the practitioner's quality of care, treatment, and services for use in privileging and performance improvement. At a minimum, this information includes all adverse outcomes related to sentinel events* considered reviewable by the Joint Commission that result from the telemedicine services provided; and complaints about the distant site licensed independent practitioner from patients, licensed independent practitioners, or staff at the originating site.
   Note: *This occurs in a way consistent with any hospital policies or procedures intended to preserve any confidentiality or privilege of information established by applicable law.*

---

* A sentinel event is an unexpected occurrence involving death or serious physical or psychological injury, or the risk thereof. Serious injury specifically includes loss of limb or function. The phrase "or the risk thereof" includes any process variation for which a recurrence would carry a significant chance of a serious adverse outcome. *See* the "Sentinel Events" chapter in this book for additional information.

For Originating and Distant Sites
Standard MS.4.130

The medical staffs at both the originating and distant sites recommend the clinical services to be provided by licensed independent practitioners through a telemedical link at their respective sites.

Rationale for MS.4.130
Telemedicine will continue to evolve making novel services and approaches through technology more readily available. Medical staff at the originating site evaluates the organization's ability to safely provide services on an ongoing basis. Medical staff at the distant site evaluates performance of those services as part of privileging and as part of the reappraisal conducted at the time of reappointment or renewal or revision of clinical privileges.

Elements of Performance for MS.4.130

B   1. The medical staff recommends which clinical services are appropriately delivered by licensed independent practitioners through this medium.

B   2. The clinical services offered are consistent with commonly accepted quality standards.

Continuing Education

Standard MS.5.10

All licensed independent practitioners and other practitioners privileged through the medical staff process participate in continuing education.

Rationale for MS.5.10
Continuing education is an adjunct to maintaining clinical skills and current competence.

Elements of Performance for MS.5.10
Hospital-Based Education:

A   1. Hospital-sponsored educational activities are offered.

A   2. These activities relate, at least in part, to the type and nature of care, treatment, and services offered by the hospital.

A   3. The organized medical staff helps prioritize hospital-sponsored continuing education.

B   4. Education is based on the findings of performance improvement activities.

Individual-Based Education:

C Ⓜ 5. Each individual's participation in continuing education is documented.

C Ⓜ 6. Participation in continuing education is considered in decisions about reappointment to membership on the medical staff or renewal or revision of individual clinical privileges.

Nursing

Overview

The quality of a hospital's nursing services is built upon the leadership of a nurse executive and the work of a qualified staff. The nurse executive ensures the continuous and timely availability of nursing services to patients. The nurse executive also ensures the quality of nursing standards of patient care and practice by incorporating current nursing research findings, nationally recognized professional standards, and other literature into the policies and procedures governing the provision of nursing care, treatment, and services. In addition, the nurse executive develops, presents, and manages the nursing services' portion of the hospital's budget.

A qualified staff provides patient care and nursing services on a continuous basis, 24 hours a day, 7 days a week, to those patients requiring such care, treatment, and services. Nursing staff monitors each patient's status and coordinates the provision of nursing care while assisting other professionals in implementing plans of care. To achieve the goal of providing quality nursing care, treatment, and services, the nurse executive participates with hospital leaders in defining the nursing care needs of the patient population served. The nurse executive also participates with hospital leaders in providing for a sufficient number of appropriately qualified nursing staff members to assess each patient's nursing care needs, plan and provide nursing care interventions, prevent complications, promote improvement in the patient's comfort and wellness, and alert other care professionals to the patient's condition, as appropriate.

Standards

The following is a list of all standards for this function. They are presented here for your convenience without footnotes or other explanatory text. If you have a question about a term used here, please check the Glossary.

Note: *A revised standard numbering system is being used with the reformatted standards. The revised numbering system will allow for more flexibility to add standards while maintaining the current number for each standard.*

NR.1.10   A nurse executive directs the hospital's nursing services.

NR.2.10   The nurse executive is a licensed professional registered nurse qualified by advanced education and management experience.

NR.3.10   The nurse executive establishes nursing policies and procedures, nursing standards of patient care, treatment, and services, and standards of nursing practice.

Understanding the Parts of This Chapter

To help you navigate this reformatted standards chapter, it may be helpful to think of its parts this way:
- The **standard** is the "goal."
- The **rationale** explains why it's important to achieve this goal.
- The **elements of performance** identify the step(s) needed to achieve this goal.

These parts are defined as follows.

Standard A statement that defines the performance expectations and/or structures or processes that must be in place in order for a hospital to provide safe, high-quality care, treatment, and services. A hospital is either "compliant" or "not compliant" with a standard.

Accreditation decisions are based on simple counts of the standards that are determined to be "not compliant."

Rationale A statement that provides background, justification, or additional information about a standard. A standard's rationale is not scored. In some instances, the rationale for a standard is self-evident. Therefore, not every standard has a written rationale.

Elements of performance (EPs) The specific performance expectations and/or structures or processes that must be in place in order for a hospital to provide safe, high-quality care, treatment, and services. The scoring of EP compliance determines a hospital's overall compliance with a standard. EPs are evaluated on the following scale:

    0 Insufficient compliance
    1 Partial compliance
    2 Satisfactory compliance
   NA Not applicable

You will find a **measure of success** icon—Ⓜ—next to some EPs. Measures of success (MOS) need to be developed for certain EPs when a standard is judged to be out of compliance through either the Periodic Performance Review (PPR) or the onsite survey. An MOS is defined as a quantifiable measure, usually related to an audit, that can be used to determine whether an action has been effective and is being sustained.*

Assessing Your Compliance

Once you are familiar with the parts of this chapter, you can begin to assess your compliance with its requirements. The scoring category for each EP is noted next to the EP. If you would like to assess your hospital's performance, mark your scores for the EPs and the standards by following the simple steps described below.

---

*For more information about measures of success, *see* the "The New Joint Commission Accreditation Process" chapter in this book.

Two components are scored for each EP: (1) compliance with the requirement itself **and** (2) compliance with the track record* for that requirement. Scoring has been simplified, and track record achievements (which have always been part of the scoring) have been appropriately modified.

Note: *Some standards and EPs do not apply to a particular type of organization; these standards and EPs are marked "not applicable" and the related text is not included. Your hospital is not expected to comply with standards and EPs marked "not applicable."*

In addition, some standards and EPs that do apply to organizations may not apply to the specific care, treatment, and services that your individual hospital provides. Although these standards and EPs are included in the manual, you are not expected to comply with them. If you are unsure about the standards or EPs that apply to your hospital, please contact the Joint Commission's Standards Interpretation Group at 630/792-5900.

Step 1: Score Your Compliance with Each Element of Performance

Before you can determine your compliance with the standards, you must score your compliance with each EP. There are three scoring criterion categories: A, B, and C (described below). Please note that for each EP scoring criterion category, your hospital must meet the performance requirement itself and the track record achievements (*see* "Track Record Achievements").

Category A

These EPs relate to the presence or absence of the requirement(s) and are scored either yes (2) or no (0); however, score 1 for partial compliance is also possible based on track record achievements.

If an A EP has multiple components designated by bullets, your hospital must be compliant with all the bullets to receive a score of 2. If your hospital does not meet one or more requirements in the bullets, you will receive a score of 0.

Category B

Category B EPs are scored in two steps:
1. As with category A EPs, category B EPs relate to the presence or absence of the requirement(s). If your hospital *does not meet* the requirement(s), the EP is scored 0; there is no need to assess your compliance with the principles of good process design.
2. If your hospital *does meet* the requirement(s), but there is concern about the quality or comprehensiveness of the effort, then and only then should you assess the qualitative aspect of the EP. That is, review the applicable principles of good process design and ask how the principles were applied in the situation under discussion. Good process design has the following characteristics:

---

* **Track record** The amount of time that an organization has been in compliance with a standard, element of performance, or other requirement.

- Is consistent with your hospital's mission, values, and goals
- Meets the needs of patients
- Reflects the use of currently accepted practices (doing the right thing, using resources responsibly, using practice guidelines)
- Incorporates current safety information and knowledge such as sentinel event data and National Patient Safety Goals
- Incorporates relevant performance improvement results

This two-part evaluation applies to both simple and bulleted B EPs. First, the EPs are assessed to determine if the requirements are present. If the EP has multiple components designated by bullets, as with the category A EPs, your hospital must meet the requirements in *all* the bulleted items to get a score of 2. If your hospital meets *none* of the requirements in the bullets, it receives a score of 0. If your hospital meets *at least one, but not all*, of the bulleted requirements, it will receive a score of 1 for the EPs.

Use the following rules to determine your EP score:
- Your EP score is 0 if your hospital does not meet the requirement(s); you *do not* need to assess your compliance with the preceding applicable principles of good process design
- Your EP score is 1 if your hospital does meet the requirement(s), but considered only *some* of the preceding applicable principles of good process design
- Your EP score is 2 if your hospital does meet the requirement(s) *and* considered *all* the preceding principles of good process design

Category C

C EPs are scored 0, 1, or 2 based on the number of times your hospital does not meet the EP. These EPs are frequency based and require totaling the number of occurrences (that is, results of performance or nonperformance) related to a particular EP. Each situation discovered by a surveyor(s) will be counted as a separate occurrence.

Note: *Multiple events of the same type related to a single patient and single practitioner/staff member are counted as* one occurrence only.

Use the following rules to determine your EP score:
- Your EP score is 2 if you find one or fewer occurrences of noncompliance with the EP
- Your EP score is 1 if you find two occurrences of noncompliance with the EP
- Your EP score is 0 if you find three or more occurrences of noncompliance with the EP

If an EP in the C category has multiple requirements designated by bullets, the following scoring guidelines apply:
- If there are fewer than 2 findings in all bullets, the EP is scored 2
- If there are three or more findings in all bullets, the EP is scored 0
- In all other combinations of findings, the EP is scored 1

Track Record Achievements

In addition to meeting the requirement(s) in each EP, regardless of category, your hospital must also meet the following track record achievements:

Score	Initial Survey	Full Survey
2	4 months or more	12 months or more
1	2 to 3 months	6 to 11 months
0	Fewer than 2 months	Fewer than 6 months

Sample Sizes

If during an onsite survey, your hospital has been found to be not compliant with one or more standards, you must demonstrate Evidence of Standards Compliance (ESC) for each standard that is not compliant. The ESC must address compliance at the EP level; when an EP within a noncompliant standard requires an MOS, your hospital must demonstrate achievement with the MOS when completing the ESC.

Note: *Not every EP requires an MOS. EPs that do require an MOS are clearly marked in this chapter. Organizations are required to demonstrate achievement with an MOS only for EPs within a noncompliant standard that require an MOS. Organizations do not need to demonstrate achievement with an MOS for any EP within a compliant standard.*

When demonstrating achievement with the MOS during the ESC process, your hospital is **required** to use the following sample sizes, which were established because of their statistical significance, their relative simplicity in application, and their sensitivity to an organization's population size:
- For a population size of fewer than 30 cases, sample 100% of available cases
- For a population size of 30 to 100 cases, sample 30 cases
- For a population size of 101 to 500 cases, sample 50 cases
- For a population size greater than 500 cases, sample 70 cases

Note: *Hospitals are encouraged, but not required, to follow this sample size when demonstrating achievement with an MOS for an EP within a noncompliant standard after conducting a full, Option 1, or Option 2 Periodic Performance Review (PPR).*

When conducting PPR (optional use) or demonstrating an ESC (mandatory use), use the following percentages to determine your score: 90% through 100% of your sample size is in compliance = score 2; 80% through 89% (two instances of noncompliance) of your sample size is in compliance = score 1; less than 80% (three or more instances of noncompliance) of your sample size is in compliance = score 0.

In addition, the following information should govern your hospital's selection of samples:
- The appropriate sample size should be determined by the specific population related to the survey findings
- The sampling approach should involve either systematic random sampling (for example, your hospital selects every second or third case for review) or simple random sampling (for example, your hospital uses a series of random numbers generated by a computer to identify the cases to be reviewed)

- If your hospital chooses not to use these sample sizes while conducting PPR options 1 or 2, you should make sure that your sample size is sufficiently large enough to ensure statistical significance
- When submitting a clarifying ESC, if your hospital selects records as part of its sample, the records should be from a period of no more than three months before the last date of the survey
- Assessment of MOS compliance is conducted for a four-month period following the date of ESC approval. Your hospital should select records as a part of your sample following the date of ESC approval and use the required sample sizes. MOS percentage compliance rates are derived from the average of all four months.

Step 2: Use Your EP Scores to Gauge Your Compliance with the Standards

Now that you have evaluated and scored each EP for a particular standard, use these simple rules to determine your compliance with the standard itself:

- Your hospital is not in compliance (that is, "not compliant") with the standard if any EP is scored 0
- Otherwise, your hospital is in compliance with a standard if 65% or more of its EPs are scored 2

2005 Hospital Accreditation Standards

Standards, Rationales, Elements of Performance, and Scoring

Standard NR.1.10
A nurse executive directs the hospital's nursing services.

Elements of Performance for NR.1.10

B   1. An identified nurse leader at the executive level coordinates the following functions:
- Development of hospitalwide patient care programs, policies, and procedures that describe how patients' nursing care needs, or the needs of patient populations receiving nursing care, treatment, and services, are assessed, evaluated, and met
- Development and implementation of the hospital's plans for providing nursing care, treatment, and services to those patients requiring nursing care, treatment, and services
- Participation with governing body, management, medical staff, and clinical leaders in the hospital's decision-making structures and processes
- Implementation of an effective, ongoing program to measure, assess, and improve the quality of nursing care, treatment, and services delivered to patients

A   2. The nurse executive's authority and responsibility are defined in a contract, a written agreement, a letter, a memorandum, a job or position description, or other document.

A   3. The nurse executive or a designee(s) approves nursing policies and procedures, nursing standards of patient care, treatment, and services, and standards of nursing practice before implementation.

B   4. Decentralized hospital structures with geographically distant sites have an established process for selecting, electing, or appointing one appropriately prepared nurse as its nurse executive.

B   5. The nurse executive functions at the executive level to provide effective and coordinated leadership to deliver nursing care, treatment, and services.

A   6. The nurse executive participates in defined and established meetings of the hospital's corporate leaders (when such leaders exist) and with other clinical and managerial leaders.

A   7. The nurse executive has the authority to speak on behalf of nursing to the same extent that other hospital leaders speak for their respective disciplines or departments.

Standard NR.2.10

The nurse executive is a licensed professional registered nurse qualified by advanced education and management experience.

Rationale for NR.2.10

A nurse who possesses the requisite education to become a nurse executive has acquired extensive and valuable knowledge of the nursing profession.

Elements of Performance for NR.2.10

A   1.   The nurse executive is currently licensed as a registered professional nurse in the state, commonwealth, or territory as required by law.

The following factors are considered when appointing the nurse executive:

B   2.   Whether the prospective nurse executive possesses the knowledge and skills associated with a master's degree in nursing or a related field or another appropriate postgraduate degree, or has a written plan to obtain these qualifications

B   3.   The hospital's scope and complexity and the position's authority and responsibility

B   4.   The scope and complexity of the nursing care needs of the major patient population(s) served

B   5.   The availability of adequate nursing support staff and services to help the nurse executive address the responsibilities required in this chapter

B   6.   The education and experience required for peer leadership positions*

Standard NR.3.10

The nurse executive establishes nursing policies and procedures, nursing standards of patient care, treatment, and services, and standards of nursing practice.

Elements of Performance for NR.3.10

A   1.   The nurse executive, registered nurses, and other designated nursing staff members write nursing policies and procedures; nursing standards of patient care, treatment, and services; standards of nursing practice; and standards to measure, assess, and improve patient outcomes.

A   2.   The nurse executive is responsible for ensuring that nursing policies, procedures, and standards describe and guide how the nursing staff provides the nursing care, treatment, and services required by all patients and patient populations served by the hospital and as defined in the hospital's plan(s) for providing nursing care, treatment, and services.

---

* For example, when leadership peers are expected to have a masters or doctoral degree or appropriate professional certification, the nurse executive possesses similar qualifications.

A 3. All nursing policies, procedures, and standards are defined, documented, and accessible to the nursing staff in written or electronic format.

A 4. The nurse executive or a designee(s) exercises final authority over those associated with providing nursing care, treatment, and services.

Crosswalks of Standards

Crosswalk of Previous Patient Rights and Organization Ethics Standards for Hospitals to Current Ethics, Rights, and Responsibilities Standards for Hospitals

This crosswalk is designed to show where the previous Patient Rights and Organization Ethics (RI) standards requirements appear in the reformatted RI standards. The left column (Previous Standards) lists consecutively each previous RI standard; standards from other functional chapters might also be included in this column, as appropriate. The middle column, Current Standards, indicates the RI standards with revised numbers. Standards from other functional chapters might also be included in this column, as appropriate. The right column, Comments, identifies what changes have occurred between the previous standards and the current standards.

Previous Standards	Current Standards	Comments
RI.1 The hospital addresses ethical issues in providing patient care.	RI.2.10 The hospital respects the rights of patients. RI.2.30 Patients are involved in decisions about care, treatment, and services provided. RI.2.80 The hospital addresses the wishes of the patient relating to end-of-life decisions. RI.2.90 Patients and, when appropriate, their families are informed about the outcomes of care, treatment, and services, including unanticipated outcomes. RI.2.130 The hospital respects the needs of patients for confidentiality, privacy, and security. RI.2.170 Patients have a right to access protective and advocacy services. RI.2.180 The hospital protects research subjects and respects their rights during research, investigation, and clinical trials involving human subjects. HR.2.10 Orientation provides initial job training and information.	Reformatted, renumbered, and rewritten to be consistent across accreditation programs.
RI.1.1 The patient's right to treatment or services is respected and supported.	RI.2.10 The hospital respects the rights of patients.	Reformatted, renumbered, and rewritten to be consistent across accreditation programs.
RI.1.2 Patients are involved in all aspects of their care.	RI.2.30 Patients are involved in decisions about care, treatment, and services provided.	Reformatted, renumbered, and rewritten to be consistent across accreditation programs.
RI.1.2.1 Informed consent is obtained.	RI.2.40 Informed consent is obtained. RI.2.60 Patients receive adequate information about the person(s) responsible for the delivery of their care, treatment, and services.	Reformatted, renumbered, and rewritten to be consistent across accreditation programs.
RI.1.2.1.1 All patients asked to participate in a research project are given a description of the expected benefit.	RI.2.180 The hospital protects research subjects and respects their rights during research, investigation, and clinical trials involving human subjects.	Requirements added to RI.2.180 to address confidentiality and inclusion of research information in the medical record.
RI.1.2.1.2 All patients asked to participate in a research project are given a description of the potential discomforts and risks.	RI.2.180 The hospital protects research subjects and respects their rights during research, investigation, and clinical trials involving human subjects.	Reformatted, renumbered, and rewritten to be consistent across accreditation programs.

Previous Standards	Current Standards	Comments
RI.1.2.1.3 All patients asked to participate in a research project are given a description of alternative services that might also prove advantageous to them.	RI.2.180 The hospital protects research subjects and respects their rights during research, investigation, and clinical trials involving human subjects.	Reformatted, renumbered, and rewritten to be consistent across accreditation programs.
RI.1.2.1.4 All patients asked to participate in a research project are given a full explanation of the procedures to be followed, especially those that are experimental in nature.	RI.2.180 The hospital protects research subjects and respects their rights during research, investigation, and clinical trials involving human subjects.	Reformatted, renumbered, and rewritten to be consistent across accreditation programs.
RI.1.2.1.5 All patients asked to participate in a research project are told that they may refuse to participate, and that their refusal will not compromise their access to services.	RI.2.180 The hospital protects research subjects and respects their rights during research, investigation, and clinical trials involving human subjects.	Reformatted, renumbered, and rewritten to be consistent across accreditation programs.
RI.1.2.2 Patients and, when appropriate, their families are informed about the outcomes of care, including unanticipated outcomes.	RI.2.90 Patients and, when appropriate, their families are informed about the outcomes of care, treatment, and services, including unanticipated outcomes.	Reformatted, renumbered, and rewritten to be consistent across accreditation programs.
RI.1.2.3 The family participates in care decisions.	RI.2.30 Patients are involved in decisions about care, treatment, and services provided.	Reformatted, renumbered, and rewritten to be consistent across accreditation programs.
RI.1.2.4 Patients are involved in resolving dilemmas about care decisions.	RI.2.30 Patients are involved in decisions about care, treatment, and services provided.	Reformatted, renumbered, and rewritten to be consistent across accreditation programs.
RI.1.2.5 The hospital addresses advance directives.	RI.2.80 The hospital addresses the wishes of the patient relating to end-of-life decisions.	Reformatted, renumbered, and rewritten to be consistent across accreditation programs.
RI.1.2.6 The hospital addresses withholding resuscitative services.	RI.2.80 The hospital addresses the wishes of the patient relating to end-of-life decisions.	Reformatted, renumbered, and rewritten to be consistent across accreditation programs.
RI.1.2.7 The hospital addresses forgoing or withdrawing life-sustaining treatment.	RI.2.80 The hospital addresses the wishes of the patient relating to end-of-life decisions.	Reformatted, renumbered, and rewritten to be consistent across accreditation programs.
RI.1.2.8 The hospital addresses care at the end of life.	PC.8.70 Comfort and dignity are optimized during end-of-life care.	Reformatted, renumbered, and rewritten to be consistent across accreditation programs.
RI.1.2.9 Patients have the right to appropriate assessment and management of pain.	RI.2.160 Patients have the right to pain management.	Reformatted, renumbered, and rewritten to be consistent across accreditation programs.
RI.1.3 *The hospital demonstrates respect for the following patient needs:* RI.1.3.1 confidentiality	RI.2.130 The hospital respects the needs of patients for confidentiality, privacy, and security.	Reformatted, renumbered, and rewritten to be consistent across accreditation programs.
RI.1.3 *The hospital demonstrates respect for the following patient needs:* RI.1.3.2 privacy	RI.2.130 The hospital respects the needs of patients for confidentiality, privacy, and security.	Reformatted, renumbered, and rewritten to be consistent across accreditation programs.
RI.1.3 *The hospital demonstrates respect for the following patient needs:* RI.1.3.3 security	RI.2.130 The hospital respects the needs of patients for confidentiality, privacy, and security.	Reformatted, renumbered, and rewritten to be consistent across accreditation programs.
RI.1.3 *The hospital demonstrates respect for the following patient needs:* RI.1.3.4 resolution of complaints.	RI.2.120 The hospital addresses the resolution of complaints from patients and their families.	Reformatted, renumbered, and rewritten to be consistent across accreditation programs.
RI.1.3 *The hospital demonstrates respect for the following patient needs:* RI.1.3.5 pastoral care and other spiritual services;	RI.2.10 The hospital respects the rights of patients.	Reformatted, renumbered, and rewritten to be consistent across accreditation programs.
RI.1.3 *The hospital demonstrates respect for the following patient needs:* RI.1.3.6 communication.	RI.2.100 The hospital respects the patient's right to and need for effective communication.	Reformatted, renumbered, and rewritten to be consistent across accreditation programs.
RI.1.3.6.1 When the hospital restricts a patient's visitors, mail, telephone calls, or other forms of communication, the restrictions are evaluated for their therapeutic effectiveness.	RI.2.100 The hospital respects the patient's right to and need for effective communication.	Reformatted, renumbered, and rewritten to be consistent across accreditation programs.
RI.1.3.6.1.1 Any restrictions on communication are fully explained to the patient and family, and are determined with their participation.	RI.2.100 The hospital respects the patient's right to and need for effective communication.	Reformatted, renumbered, and rewritten to be consistent across accreditation programs.

Crosswalks of Standards

Previous Standards	Current Standards	Comments
RI.1.4 Each patient receives a written statement of his or her rights.	RI.2.20 Patients receive information about their rights.	Requirement added to RI.2.20 to address the patient's right to access, request amendment, and receive an accounting of disclosures regarding his or her health information.
RI.1.5 The hospital supports the patient's rights to access protective services.	RI.2.170 Patients have a right to access protective and advocacy services.	Reformatted, renumbered, and rewritten to be consistent across accreditation programs.
RI.2 The hospital implements policy and procedures, developed with the medical staff's participation, for the procuring and donations of organs and other tissues.	LD.3.110 The hospital implements policies and procedures developed with the medical staff's participation for procuring and donating organs and other tissues.	Reformatted, renumbered, and rewritten to be consistent across accreditation programs.
RI.3 The hospital protects patients and respects their rights during research, investigation, and clinical trials involving human subjects.	RI.2.180 The hospital protects research subjects and respects their rights during research, investigation, and clinical trials involving human subjects.	Reformatted, renumbered, and rewritten to be consistent across accreditation programs.
RI.3.1 All consent forms address the information specified in RI.1.2.1.1 through RI.1.2.1.5; indicate the name of the person who provided the information and the date the form was signed; and address the participant's right to privacy, confidentiality, and safety.	RI.2.180 The hospital protects research subjects and respects their rights during research, investigation, and clinical trials involving human subjects.	Reformatted, renumbered, and rewritten to be consistent across accreditation programs.
RI.4 The hospital operates according to a code of ethical behavior.	RI.1.10 The hospital follows ethical behavior in its care, treatment, and services and business practices.	Part of the concept of LD.1.6 was moved to RI.1.10. In addition, HR.6, HR.6.1, and HR.6.2 were moved to RI.1.10.
RI.4.1 The code addresses marketing, admission, transfer and discharge, and billing practices.	RI.1.10 The hospital follows ethical behavior in its care, treatment, and services and business practices.	Reformatted, renumbered, and rewritten to be consistent across accreditation programs.
RI.4.2 The code addresses the relationship of the hospital and its staff members to other health care providers, educational institutions, and payers.	RI.1.20 The hospital addresses conflicts of interest.	Reformatted, renumbered, and rewritten to be consistent across accreditation programs.
RI.4.3 In hospitals with longer lengths of stay, the code addresses a patient's right to perform or refuse to perform tasks in or for the hospital.	RI.2.190 In hospitals that provide opportunities for work, a defined policy addresses situations in which patients work.	Reformatted, renumbered, and rewritten to be consistent across accreditation programs.
RI.4.4 The hospital's code of ethical business and professional behavior protects the integrity of clinical decision making, regardless of how the hospital compensates or shares financial risk with its leaders, managers, clinical staff, and licensed independent practitioners.	RI.1.30 The integrity of decisions is based on identified care, treatment, and service needs of the patients.	Reformatted, renumbered, and rewritten to be consistent across accreditation programs.
CC.6 An established procedure(s) is used to resolve denial-of-care conflicts. When care or services are subject to internal or external review that results in the denial of care, services or payment, the hospital makes decisions regarding the provision of ongoing care or discharge based on the assessed needs of the patient.	RI.1.40 When care, treatment, and services are subject to internal or external review that results in the denial of care, treatment, services or payment, the hospital makes decisions regarding the provision of ongoing care, treatment, services, or discharge based on the assessed needs of the patients.	Reformatted, renumbered, and rewritten to be consistent across accreditation programs.
	RI.2.50 Consent is obtained for recording or filming made for purposes other than the identification, diagnosis, or treatment of the patients.	New standard based on a Joint Commission standards clarification/frequently asked question.
	RI.2.70 Patients have the right to refuse care, treatment, and services in accordance with law and regulation.	New standard added to more explicitly state this concept.

Previous Standards	Current Standards	Comments
EC.3.1 The hospital establishes an environment that meets the needs of patients, encourages a positive self-image, and respects their human dignity. **EC.3.2** The hospital provides an environment with appropriate space and equipment.	**RI.2.140** Patients have a right to an environment that preserves dignity and contributes to a positive self-image.	Reformatted, renumbered, and rewritten to be consistent across accreditation programs.
	RI.2.150 Patients have the right to be free from mental, physical, sexual, and verbal abuse, neglect, and exploitation.	New standard added to more specifically address safety and security of patients.
PF.3.7 Education includes information about patient responsibilities in the patient's care.	**RI.3.10** Patients are given information about their responsibilities while receiving care, treatment, and services.	Reformatted, renumbered, and rewritten to be consistent across accreditation programs.

Crosswalks of Standards

Crosswalk of Previous Standards for Hospitals to Current Provision of Care, Treatment, and Services Standards for Hospitals

This crosswalk is designed to show where the previous Assessment of Patients (PE), Care of Patients (TX), Education (PF), and Continuum of Care (CC) standards requirements appear in the new PC standards. The left column (Previous Standards) lists consecutively each previous PE, TX, PF, and CC standard. The middle column, Current Standards, indicates the new PC standards. The right column, Comments, identifies what changes have occurred between the previous standards and the current standards.

Previous Standards	Current Standards	Comments
CC.1 Within its capability, the hospital has a process to provide access to the appropriate level of care and services based on the patient's assessed needs.	**PC.1.10** The hospital accepts for care, treatment, and services only those patients whose identified care, treatment, and service needs it can meet.	Reformatted, renumbered, and rewritten to be consistent across accreditation programs.
CC.2 A patient is accepted to appropriate care and services based on the hospital's assessment procedures.	**PC.1.10** The hospital accepts for care, treatment, and services only those patients whose identified care, treatment, and service needs it can meet.	Reformatted, renumbered, and rewritten to be consistent across accreditation programs.
CC.2.1 Criteria define the information necessary to determine the appropriate care, service, and setting.	**PC.1.10** The hospital accepts for care, treatment, and services only those patients whose identified care, treatment, and service needs it can meet.	Reformatted, renumbered, and rewritten to be consistent across accreditation programs.
CC.3 The hospital provides for continuity over time among the care and services provided to a patient.	**PC.5.60** The hospital coordinates the care, treatment, and services provided to a patient as part of the plan for care, treatment, and services and consistent with the hospital's scope of care, treatment, and services.	Reformatted, renumbered, and rewritten to be consistent across accreditation programs.
CC.3.1 The hospital provides for coordination of care and services among health professionals and settings.	**PC.5.60** The hospital coordinates the care, treatment, and services provided to a patient as part of the plan for care, treatment, and services and consistent with the hospital's scope of care, treatment, and services.	Reformatted, renumbered, and rewritten to be consistent across accreditation programs.
CC.4 Referral, transfer, discontinuation of services, or discharge of a patient to other levels of care, health professionals, or settings is based on the patient's assessed needs and each hospital's capability to provide needed care and services.	**PC.15.20** A patient's transfer or discharge to another level of care, treatment, and services, different professionals, or different settings is based on the patient's assessed needs and the hospital's capabilities.	Reformatted, renumbered, and rewritten to be consistent across accreditation programs.
CC.4.1 The follow-up process provides for continuing care to meet the patient's needs.	**PC.15.10** A process addresses the needs for continuing care, treatment, and services after discharge or transfer.	Reformatted, renumbered, and rewritten to be consistent across accreditation programs.
CC.4.1.1 The patient is informed in a timely manner of the need for planning for discharge or transfer to another organization or level of care.	**PC.15.20** A patient's transfer or discharge to another level of care, treatment, and services, different professionals, or different settings is based on the patient's assessed needs and the hospital's capabilities.	Reformatted, renumbered, and rewritten to be consistent across accreditation programs.
CC.5 Appropriate information related to the care and services provided is exchanged when a patient is accepted, referred, transferred, discontinued service, or discharged to receive further care or services.	**PC.15.30** When patients are transferred or discharged, appropriate information related to the care, treatment, and services provided is exchanged with other providers.	Reformatted, renumbered, and rewritten to be consistent across accreditation programs.

Previous Standards	Current Standards	Comments
CC.6 An established procedure(s) is used to resolve denial-of-care conflicts. When care or services are subject to internal or external review that results in a denial of care, services, or payment, the hospital makes decisions regarding the provision of ongoing care or discharge based on the assessed needs of the patient.		Moved to standard **RI.1.40**.
PE.1 Each patient's physical, psychological, and social status are assessed.	**PC.2.20** The hospital defines in writing the data and information gathered during assessment and reassessment. **PC.2.130** Initial assessments are performed as defined by the hospital.	Reformatted, renumbered, and rewritten to be consistent across accreditation programs.
PE.1.1 The scope and intensity of any further assessment are based on the patient's diagnosis, the care setting, the patient's desire for care, and the patient's response to any previous care.	**PC.2.20** The hospital defines in writing the data and information gathered during assessment and reassessment. **PC.8.70** Comfort and dignity are optimized during end-of-life care.	Reformatted, renumbered, and rewritten to be consistent across accreditation programs.
PE.1.2 Nutritional status is assessed when warranted by the patient's needs or condition.		Addressed in the assessment standards **PC.2.20**, **PC.2.120**, **PC.2.130**, and **PC.2.150**.
PE.1.3 Functional status is assessed when warranted by the patient's needs or condition.		Addressed in the assessment standards **PC.2.20**, **PC.2.120**, **PC.2.130**, and **PC.2.150**.
PE.1.3.1 All patients referred for rehabilitation services receive a functional assessment.		Addressed in the assessment standards **PC.2.20**, **PC.2.120**, **PC.2.130**, and **PC.2.150**.
PE.1.4 Pain is assessed in all patients.	**PC.8.10** When pain is identified, the patient is assessed and treated by the hospital or referred for treatment.	Reformatted, renumbered, and rewritten to be consistent across accreditation programs.
PE.1.5 Diagnostic testing necessary for determining the patient's health care needs is performed.	**PC.3.230** Diagnostic testing necessary for determining the patient's health care needs is performed.	Reformatted, renumbered, and rewritten to be consistent across accreditation programs.
PE.1.5.1 When a test report requires clinical interpretation, any relevant clinical information is provided with the request.	**PC.3.230** Diagnostic testing necessary for determining the patient's health care needs is performed.	Reformatted, renumbered, and rewritten to be consistent across accreditation programs.
PE.1.6 The need for a discharge planning assessment is determined.	**PC.15.20** A patient's transfer or discharge to another level of care, treatment, and services, different professionals, or different settings is based on the patient's assessed needs and the hospital's capabilities.	Reformatted, renumbered, and rewritten to be consistent across accreditation programs.
PE.1.7 Each admitted patient's initial assessment is conducted within a time frame specified by hospital policy.	**PC.2.120** The hospital defines in writing the time frame(s) for conducting the initial assessment(s).	Reformatted, renumbered, and rewritten to be consistent across accreditation programs.
PE.1.7.1 The patient's history and physical examination, nursing assessment, and other screening assessments are completed within 24 hours of admission as an inpatient.	**PC.2.120** The hospital defines in writing the time frame(s) for conducting the initial assessment(s).	Reformatted, renumbered, and rewritten to be consistent across accreditation programs.
PE.1.7.1.1 If a history and a physical examination have been performed within 30 days before admission, a durable, legible copy of this report may be used in the patient's medical record, provided any changes that may have occurred are recorded in the medical record at the time of admission.	**PC.2.120** The hospital defines in writing the time frame(s) for conducting the initial assessment(s).	Reformatted, renumbered, and rewritten to be consistent across accreditation programs.
PE.1.8 Before surgery, the patient's physical examination and medical history, any indicated diagnostic tests, and a preoperative diagnosis are completed and recorded in the patient's medical record.		Addressed in **IM.6.30**.

Crosswalks of Standards

Previous Standards	Current Standards	Comments
PE.1.8.1 Any patient for whom moderate or deep sedation or anesthesia is contemplated receives a presedation or preanesthesia assessment.	**PC.13.20** Operative or other procedures and/or the administration of moderate or deep sedation or anesthesia are planned.	Reformatted, renumbered, and rewritten to be consistent across accreditation programs.
PE.1.8.2 Before anesthesia, the patient is determined to be an appropriate candidate for the planned anesthesia.	**PC.13.20** Operative or other procedures and/or the administration of moderate or deep sedation or anesthesia are planned.	Reformatted, renumbered, and rewritten to be consistent across accreditation programs.
PE.1.8.3 The patient is reevaluated immediately before moderate or deep sedation use and before anesthesia induction.	**PC.13.20** Operative or other procedures and/or the administration of moderate or deep sedation or anesthesia are planned.	Reformatted, renumbered, and rewritten to be consistent across accreditation programs.
PE.1.8.4 The patient's postoperative status is assessed on admission to and discharge from the postanesthesia recovery area.	**PC.13.30** Patients are monitored during the procedure and/or administration of moderate or deep sedation or anesthesia.	Reformatted, renumbered, and rewritten to be consistent across accreditation programs.
PE.1.9 Possible victims of abuse are identified using criteria developed by the hospital.	**PC.3.10** Patients who may be victims of abuse or neglect are assessed (see standard RI.2.150).	Reformatted, renumbered, and rewritten to be consistent across accreditation programs.
PE.1.10 Pathology and clinical laboratory services and consultation are readily available to meet patients' needs.		Addressed in **LD.3.10**.
PE.1.10.1 The hospital provides for prompt performance of adequate examinations in anatomic pathology, hematology, chemistry, microbiology, clinical microscopy, parasitology, immunohematology, serology, virology, and nuclear medicine related to pathology and clinical laboratory services.		Addressed in **LD.3.10**.
PE.1.10.2 While the patient is under the hospital's care, all laboratory testing is done in the hospital's laboratories or approved reference laboratories.		Addressed in **LD.3.50**.
PE.1.10.2.1 When organized central pathology and clinical laboratory services are not offered, the hospital identifies acceptable reference or contract laboratory services.		Addressed in **LD.3.50**.
PE.1.10.2.2 Reference and contract laboratory services meet applicable federal standards for clinical laboratories.		Addressed in **LD.3.50**.
PE.1.11 The hospital defines the extent to which the test results are used in an individual's care (definitive or used only as a screen).	**PC.16.10** The hospital defines the extent to which waived test results are used in patient care, treatment, and services (definitively or only as a screen).	Reformatted, renumbered, and rewritten to be consistent across accreditation programs.
PE.1.12 The hospital identifies the staff members responsible for performing and supervising waived testing.	**PC.16.20** The hospital identifies the staff responsible for performing and supervising waived testing.	Reformatted, renumbered, and rewritten to be consistent across accreditation programs.
PE.1.13 Those performing tests have adequate, specific training and orientation to perform the tests, and demonstrate satisfactory levels of competence.	**PC.16.30** Staff performing tests has adequate, specific training and orientation to perform the tests and demonstrates satisfactory levels of competence.	Reformatted, renumbered, and rewritten to be consistent across accreditation programs.
PE.1.14 Policies and procedures governing specific testing-related processes are current and readily available.	**PC.16.40** Approved policies and procedures governing specific testing-related processes are current and readily available.	Reformatted, renumbered, and rewritten to be consistent across accreditation programs.
PE.1.15 Quality control checks, as defined by the hospital, are conducted on each procedure.	**PC.16.50** Quality control checks, as defined by the hospital, are conducted on each procedure.	Reformatted, renumbered, and rewritten to be consistent across accreditation programs.
PE.1.15.1 At a minimum, manufacturers' instructions are followed.	**PC.16.50** Quality control checks, as defined by the hospital, are conducted on each procedure.	Reformatted, renumbered, and rewritten to be consistent across accreditation programs.
PE.1.15.2 Appropriate quality control and test records are maintained.	**PC.16.60** Appropriate quality control and test records are maintained.	Reformatted, renumbered, and rewritten to be consistent across accreditation programs.
PE.2 Each patient is reassessed at points designated in hospital policy.	**PC.2.150** Patients are reassessed as needed.	Reformatted, renumbered, and rewritten to be consistent across accreditation programs.

Previous Standards	Current Standards	Comments
PE.2.1 Reassessment occurs at regular intervals in the course of care.	PC.2.150 Patients are reassessed as needed.	Reformatted, renumbered, and rewritten to be consistent across accreditation programs.
PE.2.2 Reassessment determines a patient's response to care.	PC.2.150 Patients are reassessed as needed.	Reformatted, renumbered, and rewritten to be consistent across accreditation programs.
PE.2.3 Significant change in a patient's condition results in reassessment.	PC.2.150 Patients are reassessed as needed.	Reformatted, renumbered, and rewritten to be consistent across accreditation programs.
PE.2.4 Significant change in a patient's diagnosis results in reassessment.	PC.2.150 Patients are reassessed as needed.	Reformatted, renumbered, and rewritten to be consistent across accreditation programs.
PE.3 Staff members integrate the information from various assessments of the patient to identify and assign priorities to his or her care needs.	PC.4.10 Development of a plan for care, treatment, and services is individualized and appropriate to the patient's needs, strengths, limitations and goals.	Reformatted, renumbered, and rewritten to be consistent across accreditation programs.
PE.3.1 Staff members base care decisions on the identified patient needs and care priorities.	PC.4.10 Development of a plan for care, treatment, and services is individualized and appropriate to the patient's needs, strengths, limitations, and goals.	Reformatted, renumbered, and rewritten to be consistent across accreditation programs.
PE.4 The hospital has defined patient assessment activities in writing.	PC.2.20 The hospital defines in writing the data and information gathered during assessment and reassessment.	Reformatted, renumbered, and rewritten to be consistent across accreditation programs.
PE.4.1 The hospital defines the scope of assessment performed by each discipline.	PC.2.20 The hospital defines in writing the data and information gathered during assessment and reassessment.	Reformatted, renumbered, and rewritten to be consistent across accreditation programs.
PE.4.2 A licensed independent practitioner with appropriate clinical privileges determines the scope of assessment and care for patients in need of emergency care.		Addressed in assessment standards and PC.2.20 and MS 2.20.
PE.4.3 A registered nurse assesses the patient's need for nursing care in all settings where nursing care is provided.	PC.2.130 Initial assessments are performed as defined by the hospital.	Reformatted, renumbered, and rewritten to be consistent across accreditation programs.
PE.5 The assessment process for an infant, child, or adolescent patient is individualized.		Addressed in the assessment standards PC.2.20, PC.2.120, PC.2.130, and PC.2.150.
PE.6 The special needs of patients who are receiving treatment for emotional or behavioral disorders are addressed by the assessment process.	PC.3.130 The needs of patients receiving treatment for emotional or behavioral disorders are assessed.	Reformatted, renumbered, and rewritten to be consistent across accreditation programs.
PE.7 The special needs of patients who are receiving treatment for alcoholism or other drug dependencies are addressed by the assessment process.	PC.3.120 The needs of patients receiving psychosocial services to treat alcoholism or other substance use disorders are assessed.	Reformatted, renumbered, and rewritten to be consistent across accreditation programs.
PE.8 Patients who are possible victims of alleged or suspected abuse or neglect have special needs relative to the assessment process.	PC.3.10 Patients who may be victims of abuse or neglect are assessed (see standard RI.2.150).	Reformatted, renumbered, and rewritten to be consistent across accreditation programs.
TX.1 Care, treatment, and rehabilitation are planned to ensure that they are appropriate to the patient's needs and severity of disease, condition, impairment, or disability.	PC.4.10 Development of a plan for care, treatment, and services is individualized and appropriate to the patient's needs, strengths, limitations, and goals.	Reformatted, renumbered, and rewritten to be consistent across accreditation programs.
TX.1.1 Settings and services required to meet patient care goals are identified, planned, and provided if appropriate.	PC.4.10 Development of a plan for care, treatment, and services is individualized and appropriate to the patient's needs, strengths, limitations, and goals.	Reformatted, renumbered, and rewritten to be consistent across accreditation programs.
TX.1.1.1 When care is not planned to meet all identified needs, this is documented in the medical record.		This standard has been deleted.
TX.1.2 Care is planned and provided in an interdisciplinary, collaborative manner by qualified individuals.	PC.5.50 Care, treatment, and services are provided in an interdisciplinary, collaborative manner.	Reformatted, renumbered, and rewritten to be consistent across accreditation programs.

Crosswalks of Standards

Previous Standards	Current Standards	Comments
TX.1.2.1 Patient care procedures (such as bathing) are performed in a manner that respects privacy.		Privacy is addressed at RI.2.130.
TX.1.3 Patients' progress is periodically evaluated against care goals and the plan of care and when indicated, the plan or goals are revised.	PC.4.10 Development of a plan for care, treatment, and services is individualized and appropriate to the patient's needs, strengths, limitations, and goals.	Reformatted, renumbered, and rewritten to be consistent across accreditation programs.
TX.2 Moderate or deep sedation and anesthesia are provided by qualified individuals.	PC.13.20 Operative or other procedures and/or the administration of moderate or deep sedation or anesthesia are planned.	Reformatted, renumbered, and rewritten to be consistent across accreditation programs.
TX.2.1 A presedation or preanesthesia assessment is performed for each patient before beginning moderate or deep sedation and before anesthesia induction.	PC.13.20 Operative or other procedures and/or the administration of moderate or deep sedation or anesthesia are planned.	Reformatted, renumbered, and rewritten to be consistent across accreditation programs.
TX.2.1.1 Each patient's moderate or deep sedation and anesthesia care is planned.	PC.13.20 Operative or other procedures and/or the administration of moderate or deep sedation or anesthesia are planned.	Reformatted, renumbered, and rewritten to be consistent across accreditation programs.
TX.2.2 Sedation and anesthesia options and risks are discussed with the patient and family prior to administration.		Addressed in RI.2.40.
TX.2.3 Each patient's physiological status is monitored during sedation or anesthesia administration.	PC.13.30 Patients are monitored during the procedure and/or administration of moderate or deep sedation or anesthesia.	Reformatted, renumbered, and rewritten to be consistent across accreditation programs.
TX.2.4 The patient's postprocedure status is assessed on admission to and before discharge from the postsedation or postanesthesia recovery area.	PC.13.40 Patients are monitored during the period immediately after the procedure and/or administration of moderate or deep sedation or anesthesia.	Reformatted, renumbered, and rewritten to be consistent across accreditation programs.
TX.2.4.1 Patients are discharged from the postsedation or postanesthesia recovery area and the hospital by a qualified licensed independent practitioner or according to criteria approved by the medical staff.	PC.13.40 Patients are monitored during the period immediately after the procedure and/or administration of moderate or deep sedation or anesthesia.	Reformatted, renumbered, and rewritten to be consistent across accreditation programs.
TX.3 Medication use processes are organized and systematic throughout the hospital.		Concept embedded throughout MM chapter.
TX.3.1 The hospital identified an appropriate selection of medications available for prescribing or ordering.		Moved to MM.2.10.
TX.3.2 The hospital addressed prescribing or ordering and procuring medications not available in the hospital.		Moved to MM.2.10.
TX.3.3 Policies and procedures support safe medication prescription or ordering.		Addressed in MM.2.20, MM.3.10, MM.5.10, MM.7.10, and MM.7.40.
TX.3.4 Preparing and dispensing medication(s) adhere to law, regulation, licensure, and professional standards of practice.		Addressed in MM.4.20, MM.4.30, and MM.4.40.
TX.3.5 Preparation and dispensing of medication(s) is appropriately controlled.		Addressed in MM.4.20 and MM.4.40.
TX.3.5.1 A patient medication dose system is implemented.		Addressed in MM.4.30 and MM.4.40.
TX.3.5.2 Pharmacists review all prescriptions or orders.		Addressed in MM.4.10.
TX.3.5.3 When preparing and dispensing a medication(s) for a patient, important patient medication information is considered.		Addressed in MM.1.10.
TX.3.5.4 Pharmacy services are available when the pharmacy department is closed or not available.		Addressed in MM.4.50.

Previous Standards	Current Standards	Comments
TX.3.5.5 Emergency medications are consistently available, controlled, and secure in the pharmacy and patient care areas.		Addressed in MM.2.30.
TX.3.5.6 A medication recall system provides for retrieval and safe disposition of discontinued and recalled medications.		Addressed in MM.4.70.
TX.3.6 Prescriptions or orders are verified and patients are identified before medication is administered.		Addressed in MM.5.10.
TX.3.7 The hospital has alternative medication administration systems.		Addressed in MM.2.40 and MM.5.20.
TX.3.8 Investigational medications are safely controlled, administered, and destroyed.		Addressed in MM.7.40.
TX.3.9 Medication effects on patients are continually monitored.		Addressed in MM.3.20, MM.4.80, MM.6.10, MM.6.20, and MM.8.10.
TX.4 Each patient's nutrition care is planned.		Addressed in the care planning standard PC.4.10.
TX.4.1 An interdisciplinary nutrition therapy plan is developed and periodically updated for patients at nutritional risk.		Addressed in the care planning standard PC.4.10.
TX.4.1.1 When appropriate to the patient groups served by a unit, meals and snacks support program goals.	PC.7.10 The hospital has a process for preparing and/or distributing food and nutrition products as appropriate to the care, treatment, and services provided.	Reformatted, renumbered, and rewritten to be consistent across accreditation programs.
TX.4.2 Authorized individuals prescribe or order food and nutrition products in a timely manner.	PC.7.10 The hospital has a process for preparing and/or distributing food and nutrition products as appropriate to the care, treatment, and services provided.	Reformatted, renumbered, and rewritten to be consistent across accreditation programs.
TX.4.3 Responsibilities are assigned for all activities involved in safe and accurate provision of food and nutrition products.	PC.7.10 The hospital has a process for preparing and/or distributing food and nutrition products as appropriate to the care, treatment, and services provided.	Reformatted, renumbered, and rewritten to be consistent across accreditation programs.
TX.4.4 Food and nutrition products are distributed and administered in a safe, accurate, timely, and acceptable manner.	PC.7.10 The hospital has a process for preparing and/or distributing food and nutrition products as appropriate to the care, treatment, and services provided.	Reformatted, renumbered, and rewritten to be consistent across accreditation programs.
TX.4.5 Each patient's response to nutrition care is monitored.		Addressed in the care planning standard PC.4.10.
TX.4.6 The nutrition care service meets patients' needs for special diets and accommodates altered diet schedules.	PC.7.10 The hospital has a process for preparing and/or distributing food and nutrition products as appropriate to the care, treatment, and services provided.	Reformatted, renumbered, and rewritten to be consistent across accreditation programs.
TX.4.7 Nutrition care practices are standardized throughout the hospital.		Addressed in care planning standard PC.4.10, as well as PC.5.50 and LD.3.30.
TX.5 The medical staff defines the scope of assessment for operative and other procedures.	PC.13.20 Operative or other procedures and/or the administration of moderate or deep sedation or anesthesia are planned.	Reformatted, renumbered, and rewritten to be consistent across accreditation programs.
TX.5.1 Determining the appropriateness of a procedure for each patient is based, in part, on a review of		This standard is less specific, but the topic is still addressed in PC.13.20.
TX.5.1.1 the patient's history;		This standard is less specific, but the topic is still addressed in PC.13.20.
TX.5.1.2 the patient's physical status;		This standard is less specific, but the topic is still addressed in PC.13.20.
TX.5.1.3 diagnostic data;		This standard is less specific, but the topic is still addressed in PC.13.20.
TX.5.1.4 the risks and benefits of procedures; and		This standard is less specific, but the topic is still addressed in PC.13.20.

Crosswalks of Standards

Previous Standards	Current Standards	Comments
TX.5.1.5 the need to administer blood or blood components.		This standard is less specific, but the topic is still addressed in PC.13.20.
TX.5.2 Before obtaining informed consent, the risks, benefits, and potential complications associated with procedures are discussed with the patient and family.		Addressed in RI.2.40.
TX.5.2.1 Alternative options are considered.		Addressed in RI.2.40.
TX.5.2.2 Discussions with the patient and family about the need for, risk of, and alternatives to blood transfusion when blood or blood components may be needed are considered.		Addressed in RI.2.40.
TX.5.3 Plans of care are developed and documented in the patient's medical record before the operative or other procedure is performed.		Addressed in IM.6.30.
TX.5.4 The patient is monitored during the postprocedure period.	PC.13.40 Patients are monitored during the period immediately after the procedure and/or administration of moderate or deep sedation or anesthesia.	Reformatted, renumbered, and rewritten to be consistent across accreditation programs.
TX.6 Functional rehabilitation status is assessed to determine the current level of functioning, self-care, self-responsibility, independence, and quality of life.		Addressed in the assessment standards PC.2.20, PC.2.120, PC.2.130, and PC.2.150.
TX.6.1 Qualified rehabilitation professionals determine the scope of the functional rehabilitation assessment; provide rehabilitation services consistent with professional licensure laws, regulations, registration, and certification; and implement the rehabilitation plan with the patient and his or her family, social network, or support system.		Addressed in the assessment standards PC.2.20, PC.2.120, PC.2.130, and PC.2.150.
TX.6.1.1 Discharge planning from rehabilitation services is integrated into the functional rehabilitation assessment.		Addressed in the assessment standards PC.2.20, PC.2.120, PC.2.130, and PC.2.150.
TX.6.2 Reassessment of the patient receiving rehabilitation services is an ongoing process.		Addressed in the assessment standards PC.2.20, PC.2.120, PC.2.130, and PC.2.150.
TX.6.3 An interdisciplinary rehabilitation plan and goals, developed by qualified professionals, in conjunction with the patient and/or his or her family social network, or support system, and based on a functional assessment of patient needs, guide the provision of rehabilitation services, appropriate to the patient's environment.		Addressed in the care planning standard PC.4.10.
TX.6.4 Rehabilitation services are appropriate to the patient's needs and severity of disease, condition, impairment, or disability.		Addressed in the care planning standard PC.4.10.
TX.6.5 Rehabilitation outcomes are restoration, improvement, or maintenance of the patient's optimal level of functioning, self-care, self-responsibility, independence, and quality of life.		Addressed in the care planning standard PC.4.10.
TX.7 The hospital ensures that special interventions are safely and appropriately used.		Addressed in LD.3.90.
TX.7.1 The leaders establish and communicate the hospital's philosophy on the use of restraint and seclusion to all staff who have direct care responsibility.	PC.12.10 The leaders establish and communicate the hospital's philosophy on the use of restraint and seclusion to all staff with direct care responsibility.	Reformatted, renumbered, and rewritten to be consistent across accreditation programs.

Previous Standards	Current Standards	Comments
TX.7.1.1 Staffing levels and assignments are set to minimize circumstances that give rise to restraint or seclusion use and to maximize safety when restraint and seclusion are used.	PC.12.20 Staffing levels and assignments are set to minimize circumstances that give rise to restraint or seclusion use and to maximize safety when restraint and seclusion are used.	Reformatted, renumbered, and rewritten to be consistent across accreditation programs.
TX.7.1.2 Staff are trained and competent to minimize the use of restraint and seclusion, and when their use is indicated, to use them safely.	PC.12.30 Staff is trained and competent to minimize the use of restraint and seclusion, and, when use is indicated, to use restraint or seclusion safely.	Reformatted, renumbered, and rewritten to be consistent across accreditation programs.
TX.7.1.3 The initial assessment of each patient at the time of admission or intake assists in obtaining information about the patient that could help minimize the use of restraint or seclusion.	PC.12.40 The initial assessment of each patient at admission or intake assists in obtaining information about the patient that could help minimize the use of restraint or seclusion.	Reformatted, renumbered, and rewritten to be consistent across accreditation programs.
TX.7.1.4 Nonphysical techniques are the preferred intervention in the management of behavior.	PC.12.50 Nonphysical techniques are the preferred intervention in behavior management.	Reformatted, renumbered, and rewritten to be consistent across accreditation programs.
TX.7.1.4.1 Restraint or seclusion use is limited to emergencies in which there is an imminent risk of a patient physically harming himself or herself, staff, or others, and nonphysical interventions would not be effective.	PC.12.60 Restraint or seclusion is limited to emergencies in which there is an imminent risk of a patient physically harming himself or herself, staff, or others, and nonphysical interventions would not be effective.	Reformatted, renumbered, and rewritten to be consistent across accreditation programs.
TX.7.1.5 A licensed independent practitioner orders the use of restraint or seclusion.	PC.12.70 A licensed independent practitioner orders the use of restraint or seclusion.	Reformatted, renumbered, and rewritten to be consistent across accreditation programs.
TX.7.1.5.1 The patient's family is notified promptly of the initiation of restraint or seclusion.	PC.12.80 The patient's family is notified promptly of the initiation of restraint or seclusion.	Reformatted, renumbered, and rewritten to be consistent across accreditation programs.
TX.7.1.6 A licensed independent practitioner sees and evaluates the patient in person.	PC.12.90 A licensed independent practitioner sees and evaluates the patient in person.	Reformatted, renumbered, and rewritten to be consistent across accreditation programs.
TX.7.1.7 Written or verbal orders for initial and continuing use of restraint and seclusion are time limited.	PC.12.100 Written or verbal orders for initial and continuing use of restraint and seclusion are time limited.	Reformatted, renumbered, and rewritten to be consistent across accreditation programs.
TX.7.1.8 Patients who are in restraint or seclusion are regularly reevaluated.	PC.12.110 Patients in restraint or seclusion are regularly reevaluated.	Reformatted, renumbered, and rewritten to be consistent across accreditation programs.
TX.7.1.9 Clinical leadership is informed of instances in which patients experience extended, or multiple episodes of, restraint or seclusion.	PC.12.120 Clinical leaders are told of instances in which patients experience extended or multiple episodes of restraint or seclusion.	Reformatted, renumbered, and rewritten to be consistent across accreditation programs.
TX.7.1.10 Patients in restraint or seclusion are assessed and assisted.	PC.12.130 Patients in restraint or seclusion are assessed and assisted.	Reformatted, renumbered, and rewritten to be consistent across accreditation programs.
TX.7.1.11 Patients in restraint or seclusion are monitored.	PC.12.140 Patients in restraint or seclusion are monitored.	Reformatted, renumbered, and rewritten to be consistent across accreditation programs.
TX.7.1.12 Restraint and seclusion use are discontinued when the patient meets the behavior criteria for their discontinuation.	PC.12.150 Restraint and seclusion are discontinued when the patient meets the behavior criteria for their discontinuation.	Reformatted, renumbered, and rewritten to be consistent across accreditation programs.
TX.7.1.13 The patient and staff participate in a debriefing about the restraint or seclusion episode.	PC.12.160 The patient and staff participate in a debriefing about the restraint or seclusion episode.	Reformatted, renumbered, and rewritten to be consistent across accreditation programs.
TX.7.1.14 Medical records document that the use of restraint or seclusion is consistent with hospital policy.	PC.12.170 Medical records document that the use of restraint or seclusion is consistent with hospital policy.	Reformatted, renumbered, and rewritten to be consistent across accreditation programs.
TX.7.1.15 The hospital collects data on the use of restraint and seclusion in order to monitor and improve its performance of processes that involve risks or may result in sentinel events.	PC.12.180 The hospital collects data on the use of restraint and seclusion.	Reformatted, renumbered, and rewritten to be consistent across accreditation programs.
TX.7.1.16 Hospital policy(ies) and procedure(s) address the prevention of the use of restraint and seclusion and, when employed, guide their use.	PC.12.190 Hospital policies and procedures address prevention of restraint and seclusion and, when employed, guide their use.	Reformatted, renumbered, and rewritten to be consistent across accreditation programs.

Crosswalks of Standards

Previous Standards	Current Standards	Comments
TX.7.2 Electroconvulsive and other forms of convulsive therapy are used with adequate justification, documentation, and regard for patient safety.	**PC.13.50** Electroconvulsive therapy is used with adequate justification, documentation, and regard for patient safety.	Reformatted, renumbered, and rewritten to be consistent across accreditation programs.
TX.7.3 Psychosurgery or other surgical treatments for emotional, mental, or behavioral disorders are performed with adequate justification, documentation, and regard for patient safety.	**PC.13.60** Psychosurgery or other surgical treatments for emotional, mental, or behavioral disorders are performed with adequate justification, documentation, and regard for patient safety.	Reformatted, renumbered, and rewritten to be consistent across accreditation programs.
TX.7.4 Use of behavior-management procedures conforms to the patient's treatment plan and hospital policy.	**PC.13.70** Use of behavior management procedures conforms to the patient's treatment plan and hospital policy.	Reformatted, renumbered, and rewritten to be consistent across accreditation programs.
TX.7.4.1 Qualified staff review, evaluate, and approve all behavior-management procedures.	**PC.13.70** Use of behavior management procedures conforms to the patient's treatment plan and hospital policy.	Reformatted, renumbered, and rewritten to be consistent across accreditation programs.
TX.7.5 The hospital's leaders determine the hospital's approach to the use of restraint in the care of nonpsychiatric patients, which limits its use to those situations where there is appropriate clinical justification.	**PC.11.10** The hospital's leaders determine the hospital's approach to the use of restraint for nonpsychiatric patients and limit its use to those situations where there is appropriate clinical justification.	Reformatted, renumbered, and rewritten to be consistent across accreditation programs.
TX.7.5.1 Performance improvement processes seek to identify opportunities to reduce the risks associated with restraint use through the introduction of preventive strategies, innovative alternatives, and process improvements.	**PC.11.20** Performance improvement processes seek to identify opportunities to reduce the risks associated with restraint use through preventive strategies, innovative alternatives, and process improvements.	Reformatted, renumbered, and rewritten to be consistent across accreditation programs.
TX.7.5.2 Hospital policy(ies) and procedure(s) guide appropriate and safe use of restraint.	**PC.11.30** Hospital policies and procedures guide appropriate and safe use of restraint.	Reformatted, renumbered, and rewritten to be consistent across accreditation programs.
TX.7.5.3 Any use of restraint (to which these standards apply) is initiated pursuant to either an individual order (standard **TX.7.5.3.1**) or an approved protocol (standard **TX.7.5.3.2**), the use of which is authorized by an individual order.	**PC.11.40** Any use of restraint (to which these standards apply) is initiated pursuant to either an individual order (standard **PC.11.50**) or an approved protocol (standard **PC.11.60**), the use of which is authorized by an individual order.	Reformatted, renumbered, and rewritten to be consistent across accreditation programs.
TX.7.5.3.1 Individual orders for initiation and renewal of restraint are consistent with hospital policy(ies) and procedure(s), and are consistent with the patient's needs and clinical condition.	**PC.11.50** Individual orders for initiating and renewing restraint are consistent with hospital policies and procedures and with the patient's needs and clinical condition.	Reformatted, renumbered, and rewritten to be consistent across accreditation programs.
TX.7.5.3.2 Protocols for restraint use contain criteria to ensure only clinically justified use.	**PC.11.60** Protocols for restraint use contain criteria to ensure only clinically justified use.	Reformatted, renumbered, and rewritten to be consistent across accreditation programs.
TX.7.5.4 Patients in restraint are monitored.	**PC.11.70** Patients in restraint are monitored.	Reformatted, renumbered, and rewritten to be consistent across accreditation programs.
TX.7.5.5 Each episode of restraint use is documented in the patient's medical record, consistent with hospital policy(ies) and procedure(s).	**PC.11.100** Each episode of restraint use is documented in the patient's medical record, consistent with hospital policies and procedures.	Reformatted, renumbered, and rewritten to be consistent across accreditation programs.
TX.8 Effective resuscitation services are systematically available throughout the hospital.	**PC.9.30** Resuscitation services are available throughout the hospital.	Reformatted, renumbered, and rewritten to be consistent across accreditation programs.
PF.1 The hospital plans for and supports the provision and coordination of patient education activities.		Addressed in **LD.3.120**.
PF.1.1 The hospital identifies and provides the resources necessary for achieving educational objectives.		Addressed in **LD.3.120**.
PF.2 The patient education process is coordinated among appropriate staff or disciplines who are providing care or services.	**PC.6.30** The patient receives education and training specific to the patient's abilities as appropriate to the care, treatment, and services provided by the hospital.	Reformatted, renumbered, and rewritten to be consistent across accreditation programs.

Previous Standards	Current Standards	Comments
PF.3 The patient receives education and training specific to the patient's assessed needs, abilities, learning preferences, and readiness to learn as appropriate to the care and services provided by the hospital.	PC.6.10 The patient receives education and training specific to the patient's needs and as appropriate to the care, treatment, and services provided.	Reformatted, renumbered, and rewritten to be consistent across accreditation programs.
PF.3.1 Based on assessed needs, the patient is educated about how to safely and effectively use medications, according to law and regulation, and the hospital's scope of services, as appropriate.	PC.6.10 The patient receives education and training specific to the patient's needs and as appropriate to the care, treatment, and services provided.	Reformatted, renumbered, and rewritten to be consistent across accreditation programs.
PF.3.2 The patient is educated about nutrition interventions, modified diets, or oral health, when applicable.	PC.6.10 The patient receives education and training specific to the patient's needs and as appropriate to the care, treatment, and services provided.	Reformatted, renumbered, and rewritten to be consistent across accreditation programs.
PF.3.3 The hospital assures that the patient is educated about how to safely and effectively use medical equipment or supplies, as appropriate.	PC.6.10 The patient receives education and training specific to the patient's needs and as appropriate to the care, treatment, and services provided.	Reformatted, renumbered, and rewritten to be consistent across accreditation programs.
PF.3.4 Patients are educated about pain and managing pain as part of treatment, as appropriate.	PC.6.10 The patient receives education and training specific to the patient's needs and as appropriate to the care, treatment, and services provided.	Reformatted, renumbered, and rewritten to be consistent across accreditation programs.
PF.3.5 Patients are educated about habilitation or rehabilitation techniques to help them be more functionally independent, as appropriate.	PC.6.10 The patient receives education and training specific to the patient's needs and as appropriate to the care, treatment, and services provided.	Reformatted, renumbered, and rewritten to be consistent across accreditation programs.
PF.3.6 The patient is educated about other available resources, and when necessary, how to obtain further care, services, or treatment to meet his or her identified needs.	PC.15.20 A patient's transfer or discharge to another level of care, treatment, and services, different professionals, or different settings is based on the patient's assessed needs and the hospital's capabilities.	Reformatted, renumbered, and rewritten to be consistent across accreditation programs.
PF.3.7 Education includes information about patient responsibilities in the patient's care.		Moved to RI.3.10.
PF.3.8 Education includes self-care activities, as appropriate.		Addressed in PC.6.10.
PF.3.9 Discharge instructions are given to the patient and those responsible for providing continuing care.	PC.15.20 A patient's transfer or discharge to another level of care, treatment, and services, different professionals, or different settings is based on the patient's assessed needs and the hospital's capabilities.	Reformatted, renumbered, and rewritten to be consistent across accreditation programs.
PF.3.10 Academic education is provided to children and adolescents either directly by the hospital or through other arrangements, when appropriate.	PC.6.50 The hospital provides academic education to children and youth as needed.	Reformatted, renumbered, and rewritten to be consistent across accreditation programs.
	PC.5.10 The hospital provides care, treatment, and services for each patient according to the plan for care, treatment, and services.	This standard is implicit in multiple standards, but has been newly defined here.
	PC.8.50 Unless contraindicated, the hospital accommodates patients' needs to be outdoors when patients experience long lengths of stay.	This requirement was moved to the PC chapter from previous standard EC.3.2. The other requirements of EC.3.2 remain in the renumbered standard EC.8.10.
	PC.8.60 In accordance with the patients' needs, good standards of personal hygiene and grooming are taught and maintained, particularly bathing, brushing teeth, caring for hair and nails, and using the toilet, with due regard for privacy.	New requirement applicable only to hospitals with behavioral health units.

Crosswalk of Previous Standards for Hospitals to Current Medication Management Standards for Hospitals

This crosswalk is designed to show where the previous Care of Patients (TX) standards requirements appear in the new Medication Management (MM) standards. The left column (Previous Standards) lists consecutively each previous TX standard; a standard appearing in italics in this column indicates that the standard was previously not scorable. The middle column, Current Standards, indicates the new MM standards. The right column, Comments, identifies what changes have occurred between the previous standards and the current standards.

Previous Standards	Current Standards	Comments
TX.3 *Medication use processes are organized and systematic throughout the hospital.*		Concept embedded throughout chapter.
TX.3.1 The hospital identified an appropriate selection of medications available for prescribing or ordering.	MM.2.10 Medications available for dispensing or administration are selected, listed, and procured based on criteria.	Reformatted, renumbered, and rewritten to be consistent across accreditation programs.
TX.3.2 The hospital addressed prescribing or ordering and procuring medications not available in the hospital.	MM.2.10 Medications available for dispensing or administration are selected, listed, and procured based on criteria.	Reformatted, renumbered, and rewritten to be consistent across accreditation programs.
TX.3.3 Policies and procedures support safe medication prescription or ordering.	MM.2.20 Medications are properly and safely stored throughout the hospital. MM.3.10 Only medications needed to treat the patient's condition are ordered. MM.5.10 Medications are safely and accurately administered. MM.7.10 The hospital develops processes for managing high-risk or high-alert medications. MM.7.40 Investigational medications are safely controlled and administered.	Reformatted, renumbered, and rewritten to be consistent across accreditation programs.
TX.3.4 Preparing and dispensing medication(s) adhere to law, regulation, licensure, and professional standards of practice.	MM.4.20 Medications are prepared safely. MM.4.30 Medications are appropriately labeled. MM.4.40 Medications are dispensed safely.	Reformatted, renumbered, and rewritten to be consistent across accreditation programs.
TX.3.5 Preparation and dispensing of medication(s) is appropriately controlled.	MM.4.20 Medications are prepared safely. MM.4.40 Medications are dispensed safely.	Reformatted, renumbered, and rewritten to be consistent across accreditation programs.
TX.3.5.1 A patient medication dose system is implemented.	MM.4.30 Medications are appropriately labeled. MM.4.40 Medications are dispensed safely.	Reformatted, renumbered, and rewritten to be consistent across accreditation programs.
TX.3.5.2 Pharmacists review all prescriptions or orders.	MM.4.10 All prescriptions or medication orders are reviewed for appropriateness.	Reformatted, renumbered, and rewritten to be consistent across accreditation programs.
TX.3.5.3 When preparing and dispensing a medication(s) for a patient, important patient medication information is considered.	MM.1.10 Patient-specific information is readily accessible to those involved in the medication management system.	Reformatted, renumbered, and rewritten to be consistent across accreditation programs.
TX.3.5.4 Pharmacy services are available when the pharmacy department is closed or not available.	MM.4.50 The hospital has a system for safely providing medications to meet patient needs when the pharmacy is closed.	Reformatted, renumbered, and rewritten to be consistent across accreditation programs.
TX.3.5.5 Emergency medications are consistently available, controlled, and secure in the pharmacy and patient care areas.	MM.2.30 Emergency medications and/or supplies, if any, are consistently available, controlled, and secure in the hospital's patient care areas.	Reformatted, renumbered, and rewritten to be consistent across accreditation programs.
TX.3.5.6 A medication recall system provides for retrieval and safe disposition of discontinued and recalled medications.	MM.4.70 Medications dispensed by the hospital are retrieved when recalled or discontinued by the manufacturer or the Food and Drug Administration for safety reasons.	Reformatted, renumbered, and rewritten to be consistent across accreditation programs.
TX.3.6 Prescriptions or orders are verified and patients are identified before medication is administered.	MM.5.10 Medications are safely and accurately administered.	Reformatted, renumbered, and rewritten to be consistent across accreditation programs.

Previous Standards	Current Standards	Comments
TX.3.7 The hospital has alternative medication administration systems.	MM.2.40 A process is established to safely manage medications brought into the hospital by patients or their families.	Reformatted, renumbered, and rewritten to be consistent across accreditation programs.
	MM.5.20 Self-administered medications are safely and accurately administered.	
TX.3.8 Investigational medications are safely controlled, administered, and destroyed.	MM.7.40 Investigational medications are safely controlled and administered.	Reformatted, renumbered, and rewritten to be consistent across accreditation programs.
TX.3.9 Medication effects on patients are continually monitored.	MM.6.10 The effects of medication(s) on patients are monitored.	Reformatted, renumbered, and rewritten to be consistent across accreditation programs.
	MM.3.20 Medication orders are written clearly and transcribed accurately.	New, detailed requirements, formerly appearing in TX.3.3.
	MM.4.80 Medications returned to the pharmacy are appropriately managed.	New requirement.
	MM.6.20 The hospital responds appropriately to actual or potential adverse drug events and medication errors.	Moved to this chapter from previous PI.4.3.
	MM.8.10 The hospital evaluates its medication management system.	Moved to this chapter from previous PI.3.1.1.

Crosswalk of 2004 Surveillance, Prevention, and Control of Infection Standards for Hospitals to 2005 Surveillance, Prevention, and Control of Infection Standards for Hospitals

This crosswalk is designed to show where the 2004 "Surveillance, Prevention, and Control of Infection" (IC) requirements appear in the reformatted IC standards and elements of performance (EPs) for 2005. The left column, "2004 IC Standards and EPs," lists consecutively each standard that was effective in 2004. The right column, "2005 IC Standards and EPs," identifies where the 2004 requirements are located within the new 2005 IC requirements.

2004 IC Standards and EPs	2005 IC Standards and EPs
IC.1.10	
EP 1	IC.1.10, IC.2.10, IC.4.10
EP 2	IC.2.10, EP 1
	IC.4.10, EP 1
EP 3	IC.2.10, EP 3
EP 4	IC.1.10, EP 5
IC.1.20	
EP 1	IC.7.10, EP 1
IC.2.10	
EP 1	IC.1.10, IC.2.10, IC.5.10
EP 2	IC.2.10, EP 1
EP 3	IC.2.10, EP 3, IC.3.10, EP 1
IC.3.10	
EP 1	IC.1.10, EP 5
IC.4.10	
EP 1	IC.4.10, EP 3
	IC.4.10, EP 4
	IC.4.10, EP 5
	IC.4.10, EP 6
	IC.4.10, EP 7
	IC.4.10, EP 8
EP 2	IC.4.10, EP 1
	IC.5.10, EP 7
EP 3	IC.2.10, EP 1
IC.5.10	
EP 1	IC.1.10, EP 6
IC.6.10	IC.2.10, EP 1
EP 1	IC.4.10, EP 3
	IC.4.10, EP 5
	IC.4.10, EP 6
	IC.4.10, EP 7
	IC.4.10, EP 8
EP 2	IC.2.10, EP 1
EP 3	IC.9.10, EP 1
EP 4	IC.4.10, EP 3
	IC.4.10, EP 4
	IC.4.10, EP 5
	IC.4.10, EP 6
	IC.4.10, EP 7
	IC.4.10, EP 8
IC.6.20	
EP 1	IC.9.10, EP 2
	IC.9.10, EP 3
	IC.9.10, EP 4
EP 2	IC.2.10, EP 1
	IC.2.10, EP 3
IC.6.30	
EP 1	IC.4.10

Crosswalk of Previous Improving Organization Performance Standards for Hospitals to Current Improving Organization Performance Standards for Hospitals

This crosswalk is designed to show where the Current Improving Organization Performance (PI) standards requirements appear in the reformatted PI standards. The left column (Previous Standards) lists consecutively each previous PI standard. The middle column, Current Standards, indicates the PI standards with revised numbers. The right column, Comments, identifies what changes have occurred between the previous standards and the current standards.

Previous Standards	Current Standards	Comments
PI.1 The leaders establish a planned, systematic, organizationwide approach to process design and performance measurement, analysis, and improvement.		This standard is now located in the LD chapter.
PI.1.1 The activities are planned in a collaborative and interdisciplinary manner.		This standard is now Element of Performance (EP) 5 at **LD.4.10**.
PI.2 New or modified processes are designed well.		This standard is now located at **LD.4.20**.
PI.2.1 Performance expectations are established for new and modified processes.		This standard has been deleted.
PI.2.2 The performance of new and modified processes is measured.		This standard has been deleted.
PI.3 Data are collected to monitor the stability of existing processes, identify opportunities for improvement, identify changes that will lead to improvement, or sustain improvements.	PI.1.10 The hospital collects data to monitor its performance.	Former standards PI.3–PI.3.1.3 are reflected as EPs under standards PI.2.10–PI.2.20. Standards addressing data collection were consolidated into one standard.
PI.3.1 The organization collects data to monitor its performance.	PI.1.10 The hospital collects data to monitor its performance.	
PI.3.1.1 The organization collects data to monitor the performance of processes that involve risks or may result in sentinel events.	PI.1.10 The hospital collects data to monitor its performance.	
PI.3.1.2 The organization collects data to monitor performance of areas targeted for further study.	PI.1.10 The hospital collects data to monitor its performance.	
PI.3.1.3 The organization collects data to monitor improvements in performance.	PI.1.10 The hospital collects data to monitor its performance.	
PI.4 Data are systematically aggregated and analyzed on an ongoing basis.	PI.2.10 Data are systematically aggregated and analyzed.	Reformatted, renumbered, and rewritten to be consistent across accreditation programs.
PI.4.1 Appropriate statistical techniques are used to analyze and display data.	PI.2.10 Data are systematically aggregated and analyzed.	Reformatted, renumbered, and rewritten to be consistent across accreditation programs.
PI.4.2 The organization compares its performance over time and with other sources of information.	PI.2.10 Data are systematically aggregated and analyzed.	Reformatted, renumbered, and rewritten to be consistent across accreditation programs.
PI.4.3 Undesirable patterns or trends in performance and sentinel events are intensively analyzed.	PI.2.20 Undesirable patterns or trends in performance are analyzed. PI.2.30 Processes for identifying and managing sentinel events are defined and implemented.	Reformatted, renumbered, and rewritten to be consistent across accreditation programs.
PI.4.4 The organization identifies changes that will lead to improved performance and reduce the risk of sentinel events.	PI.3.10 Information from data analysis is used to make changes that improve performance and patient safety and reduce the risk of sentinel events.	Reformatted, renumbered, and rewritten to be consistent across accreditation programs.
PI.5 Improved performance is achieved and sustained.	PI.3.10 Information from data analysis is used to make changes that improve performance and patient safety and reduce the risk of sentinel events.	Reformatted, renumbered, and rewritten to be consistent across accreditation programs.

Crosswalks of Standards

Previous Standards	Current Standards	Comments
LD.5.1 Leaders ensure that the processes for identifying and managing sentinel events are defined and implemented.	**PI.2.30** Processes for identifying and managing sentinel events are defined and implemented.	The former LD standard was moved to the PI chapter to better reflect the relationship to PI activities.
LD.5.2 Leaders ensure that an ongoing, proactive, program for identifying risks to patient safety and reducing medical/health care errors is defined and implemented.	**PI.3.20** An ongoing, proactive program for identifying and reducing adverse events and safety risks to patients is defined and implemented.	The former LD standard was moved to the PI chapter to better reflect the relationship to PI activities.

Crosswalk of Previous Standards for Hospitals to Current Leadership Standards for Hospitals

This crosswalk is designed to show where the previous Leadership (LD), Governance (GO), and Management (MA) standards requirements appear in the reformatted LD standards. The left column (Previous Standards) lists consecutively each previous standard; a standard appearing in italics in this column indicates that the standard was previously not scorable. The middle column, Current Standards, indicates the LD standards with revised numbers. The right column, Comments, identifies what changes have occurred between the previous standards and the current standards.

Previous Standards	Current Standards	Comments
GO.1 The hospital identifies how it is governed and the key individuals involved.	LD.1.10 The hospital identifies how it is governed.	Reformatted and renumbered.
GO.2 *Those responsible for governance establish policy, promote performance improvement, and provide for hospital management and planning.*	LD.1.20 Governance responsibilities are defined in writing, as applicable.	Reformatted and renumbered; standard is now scorable.
GO.2.1 The hospital's governing body or authority adopts bylaws addressing its legal accountabilities and responsibility to the patient population served.	LD.1.20 Governance responsibilities are defined in writing, as applicable.	Reformatted and renumbered.
GO.2.2 The hospital's governing body or authority provides for appropriate medical staff participation in governance.	LD.1.10 The hospital identifies how it is governed.	Reformatted and renumbered.
GO.2.2.1 The medical staff has the right to representation (through attendance and voice), by one or more medical staff at governing body meetings.	LD.1.10 The hospital identifies how it is governed.	Reformatted and renumbered.
GO.2.2.2 Medical staff members are eligible for full membership in the hospital's governing body, unless legally prohibited.	LD.1.10 The hospital identifies how it is governed.	Reformatted and renumbered.
GO.2.3 The hospital's governing body or authority establishes a criteria-based process for selecting a qualified and competent chief executive officer.	LD.1.20 Governance responsibilities are defined in writing, as applicable.	Reformatted and renumbered.
GO.2.4 The hospital's governing body or authority provides for compliance with applicable law and regulation.	LD.1.30 The hospital complies with applicable law and regulation.	Reformatted and renumbered.
GO.2.5 The hospital's governing body provides for the collaboration of leaders in developing, reviewing, and revising policies and procedures.	LD.1.20 Governance responsibilities are defined in writing, as applicable.	Reformatted and renumbered.
GO.2.6 The hospital's governing body or authority provides for conflict resolution.		Requirement deleted.
MA.1 The chief executive officer, selected by the governing body, is responsible for operating the hospital according to the authority conferred by the governing body.	LD.2.10 An individual(s) or designee(s) is responsible for operating the hospital according to the authority conferred by governance.	Reformatted and renumbered.
MA.1.1 The chief executive officer has the education and experience necessary to carry out the responsibilities of the position.	HR.1.20 The hospital has a process to ensure that a person's qualifications are consistent with his or her job responsibilities.	Addressed in HR chapter.
MA.2 The chief executive officer provides for the hospital's compliance with applicable law and regulation.	LD.1.30 The hospital complies with applicable law and regulation.	Reformatted and renumbered.
MA.2.1 The chief executive officer reviews and promptly responds to reports and recommendations from planning, regulatory, and inspecting agencies, as outlined by the governing body.	LD.2.10 An individual(s) or designee(s) is responsible for operating the hospital according to the authority conferred by governance.	Reformatted and renumbered.

Crosswalks of Standards

Previous Standards	Current Standards	Comments
MA.3 The chief executive officer, working with management, clinical, and administrative staff, provides for a well-managed hospital with clear lines of responsibility and accountability within departments and between departments and administration.	LD.2.20 Each hospital program, service, site, or department has effective leadership.	Reformatted and renumbered.
MA.4 The chief executive officer, working with management, clinical, and administrative staff, provides for internal controls protecting human, physical, financial, and information resources.	LD.2.10 An individual(s) or designee(s) is responsible for operating the hospital according to the authority conferred by governance.	Reformatted and renumbered.
LD.1 *The leaders provide for hospital planning.*	LD.3.10 The leaders engage in both short-term and long-term planning.	Reformatted, renumbered, and rewritten to be consistent across accreditation programs; standard is now scorable.
LD.1.1 Planning includes defining a mission, a vision, and values for the hospital and creating the strategic, operational, programmatic, and other plans and policies to achieve the mission and vision.	LD.3.10 The leaders engage in both short-term and long-term planning.	Reformatted, renumbered, and rewritten to be consistent across accreditation programs.
LD.1.1.1 Planning addresses at least those important patient care and hospital wide functions identified by chapter titles in this manual.		Requirement deleted; concept is inherent in the remaining planning standards.
LD.1.1.2 The leaders of the hospital that belong to a multihospital system participate in systemwide policy decisions affecting the hospital.	LD.1.20 Governance responsibilities are defined in writing, as applicable.	Reformatted, renumbered, and rewritten to be consistent across accreditation programs.
LD.1.1.3 The hospital plans for the appropriate care of patients under legal or correctional restrictions.	LD.3.150 The hospital plans for the appropriate care, treatment, and services of patients under legal or correctional restrictions.	Reformatted, renumbered, and rewritten to be consistent across accreditation programs.
LD.1.2 The leaders communicate the hospital's mission, vision, and plans.	LD.3.60 Communication is effective throughout the hospital.	Reformatted, renumbered, and rewritten to be consistent across accreditation programs.
LD.1.3 The plan(s) includes patient care services based on identified patient needs and is consistent with the hospital's mission.	LD.3.10 The leaders engage in both short-term and long-term planning. LD.4.20 New or modified services or processes are designed well.	Reformatted, renumbered, and rewritten to be consistent across accreditation programs.
LD.1.3.1 The leaders, and, as appropriate, community leaders and the leaders of other hospitals, collaborate to design services.	LD.4.20 New or modified services or processes are designed well.	Reformatted, renumbered, and rewritten to be consistent across accreditation programs.
LD.1.3.2 The design of hospitalwide patient care services is appropriate to the scope and level of care required by the patients served.	LD.4.20 New or modified services or processes are designed well.	Reformatted, renumbered, and rewritten to be consistent across accreditation programs.
LD.1.3.3 Services are designed to respond to patient and family needs and expectations.	LD.4.20 New or modified services or processes are designed well.	Reformatted, renumbered, and rewritten to be consistent across accreditation programs.
LD.1.3.3.1 *The leaders are responsible for gathering, assessing, and acting on information regarding patient and family satisfaction with the services provided.*	PI.1.10 The hospital collects data to monitor its performance.	Requirement deleted; addressed in PI chapter.
LD.1.3.4 The hospital provides services in a timely manner to meet patients' needs.	LD.3.30 A hospital demonstrates a commitment to its community by providing essential services in a timely manner.	Reformatted, renumbered, and rewritten to be consistent across accreditation programs.
LD.1.3.4.1 Patient care services are provided either directly or through referral, consultation, contractual arrangements, or other agreements.	LD.3.50 Services provided by consultation, contractual arrangements, or other agreements are provided safely and effectively. LD.3.140 In hospitals that do not primarily provide psychiatric or substance abuse services, a written plan clearly defines the care, treatment, and services or appropriate referral of patients who are emotionally ill, who become emotionally ill while in the hospital, or who suffer the results of alcoholism or drug abuse.	Reformatted, renumbered, and rewritten to be consistent across accreditation programs.

Previous Standards	Current Standards	Comments
LD.1.3.4.2 The medical staff approves sources of patient care provided outside the hospital.	LD.3.50 Services provided by consultation, contractual arrangements, or other agreements are provided safely and effectively.	Reformatted, renumbered, and rewritten to be consistent across accreditation programs.
LD.1.4 The planning process provides for setting performance improvement priorities and identifies how the hospital adjusts priorities in response to unusual or urgent events.	LD.4.50 The leaders set performance improvement priorities and identify how the hospital adjusts priorities in response to unusual or urgent events.	Reformatted, renumbered, and rewritten to be consistent across accreditation programs.
LD.1.5 The leaders develop an annual operating budget and long-term capital expenditure plan, including a strategy to monitor the plan's implementation.	LD.2.50 The leaders develop and monitor an annual operating budget and, as appropriate, a long-term capital expenditure plan.	Reformatted, renumbered, and rewritten to be consistent across accreditation programs.
LD.1.5.1 The governing body approves the annual operating budget and long-term capital expenditure plan, including a strategy to monitor the plan's implementation.	LD.2.50 The leaders develop and monitor an annual operating budget and, as appropriate, a long-term capital expenditure plan.	Reformatted, renumbered, and rewritten to be consistent across accreditation programs.
LD.1.5.2 The budget review process considers the appropriateness of the hospital's plan.	LD.2.50 The leaders develop and monitor an annual operating budget and, as appropriate, a long-term capital expenditure plan.	Reformatted, renumbered, and rewritten to be consistent across accreditation programs.
LD.1.5.3 An independent public accountant conducts an annual audit of the hospital's finances, unless otherwise provided by law.	LD.2.50 The leaders develop and monitor an annual operating budget and, as appropriate, a long-term capital expenditure plan.	Reformatted, renumbered, and rewritten to be consistent across accreditation programs.
LD.1.6 The leaders provide for the uniform performance of patient care processes.	LD.3.20 Patients with comparable needs receive the same standard of care, treatment, and services throughout the hospital.	Reformatted, renumbered, and rewritten to be consistent across accreditation programs.
LD.1.7 The scope of services provided by each department is defined in writing and is approved by the hospital's administration, medical staff, or both, as appropriate.	LD.1.20 Governance responsibilities are defined in writing, as applicable.	Reformatted, renumbered, and rewritten to be consistent across accreditation programs.
LD.1.7.1 Each department provides patient care according to its written goals and scope of services.	LD.3.90 The leaders develop and implement policies and procedures for care, treatment, and services.	Reformatted, renumbered, and rewritten to be consistent across accreditation programs.
LD.1.8 The leaders and other relevant personnel collaborate in decision making.	LD.4.20 New or modified services or processes are designed well.	Reformatted, renumbered, and rewritten to be consistent across accreditation programs.
LD.1.9 The leaders develop programs for recruitment, retention, development, and continuing education of all staff members.	LD.3.10 The leaders engage in both short-term and long-term planning. LD.3.70 The leaders define the required qualifications and competence of those staff who provide care, treatment, and services, and recommend a sufficient number of qualified and competent staff to provide care, treatment, and services.	Reformatted, renumbered, and rewritten to be consistent across accreditation programs.
LD.1.9.1 The leaders implement programs to promote staff members' job-related advancement and educational goals.	LD.3.20 Patients with comparable needs receive the same standard of care, treatment, and services throughout the hospital.	Addressed at **HR.2.30**.
LD.1.10 Clinical practice guidelines are considered for use in designing or improving processes.	LD.5.10 The hospital considers clinical practice guidelines when designing or improving processes, as appropriate.	Reformatted, renumbered, and rewritten to be consistent across accreditation programs.
LD.1.10.1 When clinical practice guidelines are used, the hospital leaders identify criteria for their selection and implementation of clinical practice guidelines.	LD.5.20 When clinical practice guidelines are used, the leaders identify criteria for their selection and implementation.	Reformatted, renumbered, and rewritten to be consistent across accreditation programs.
LD.1.10.2 Appropriate leaders, practitioners, and health care professionals in the hospital review and approve clinical practice guidelines selected for implementation.	LD.5.30 Appropriate leaders, practitioners, and health care professionals in the hospital review and approve clinical practice guidelines selected for implementation.	Reformatted, renumbered, and rewritten to be consistent across accreditation programs.

Crosswalks of Standards

Previous Standards	Current Standards	Comments
LD.1.10.3 Leaders evaluate the outcomes related to use of clinical practice guidelines and determine indicated refinements to improve pertinent processes.	LD.5.40 The leaders evaluate the outcomes related to use of clinical practice guidelines and determine steps to improve processes.	Reformatted, renumbered, and rewritten to be consistent across accreditation programs.
LD.2 Each hospital department has effective leadership.	LD.2.20 Each organizational program, service, site, or department has effective leadership.	Reformatted, renumbered, and rewritten to be consistent across accreditation programs.
LD.2.1 Directors integrate their department's services with the hospital's primary functions.	LD.2.20 Each organizational program, service, site, or department has effective leadership.	Reformatted, renumbered, and rewritten to be consistent across accreditation programs.
LD.2.2 Directors coordinate and integrate services within their department and with other departments.	LD.2.20 Each organizational program, service, site, or department has effective leadership.	Reformatted, renumbered, and rewritten to be consistent across accreditation programs.
LD.2.3 Directors develop and implement policies and procedures that guide and support the provision of services.	LD.3.90 The leaders develop and implement policies and procedures for care, treatment, and services.	Reformatted, renumbered, and rewritten to be consistent across accreditation programs.
LD.2.4 Directors recommend a sufficient number of qualified and competent persons to provide care.	LD.3.70 The leaders define the required qualifications and competence of those staff who provide care, treatment, and services, and recommend a sufficient number of qualified and competent staff to provide care, treatment, and services.	Reformatted, renumbered, and rewritten to be consistent across accreditation programs.
LD.2.5 Directors determine the qualifications and competence of department personnel who provide patient care services and who are not licensed independent practitioners.	LD.3.70 The leaders define the required qualifications and competence of those staff who provide care, treatment, and services, and recommend a sufficient number of qualified and competent staff to provide care, treatment, and services.	Reformatted, renumbered, and rewritten to be consistent across accreditation programs.
LD.2.6 *Directors continuously assess and improve their department's performance.*	LD.4.10 The leaders set expectations, plan, and manage processes to measure, assess, and improve the hospital's governance, management, clinical, and support activities.	Reformatted, renumbered, and rewritten to be consistent across accreditation programs.
LD.2.7 Directors maintain appropriate quality control programs.	PI.1.10 The hospital collects data to monitor its performance.	Addressed in the PI chapter.
LD.2.8 Directors provide for orientation, in-service training, and continuing education of all persons in the department.	HR.2.10 Orientation provides initial job training and information.	Addressed in the HR chapter.
LD.2.9 Directors recommend space and other resources needed by the department.	LD.3.80 The leaders provide for adequate space, equipment, and other resources.	Reformatted, renumbered, and rewritten to be consistent across accreditation programs.
LD.2.10 Directors participate in selecting outside sources for needed services.	LD.3.50 Services provided by consultation, contractual arrangements, or other agreements are provided safely and effectively.	Reformatted, renumbered, and rewritten to be consistent across accreditation programs.
LD.2.11 Departments that are not medical staff services that provide patient care are directed by one or more qualified professionals.	LD.2.20 Each organizational program, service, site, or department has effective leadership.	Reformatted, renumbered, and rewritten to be consistent across accreditation programs.
LD.2.11.1 Responsibility for administrative direction and clinical direction is defined in writing.	LD.2.20 Each organizational program, service, site, or department has effective leadership.	Reformatted, renumbered, and rewritten to be consistent across accreditation programs.
LD.2.11.2 A qualified professional with appropriate clinical training and experience is responsible for the clinical direction of patient care.	LD.2.20 Each organizational program, service, site, or department has effective leadership.	Reformatted, renumbered, and rewritten to be consistent across accreditation programs.
LD.2.11.3 When a department has more than one director, the responsibilities of each are clearly defined in writing.	LD.2.20 Each organizational program, service, site, or department has effective leadership.	Reformatted, renumbered, and rewritten to be consistent across accreditation programs.
LD.3 Patient care services are integrated throughout the hospital.	LD.2.20 Each organizational program, service, site, or department has effective leadership.	Reformatted, renumbered, and rewritten to be consistent across accreditation programs.
LD.3.1 The hospital's plan for the provision of patient care services describes the organization and functional relationships of departments.	LD.2.20 An individual(s) or designee(s) is responsible for operating the hospital according to the authority conferred by governance.	Reformatted, renumbered, and rewritten to be consistent across accreditation programs.

Previous Standards	Current Standards	Comments
LD.3.2 The leaders foster communication and coordination among individuals and departments.	**LD.3.60** Communication is effective throughout the hospital.	Reformatted, renumbered, and rewritten to be consistent across accreditation programs.
LD.3.3 The leaders communicate with the leaders of health care delivery organizations corporately or functionally related to the hospital.	**LD.3.60** Communication is effective throughout the hospital.	Reformatted, renumbered, and rewritten to be consistent across accreditation programs.
LD.3.4 All departments develop policies and procedures in collaboration with associated departments.	**LD.3.90** The leaders develop and implement policies and procedures for care, treatment, and services.	Reformatted, renumbered, and rewritten to be consistent across accreditation programs.
LD.3.4.1 The leaders provide for mechanisms to measure, analyze, and manage variation in the performance of defined processes that affect patient safety.	**LD.4.40** The leaders ensure that an integrated patient safety program is implemented throughout the hospital.	Reformatted, renumbered, and rewritten to be consistent across accreditation programs.
LD.4 The hospital leaders set expectations, develop plans, and manage processes to measure, assess, and improve the quality of the hospital's governance, management, clinical, and support activities.	**LD.4.10** The leaders set expectations, plan, and manage processes to measure, assess, and improve the hospital's governance, management, clinical, and support activities.	Reformatted, renumbered, and rewritten to be consistent across accreditation programs.
LD.4.1 The leaders understand the approaches to and methods of performance improvement.		Deleted as a specific requirement; concept is inherent in the standards in the **LD.4** section.
LD.4.2 The leaders adopt an approach to performance improvement.		Deleted as a specific requirement; concept is inherent in the standards in the **LD.4** section.
LD.4.3 Leaders ensure that important processes and activities are measured, assessed, and improved systematically throughout the hospital.	**LD.4.50** The leaders set performance improvement priorities and identify how the hospital adjusts priorities in response to unusual or urgent events. **LD.4.60** The leaders allocate adequate resources for measuring, assessing, and improving the hospital's performance and improving patient safety.	Reformatted, renumbered, and rewritten to be consistent across accreditation programs.
LD.4.3.1 All leaders participate in interdisciplinary, interdepartmental performance improvement activities.	**LD.4.10** The leaders set expectations, plan, and manage processes to measure, assess, and improve the hospital's governance, management, clinical, and support activities.	Reformatted, renumbered, and rewritten to be consistent across accreditation programs.
LD.4.3.2 Relevant information is forwarded to leaders and coordinators of hospitalwide performance improvement activities.	**LD.4.10** The leaders set expectations, plan, and manage processes to measure, assess, and improve the hospital's governance, management, clinical, and support activities. **LD.4.60** The leaders allocate adequate resources for measuring, assessing, and improving the hospital's performance and improving patient safety.	Reformatted, renumbered, and rewritten to be consistent across accreditation programs.
LD.4.3.3 Responsibility for acting on recommendations generated through performance improvement activities is assigned and defined in writing.		Deleted as a specific requirement; concept is inherent in the standards in the **LD.4** section.
LD.4.4 *The leaders allocate adequate resources for measuring, assessing, and improving the hospital's performance.*	**LD.4.60** The leaders allocate adequate resources for measuring, assessing, and improving the hospital's performance and improving patient safety.	Reformatted, renumbered, and rewritten to be consistent across accreditation programs; standard is now scorable.
LD.4.4.1 The leaders assign personnel needed to participate in performance Improvement activities.	**LD.4.60** The leaders allocate adequate resources for measuring, assessing, and improving the hospital's performance and improving patient safety.	Reformatted, renumbered, and rewritten to be consistent across accreditation programs.
LD.4.4.2 The leaders provide adequate time for personnel to participate in performance improvement activities.	**LD.4.60** The leaders allocate adequate resources for measuring, assessing, and improving the hospital's performance and improving patient safety.	Reformatted, renumbered, and rewritten to be consistent across accreditation programs.

Crosswalks of Standards

Previous Standards	Current Standards	Comments
LD.4.4.3 The leaders provide information systems and data management processes for ongoing performance improvement and improvement of patient safety.	LD.4.60 The leaders allocate adequate resources for measuring, assessing, and improving the hospital's performance and improving patient safety.	Reformatted, renumbered, and rewritten to be consistent across accreditation programs.
LD.4.4.4 The leaders provide for staff training in the basic approaches to and methods of performance improvement and improvement of patient safety.	LD.4.60 The leaders allocate adequate resources for measuring, assessing, and improving the hospital's performance and improving patient safety.	Reformatted, renumbered, and rewritten to be consistent across accreditation programs.
LD.4.4.5 The leaders assess the adequacy of their allocation of human, information, physical, and financial resources in support of their identified performance improvement and safety improvement priorities.	LD.4.60 The leaders allocate adequate resources for measuring, assessing, and improving the hospital's performance and improving patient safety.	Reformatted, renumbered, and rewritten to be consistent across accreditation programs.
LD.4.5 The leaders measure and assess the effectiveness of their contributions to improving performance and improvement of patient safety.	LD.4.70 The leaders measure and assess the effectiveness of the performance improvement and safety improvement activities.	Reformatted, renumbered, and rewritten to be consistent across accreditation programs.
LD.5 The leaders ensure implementation of an integrated patient safety program throughout the hospital.	LD.4.40 The leaders ensure that an integrated patient safety program is implemented throughout the hospital.	Reformatted, renumbered, and rewritten to be consistent across accreditation programs.
LD.5.1 Leaders ensure that the processes for identifying and managing sentinel events, including near misses, are defined and implemented.		Moved to PI.2.30.
LD.5.2 Leaders ensure that an ongoing, proactive program for identifying risks to patient safety and reducing medical/health care errors is defined and implemented.		Moved to PI.3.20.
LD.5.3 Leaders ensure that patient safety issues are given a high priority and addressed when processes, functions, or services are designed or redesigned.	LD.4.40 The leaders ensure that an integrated patient safety program is implemented throughout the hospital.	Reformatted, renumbered, and rewritten to be consistent across accreditation programs.
PF.1 The hospital plans for and supports the provision and coordination of patient education activities. PF.1.1 The hospital identifies and provides the resources necessary for achieving educational objectives.	LD.3.120 The leaders plan for and support the provision and coordination of patient education activities.	Moved from PF.1 and PF.1.1.
PF.3.10 Academic education is provided to children and adolescents either directly by the hospital or through other arrangements, when appropriate.	LD.3.130 Academic education is arranged for children and youth, when appropriate.	Moved from PF.3.10.
RI.2 The hospital implements policies and procedures, developed with the medical staffs' participation, for the procuring and donation of organs and other tissues.	LD.3.110 The hospital implements policies and procedures developed with the medical staff's participation for procuring and donating organs and other tissues.	Moved from RI.2.

2005 Hospital Accreditation Standards

Crosswalk of Previous Management of the Environment of Care Standards for Hospitals to Current Management of the Environment of Care Standards for Hospitals

This crosswalk is designed to show where the previous Management of the Environment of Care (EC) standards requirements appear in the reformatted EC standards. The left column (Previous Standards) lists consecutively each previous EC standard. The middle column, Current Standards, indicates the EC standards with revised numbers. The right column, Comments, identifies what changes have occurred between the previous standards and the current standards.

Previous Standards	Current Standards	Comments
EC.1 The hospital plans for a safe, accessible, effective, and efficient environment consistent with its mission, services, law, and regulation.		Concepts addressed in standards EC.1.10 through EC.7.50, and standard LD.1.30.
EC.1.1 The hospital plans for a safe environment.	EC.1.10 The hospital manages safety risks.	a. Safety planning, safety implementation, and worker safety standards have been merged into one standard. b. EC education and staff knowledge requirements have been moved to new standard HR.2.20 in the HR chapter. c. Requirements addressing reporting, monitoring, and annual evaluations have been moved to EC.9.10.
EC.1.1.1 The hospital plans for worker safety.		
EC.2.1 The hospital implements its safety plan.		
EC.1.1.2 The hospital develops a policy regarding smoking.	EC.1.30 The hospital develops and implements a policy to prohibit smoking except in specified circumstances.	This standard has been revised from requiring a "no smoking" policy that must be absolutely enforced to requiring hospitals to identify and implement monitoring processes and take corrective actions when their "no smoking" policy is ineffective.
EC.1.2 The hospital plans for a secure environment.	EC.2.10 The hospital identifies and manages its security risks.	a. Planning and implementation standards have been merged into one standard. b. EC education and staff knowledge requirements have been moved to new standard HR.2.20 in the HR chapter. c. Requirements addressing reporting, monitoring, and annual evaluations have been moved to EC.9.10. d. New requirement in EC.2.10 regarding security measures for infant or pediatric abduction.
EC.2.2 The hospital implements its security plan.		
EC.1.3 The hospital plans for managing hazardous materials and waste.	EC.3.10 The hospital manages its hazardous materials and waste risks.	
EC.2.3 The hospital implements its plan for managing hazardous materials and waste.		
EC.1.4 A plan addresses emergency management.	EC.4.10 The hospital addresses emergency management.	
EC.2.4 The hospital implements its emergency management plan.		
EC.1.5 The hospital plans for fire prevention.	EC.5.10 The hospital manages fire safety risks.	a. Planning and implementation standards have been merged into one revised standard. b. EC education and staff knowledge requirements have been moved to new standard HR.2.20 in the HR chapter. c. Requirements addressing reporting, monitoring, and annual evaluations have been moved to EC.9.10. d. ILSM requirements have been consolidated into one new standard (EC.5.50).
EC.2.5 The hospital implements its fire prevention plan.	EC.5.50 The hospital develops and implements activities to protect occupants during periods when a building does not meet the applicable provisions of the *Life Safety Code*®.	
EC.1.5.1 Newly constructed and existing environments of care are designed and maintained to comply with the *Life Safety Code*®.	EC.5.20 Newly constructed and existing environments are designed and maintained to comply with the *Life Safety Code*®.	Reformatted, renumbered, and rewritten to be consistent across accreditation programs.

CW — 26

Crosswalks of Standards

Previous Standards	Current Standards	Comments
EC.1.6 The hospital plans for managing medical equipment.	EC.6.10 The hospital manages medical equipment risks.	a. Planning and implementation standards have been merged into one revised standard.
EC.2.6 The hospital implements its medical equipment management plan.		b. EC education and staff knowledge requirements have been moved to new standard HR.2.20 in the HR chapter.
EC.1.7 The hospital plans for managing utilities.	EC.7.10 The hospital manages its utility risks.	c. Requirements addressing reporting, monitoring, and annual evaluations have been moved to EC.9.10.
EC.2.7 The hospital implements its plan for managing utility systems.		
EC.1.7.1 The hospital provides a reliable emergency power source as required by occupancy classification and services provided.	EC.7.20 The hospital provides a reliable emergency electrical power source.	Reformatted, renumbered, and rewritten to be consistent across accreditation programs.
EC.2 *The hospital provides a safe, accessible, effective, and efficient environment consistent with its mission, services, law, and regulation.*		Concepts addressed in standards EC.1.10 through EC.7.50, and standard LD.1.30.
EC.2.8 Personnel have been oriented to and educated about the environment, and possess the knowledge and skills to perform their responsibilities in the environment.	HR.2.20 Staff members, licensed independent practitioners, students, and volunteers, as appropriate, can describe or demonstrate their roles and responsibilities, based on specific job duties or responsibilities, relative to safety.	Concept was moved to new standard HR.2.20 in the HR chapter.
EC.2.9 The hospital conducts emergency drills regularly.		Concept addressed in standards EC.4.20 and EC.5.30.
EC.2.9.1 Drills are conducted regularly to test emergency preparedness.	EC.4.20 The hospital conducts drills regularly to test emergency management.	Reformatted, renumbered, and rewritten to be consistent across accreditation programs.
EC.2.9.2 Fire drills are conducted regularly.	EC.5.30 The hospital conducts fire drills regularly.	Reformatted, renumbered, and rewritten to be consistent across accreditation programs.
EC.2.10 Components and systems of the environment are maintained, tested, and inspected.		Concept addressed in standards EC.1.20, EC.5.40, EC.6.20, EC.7.30, EC.7.40 and EC.7.50.
EC.2.10.1 Safety elements of the environment of care are maintained, tested, and inspected.	EC.1.20 The hospital maintains a safe environment.	Reformatted, renumbered, and rewritten to be consistent across accreditation programs.
EC.2.10.2 Fire safety elements in the environment of care are maintained, tested, and inspected.	EC.5.40 The hospital maintains fire-safety equipment and building features.	Reformatted, renumbered, and rewritten to be consistent across accreditation programs.
EC.2.10.3 Medical equipment is maintained, tested, and inspected.	EC.6.20 Medical equipment is maintained, tested, and inspected.	Reformatted, renumbered, and rewritten to be consistent across accreditation programs.
EC.2.10.4 Utility systems are maintained, tested, and inspected.	EC.7.30 The hospital maintains, tests, and inspects its utility systems.	Consolidated medical gas and vacuum requirements have been combined into one new standard, EC.7.50.
	EC.7.50 The hospital maintains, tests, and inspects its medical gas and vacuum systems.	
EC.2.10.4.1 Emergency power systems are maintained, tested, and inspected.	EC.7.40 The hospital maintains, tests, and inspects its emergency power systems.	Reformatted, renumbered, and rewritten to be consistent across accreditation programs.
EC.3 The hospital plans and provides for other environmental concerns.		Concept addressed in standards EC.8.10 and EC.8.30.
EC.3.1 The hospital establishes an environment that meets the needs of patients, encourages a positive self-image, and respects their human dignity.	RI.2.140 Patients have a right to an environment that preserves dignity and contributes to a positive self-image.	Concepts in standard EC.3.1 (with the exception of intent statement "b") have been moved into the RI chapter. Intent statement "b" has been moved into standard EC.8.10.
	EC.8.10 The hospital establishes and maintains an appropriate environment.	
EC.3.2 The hospital provides an environment with appropriate space and equipment.	EC.8.10 The hospital establishes and maintains an appropriate environment.	Reformatted, renumbered, and rewritten to be consistent across accreditation programs.
EC.3.2.1 The hospital uses established design criteria when designing and building the environment.	EC.8.30 The hospital manages the design and building of the environment when it is renovated, altered, or newly created.	Reformatted, renumbered, and rewritten to be consistent across accreditation programs.

Previous Standards	Current Standards	Comments
EC.3.3 The built environment provides appropriate privacy to patients.	RI.2.130 The hospital respects the needs of patients for confidentiality, privacy, and security.	Concepts have been moved into the RI chapter.
EC.3.4 The built environment supports the development and maintenance of the patient's interests, skills, and opportunities for personal growth.	EC.8.10 The hospital establishes and maintains an appropriate environment.	Applicability of requirements was clarified for all hospitals versus those with long term care settings.
EC.4 The hospital evaluates and improves conditions in the environment.		Concept addressed in standards EC.9.10 through EC.9.30.
EC.4.1 The hospital collects information about deficiencies and opportunities for improvement in the environment.	EC.9.10 The hospital monitors conditions in the environment.	Requirements from EC.1–EC.1.7 addressing reporting, monitoring, and annual evaluations have been consolidated and moved to EC.9.10.
EC.4.2 The hospital analyzes identified environment issues and develops recommendations for resolving them.	EC.9.20 The hospital analyzes identified environment issues and develops recommendations for resolving them.	Reformatted, renumbered, and rewritten to be consistent across accreditation programs.
EC.4.3 The hospital works to implement recommendations to improve the environment and monitor the effectiveness of the recommendation's implementation.	EC.9.30 The hospital improves the environment.	Reformatted, renumbered, and rewritten to be consistent across accreditation programs.

Crosswalk of Previous Management of Human Resources Standards for Hospitals to Current Management of Human Resources Standards for Hospitals

This crosswalk is designed to show where the previous Management of Human Resources (HR) and Leadership (LD) standards requirements appear in the reformatted HR standards. The left column (Previous Standards) lists consecutively each previous HR and LD standard; a standard appearing in italics in this column indicates that the standard was previously not scorable. The middle column, Current Standards, indicates the HR standards with revised numbers; standards from other functional chapters might also be included in this column, as appropriate. The right column, Comments, identifies what changes have occurred between the previous standards and the current standards.

Previous Standards	Current Standards	Comments
HR.1 The hospital's leaders define the qualifications and performance expectations for all staff positions. **LD.2.5** Directors determine the qualifications and competence of department personnel who provide patient care services who are not licensed independent practitioners.	**LD.3.70** The leaders define the required qualifications and competence of those staff who provide care, treatment, and services and recommend a sufficient number of qualified and competent staff to provide care, treatment, and services. **HR.1.20** The hospital has a process to ensure that a person's qualifications are consistent with his or her job responsibilities.	EP 2 in **HR.1.20** was moved here from **LD.2.5**.
HR.2 The hospital provides an adequate number of staff members whose qualifications are consistent with job responsibilities.	**HR.1.10** The hospital provides an adequate number and mix of staff that are consistent with the hospital's staffing plan. **HR.1.20** The hospital has a process to ensure that a person's qualifications are consistent with his or her job responsibilities.	EPs 5–7 were added to **HR.1.20** to clarify what is required by this standard.
HR.2.1 The hospital uses data on clinical/service screening indicators in combination with human resource screening indicators to assess staffing effectiveness.	**HR.1.30** The hospital uses data and clinical/service screening indicators in combination with human resource screening indicators to assess staffing effectiveness.	Reformatted, renumbered, and rewritten to be consistent across accreditation programs.
HR.3 *The leaders ensure that the competence of all staff members is assessed, maintained, demonstrated, and improved continually.*	**HR.3.10** Competence to perform job responsibilities is assessed, demonstrated, and maintained.	Reformatted, renumbered, and rewritten to be consistent across accreditation programs; this standard is now scorable.
HR.3.1 The hospital encourages and supports self-development and learning for all staff.	**LD.2.10** An individual(s) or designee(s) is responsible for operating the hospital according to the authority conferred by governance. **HR.2.30** Ongoing education, including in-services, training, and other activities, maintains and improves competence.	Reformatted, renumbered, and rewritten to be consistent across accreditation programs.
HR.4 An orientation process provides initial job training and information and assesses the staff's ability to fulfill specified responsibilities.	**HR.2.10** Orientation provides initial job training and information.	Reformatted, renumbered, and rewritten to be consistent across accreditation programs.
HR.4.1 The hospital orients and educates forensic staff about their responsibilities related to patient care.	**HR.2.10** Orientation provides initial job training and information.	Age-specific competency is now addressed in **HR.1.20**, EP 4 and **HR.3.10**, EP 1.
HR.4.2 Ongoing in-service and other education and training maintain and improve staff competence and support an interdisciplinary approach to patient care.	**HR.2.30** Ongoing education, including in-services, training, and other activities, maintains and improves competence.	Reformatted, renumbered, and rewritten to be consistent across accreditation programs.
HR.4.3 The hospital regularly collects aggregate data on competence patterns and trends to identify and respond to the staff's learning needs.	**HR.2.30** Ongoing education, including in-services, training, and other activities, maintains and improves competence.	The standard no longer requires an annual report to the governing body on the levels of competence, patterns, and trends and competence maintenance activities.

Previous Standards	Current Standards	Comments
HR.5 The hospital assesses each staff member's ability to meet the performance expectations stated in his or her job description.	HR.3.10 Competence to perform job responsibilities is assessed, demonstrated, and maintained. HR.3.20 The hospital periodically conducts performance evaluations.	EPs 6 and 7 were added to HR.3.10 to clarify the requirements for this standard. Age-specific competency is now addressed in HR.1.20, EP 4 and HR.3.10, EP 1.
HR.6 The hospital addresses a staff member's request not to participate in any aspect of patient care.	RI.1.10 The hospital follows ethical behavior in its care, treatment, and services and business practices.	Reformatted, renumbered, and rewritten to be consistent across accreditation programs.
HR.6.1 The hospital ensures that a patient's care will not be negatively affected if the hospital grants a staff member's request not to participate in an aspect of patient care.	RI.1.10 The hospital follows ethical behavior in its care, treatment, and services and business practices.	Reformatted, renumbered, and rewritten to be consistent across accreditation programs.
HR.6.2 Policies and procedures specify those aspects of patient care that might conflict with staff members' cultural values or religious beliefs.	RI.1.10 The hospital follows ethical behavior in its care, treatment, and services and business practices.	Reformatted, renumbered, and rewritten to be consistent across accreditation programs.
EC.2.8 Personnel have been oriented to and educated about the environment, and possess the knowledge and skills to perform their responsibilities in the environment.	HR.2.20 Staff members, licensed independent practitioners, students, and volunteers, as appropriate, can describe or demonstrate their roles and responsibilities, based on specific job duties or responsibilities, relative to safety.	Reformatted, renumbered, and rewritten to be consistent across accreditation programs.

Crosswalk of Previous Management of Information Standards for Hospitals to Current Management of Information Standards for Hospitals

This crosswalk is designed to show where the previous Management of Information (IM) standards requirements appear in the reformatted IM standards. The left column (Previous Standards) lists consecutively each previous IM standard; a standard appearing in italics in this column indicates that the standard was previously not scorable. The middle column, Current Standards, indicates the IM standards, with revised numbers. The right column, Comments, identifies what changes have occurred between the previous standards and the current standards.

Previous Standards	Current Standards	Comments
IM.1 The hospital plans and designs information management processes to meet internal and external information needs.	IM.1.10 The hospital plans and designs information management processes to meet internal and external information needs.	Reformatted, renumbered, and rewritten to be consistent across accreditation programs.
IM.2 Confidentiality, security, and integrity of data and information are maintained.	IM.2.10 Information privacy and confidentiality are maintained.	New EPs were added to be consistent with Health Insurance Portability and Accountability Act (HIPAA).
IM.2.1 Records and information are protected against loss, destruction, tampering, and unauthorized access or use.	IM.2.20 Information security, including data integrity, is maintained. IM.2.30 The hospital has a process for maintaining continuity of information.	Some additional requirements were added to address electronic systems.
IM.3 Uniform data definitions and data capture methods are used whenever possible.	IM.3.10 The hospital has processes in place to effectively manage information, including the capturing, reporting, processing, storing, retrieving, disseminating, and displaying of clinical/service and nonclinical data and information.	Reformatted, renumbered, and rewritten to be consistent across accreditation programs.
IM.4 The necessary expertise and tools are available for the analysis and transformation of data into information.	IM.3.10 The hospital has processes in place to effectively manage information, including the capturing, reporting, processing, storing, retrieving, disseminating, and displaying of clinical/service and nonclinical data and information. IM.2.10 Information privacy and confidentiality are maintained.	Some additional requirements were added to address electronic systems.
IM.5 Transmission of data and information is timely and accurate.	IM.3.10 The hospital has processes in place to effectively manage information, including the capturing, reporting, processing, storing, retrieving, disseminating, and displaying of clinical/service and nonclinical data and information.	Reformatted, renumbered, and rewritten to be consistent across accreditation programs.
IM.5.1 The format and methods for disseminating data and information are standardized, whenever possible.	IM.3.10 The hospital has processes in place to effectively manage information, including the capturing, reporting, processing, storing, retrieving, disseminating, and displaying of clinical/service and nonclinical data and information.	Reformatted, renumbered, and rewritten to be consistent across accreditation programs.
IM.6 Adequate integration and interpretation capabilities are provided.	IM.3.10 The hospital has processes in place to effectively manage information, including the capturing, reporting, processing, storing, retrieving, disseminating, and displaying of clinical/service and nonclinical data and information. IM.4.10 The information management system provides information for use in decision making.	Reformatted, renumbered, and rewritten to be consistent across accreditation programs.
IM.7 *The hospital defines, captures, analyzes, transforms, transmits, and reports patient-specific data and information related to care processes and outcomes.*		Concepts addressed in IM.6.10–IM.6.60.

2005 Hospital Accreditation Standards

Previous Standards	Current Standards	Comments
IM.7.1 The hospital initiates and maintains a medical record for every individual assessed or treated.	IM.6.10 The hospital has a complete and accurate medical record for every patient assessed or treated.	Reformatted, renumbered, and rewritten to be consistent across accreditation programs.
IM.7.1.1 Only authorized individuals make entries in medical records.	IM.6.10 The hospital has a complete and accurate medical record for every patient assessed or treated.	Reformatted, renumbered, and rewritten to be consistent across accreditation programs.
IM.7.1.2 The hospital determines how long medical record information is retained, based on law and regulation and the information use for patient care, legal, research, and educational purposes.	IM.6.10 The hospital has a complete and accurate medical record for every patient assessed or treated.	Reformatted, renumbered, and rewritten to be consistent across accreditation programs.
IM.7.2 The medical record contains sufficient information to identify the patient, support the diagnosis, justify the treatment, document the course and results, and promote continuity of care among health care providers.	IM.6.10 The hospital has a complete and accurate medical record for every patient assessed or treated. IM.6.20 Records contain patient-specific information, as appropriate, to the care, treatment, and services provided.	Some additional requirements were added to address electronic systems.
IM.7.3 The medical record thoroughly documents operative or other procedures and the use of sedation or anesthesia.	IM.6.30 The medical record thoroughly documents operative or other procedures and the use of moderate or deep sedation or anesthesia.	Reformatted, renumbered, and rewritten to be consistent across accreditation programs; this standard is now scorable.
IM.7.3.1 A preoperative diagnosis is recorded before surgery by the licensed independent practitioner responsible for the patient.	IM.6.30 The medical record thoroughly documents operative or other procedures and the use of moderate or deep sedation or anesthesia.	Reformatted, renumbered, and rewritten to be consistent across accreditation programs.
IM.7.3.2 Operative reports dictated or written immediately after surgery record the name of the primary surgeon and assistants, findings, technical procedures used, specimens removed, and postoperative diagnosis.	IM.6.30 The medical record thoroughly documents operative or other procedures and the use of moderate or deep sedation or anesthesia.	Reformatted, renumbered, and rewritten to be consistent across accreditation programs.
IM.7.3.2.1 The completed operative report is authenticated by the surgeon and filed in the medical record as soon as possible after surgery.	IM.6.30 The medical record thoroughly documents operative or other procedures and the use of moderate or deep sedation or anesthesia.	Reformatted, renumbered, and rewritten to be consistent across accreditation programs.
IM.7.3.2.2 When the operative report is not placed in the medical record immediately after surgery, a progress note is entered immediately.	IM.6.30 The medical record thoroughly documents operative or other procedures and the use of moderate or deep sedation or anesthesia.	Reformatted, renumbered, and rewritten to be consistent across accreditation programs.
IM.7.3.3 Postoperative documentation records the patient's vital signs and level of consciousness; medications (including intravenous fluids), blood, and blood components; any unusual events or postoperative complications; and management of such events.	IM.6.30 The medical record thoroughly documents operative or other procedures and the use of moderate or deep sedation or anesthesia.	Reformatted, renumbered, and rewritten to be consistent across accreditation programs.
IM.7.3.4 *Postoperative documentation records the patient's discharge from the postsedation or postanesthesia care area by the responsible licensed independent practitioner or according to discharge criteria.*	IM.6.30 The medical record thoroughly documents operative or other procedures and the use of moderate or deep sedation or anesthesia.	Reformatted, renumbered, and rewritten to be consistent across accreditation programs; this standard is now scorable.
IM.7.3.4.1 Compliance with discharge criteria is fully documented in the patient's medical record.	IM.6.30 The medical record thoroughly documents operative or other procedures and the use of moderate or deep sedation or anesthesia.	Reformatted, renumbered, and rewritten to be consistent across accreditation programs.
IM.7.3.5 Postoperative documentation records the name of the licensed independent practitioner responsible for discharge.	IM.6.30 The medical record thoroughly documents operative or other procedures and the use of moderate or deep sedation or anesthesia.	Reformatted, renumbered, and rewritten to be consistent across accreditation programs.
IM.7.4 For patients receiving continuing ambulatory care services, the medical record contains a summary list of known significant diagnoses, conditions, procedures, drug allergies, and medications.	IM.6.40 For patients receiving continuing ambulatory care services, the medical record contains a summary list of all significant diagnoses, procedures, drug allergies, and medications.	Reformatted, renumbered, and rewritten to be consistent across accreditation programs.

Crosswalks of Standards

Previous Standards	Current Standards	Comments
IM.7.4.1 The list is initiated for each patient by the third visit and maintained thereafter.	IM.6.40 For patients receiving continuing ambulatory care services, the medical record contains a summary list of all significant diagnoses, procedures, drug allergies, and medications.	Reformatted, renumbered, and rewritten to be consistent across accreditation programs.
IM.7.5 When emergency, urgent, or immediate care is provided, the time and means of arrival are also documented in the medical record.	IM.6.10 The hospital has a complete and accurate medical record for every patient assessed or treated.	Reformatted, renumbered, and rewritten to be consistent across accreditation programs.
IM.7.5.1 The medical record notes when a patient receiving emergency, urgent, or immediate care left against medical advice.	IM.6.10 The hospital has a complete and accurate medical record for every patient assessed or treated.	Reformatted, renumbered, and rewritten to be consistent across accreditation programs.
IM.7.5.2 The medical record of a patient receiving emergency, urgent, or immediate care notes the conclusions at termination of treatment, including final disposition, condition at discharge, and instructions for follow-up care.	IM.6.10 The hospital has a complete and accurate medical record for every patient assessed or treated.	Reformatted, renumbered, and rewritten to be consistent across accreditation programs.
IM.7.5.3 When authorized by the patient or a legally authorized representative, a copy of the emergency services provided is available to the practitioner or medical organization providing follow-up care.	IM.6.10 The hospital has a complete and accurate medical record for every patient assessed or treated.	"When authorized by the patient or legally authorized representative" was deleted to be consistent with HIPAA requirements.
IM.7.6 Medical record data and information are managed in a timely manner.	IM.6.10 The hospital has a complete and accurate medical record for every patient assessed or treated.	Reformatted, renumbered, and rewritten to be consistent across accreditation programs.
IM.7.7 Verbal orders of authorized individuals are accepted and transcribed by qualified personnel who are identified by title or category in the medical staff rules and regulations.	IM.6.50 Designated qualified personnel accept and transcribe verbal orders of authorized individuals.	Reformatted, renumbered, and rewritten to be consistent across accreditation programs.
IM.7.8 Every medical record entry is dated, its author identified and, when necessary, authenticated.	IM.6.10 The hospital has a complete and accurate medical record for every patient assessed or treated.	Reformatted, renumbered, and rewritten to be consistent across accreditation programs.
IM.7.9 The hospital can quickly assemble and have access to all relevant information from components of a patient's record when the patient is admitted or is seen for ambulatory or emergency care.	IM.6.60 The hospital can provide access to all relevant information from a patient's record when needed for use in patient care, treatment, and services.	Reformatted, renumbered, and rewritten to be consistent across accreditation programs.
IM.7.10 Medical records are reviewed on an ongoing basis for completeness and timeliness of information, and action is taken to improve the quality and timeliness of documentation that impacts patient care.	IM.6.10 The hospital has a complete and accurate medical record for every individual assessed or treated.	Reformatted, renumbered, and rewritten to be consistent across accreditation programs.
IM.7.10.1 A representative sample of records is included in the review process.		Deleted; medical record review is addressed in IM.6.10 and is not specific as to sampling.
IM.8 The hospital collects and aggregates data and information to support care and service delivery and operations.	IM.4.10 The information management system provides information for use in decision making.	Reformatted, renumbered, and rewritten to be consistent across accreditation programs.
IM.9 Knowledge-based information systems, resources, and services meet the hospital's needs.	IM.5.10 Knowledge-based information resources are readily available, current, and authoritative.	Reformatted, renumbered, and rewritten to be consistent across accreditation programs.
IM.9.1 Knowledge-based information resources are available, current, and authoritative.	IM.5.10 Knowledge-based information resources are readily available, current, and authoritative.	Reformatted, renumbered, and rewritten to be consistent across accreditation programs.
IM.10 Comparative performance data and information are defined, collected, analyzed, transmitted, reported, and used.		Deleted; concepts addressed throughout the PI chapter and Accreditation Participation Requirements 5–6 for performance measurement.

…

Crosswalk of Previous Medical Staff Standards for Hospitals to Current Medical Staff Standards for Hospitals

This crosswalk is designed to show where the previous Medical Staff (MS) and Leadership (LD) standards requirements appear in the reformatted MS standards. The left column (Previous Standards) lists consecutively each previous MS standard; a standard appearing in italics in this column indicates that the standard was previously not scorable. The middle column, Current Standards, indicates the MS and LD standards, with revised numbers. The right column, Comments, identifies what changes have occurred between the previous standards and the current standards.

Previous Standards	Current Standards	Comments
MS.1 One or more organized, self-governing medical staffs have overall responsibility for the quality of the professional services provided by individuals with clinical privileges, as well as the responsibility of accounting therefore to the governing body.	MS.1.10 The hospital has an organized, self-governing medical staff that provides oversight of care, treatment, and services provided by practitioners with privileges, provides for a uniform quality of patient care, treatment, and services, and reports to and is accountable to the governing body.	Reformatted and renumbered.
MS.1.1 *Each medical staff has the following characteristics:*		This standard was not scorable and has been deleted.
MS.1.1.1 It includes fully licensed physicians and may include other licensed individuals permitted by law and by the hospital to provide patient care services independently in the hospital (both physicians and these other individuals are referred to as "licensed independent practitioners").	MS.1.10 The hospital has an organized, self-governing medical staff that provides oversight of care, treatment, and services provided by practitioners with privileges, provides for a uniform quality of patient care, treatment, and services, and reports to and is accountable to the governing body.	Reformatted and renumbered.
MS.1.1.2 *All medical staff members have delineated clinical privileges that define the scope of patient care services they may provide independently in the hospital.*	MS.1.40 There is a medical staff executive committee. MS.4.20 There is a process for granting, renewing, or revising setting-specific clinical privileges.	Addressed in MS.1.40, EP 9 and MS.4.20, EPs 1, 2, and 3; requirements are now scorable.
MS.1.1.3 All medical staff members and all others with delineated clinical privileges are subject to medical staff and departmental bylaws, rules and regulations, and policies and are subject to review as part of the organization's performance improvement activities.	MS1.20 Medical staff bylaws address self governance and accountability to the governing body. MS.3.10 The organized medical staff has a leadership role in hospital performance improvement activities to improve quality of care, treatment, and services and patient safety. MS.4.20 There is a process for granting, renewing, or revising setting-specific clinical privileges. MS.4.40 At the time of renewal of privileges, the organized medical staff evaluates individuals for their continued ability to provide quality care, treatment, and services for the privileges requested as defined in the medical staff bylaws.	Reformatted and renumbered.
MS.2 *Each medical staff develops and adopts bylaws and rules and regulations to establish a framework for self-governance of medical staff activities and accountability to the governing body.*		This standard was previously not scored; concepts are now scored in MS.1.20 and MS.1.30.

Crosswalks of Standards

Previous Standards	Current Standards	Comments
MS.2.1 Medical staff bylaws and rules and regulations are adopted by the medical staff and approved by the governing body before becoming effective. Neither body may unilaterally amend the medical staff bylaws or rules and regulations.	**MS.1.20** Medical staff bylaws address self governance and accountability to the governing body. **MS.1.30** Neither the organized medical staff nor the governing body may unilaterally amend the medical staff bylaws or rules and regulations.	Reformatted and renumbered.
MS.2.2 Medical staff bylaws and rules and regulations create a framework within which medical staff members can act with a reasonable degree of freedom and confidence.	**MS.1.10** The hospital has an organized, self-governing medical staff that provides oversight of care, treatment, and services provided by practitioners with privileges, provides for a uniform quality of patient care, treatment, and services, and reports to and is accountable to the governing body. **MS.1.40** There is a medical staff executive committee. **MS.1.20** Medical staff bylaws address self governance and accountability to the governing body. **MS.1.30** Neither the organized medical staff nor the governing body may unilaterally amend the medical staff bylaws or rules and regulations.	Specific reference to this concept is made in the chapter overview. The chapter has been reorganized to clearly indicate the requirements for a self-governing medical staff and the specific bylaw requirements.
MS.2.3 *Medical staff bylaws include provisions for at least the following:*		This standard was not scorable and has been deleted.
MS.2.3.1 An executive committee of the medical staff;	**MS.1.40** There is a medical staff executive committee.	Reformatted and renumbered.
MS.2.3.2 Fair-hearing and appellate review mechanisms for medical staff members and other individuals holding clinical privileges;	**MS.4.50** There are mechanisms including a fair hearing and appeal process for addressing adverse decisions regarding reappointment, denial, reduction, suspension, or revocation of privileges that may relate to quality of care, treatment, and services issues.	Reformatted and renumbered.
MS.2.3.3 Mechanisms for corrective action, including indications and procedures for automatic and summary suspension of an individual's medical staff membership or clinical privileges;	**MS.1.20** Medical staff bylaws address self governance and accountability to the governing body.	Addressed in **MS.1.20**, EPs 12–16.
MS.2.3.4 A description of the medical staff's organization, including categories of medical staff membership, when such exist, and appropriate officer positions, with the stipulation that each officer is a medical staff member;	**MS.1.10** The hospital has an organized, self-governing medical staff that provides oversight of care, treatment, and services provided by practitioners with privileges, provides for a uniform quality of patient care, treatment, and services, and reports to and is accountable to the governing body. **MS.1.40** There is a medical staff executive committee.	The specific requirements for descriptions of categories of membership, officer positions were deleted. These items are implicit in the general standard "a description of the medical staff's organization." Additionally, the standard used the language "when such exists," which made these references less meaningful.
MS.2.3.4.1 The bylaws define		This standard was not scorable and has been deleted.
MS.2.3.4.1.1 the method of selecting officers,	**MS.1.20** Medical staff bylaws address self governance and accountability to the governing body.	Addressed in **MS.1.20**, EP 10.
MS.2.3.4.1.2 the qualifications, responsibilities, and tenures of officers, and	**MS.1.20** Medical staff bylaws address self governance and accountability to the governing body.	Addressed in **MS.1.20**, EPs 2 and 3.
MS.2.3.4.1.3 the conditions and mechanisms for removing officers from their positions;	**MS.1.20** Medical staff bylaws address self governance and accountability to the governing body.	Addressed in **MS.1.20**, EP 10.

Previous Standards	Current Standards	Comments
MS.2.3.5 Requirements for frequency of meetings and for attendance;		Deleted; administrative requirement.
MS.2.3.6 A mechanism designed to provide for effective communication among the medical staff, hospital administration, and governing body;	MS.2.20 The management and coordination of each patient's care, treatment, and services is the responsibility of a practitioner with appropriate privileges. MS.2.30 In hospitals participating in a professional graduate education program(s), the organized medical staff has a defined process for supervision by a licensed independent practitioner with appropriate clinical privileges of each member in the program in carrying out his or her patient care responsibilities.	The issue of a comprehensive and measurable communication standard will be addressed at a future date. Communication is also addressed in LD.3.60.
MS.2.3.6.1 If there are multiple levels of governance, there is an established mechanism for the medical staff to communicate with all levels of governance involved in policy decisions affecting patient care services in the hospital.	MS.2.20 The management and coordination of each patient's care, treatment, and services is the responsibility of a practitioner with appropriate privileges.	Also addressed in LD.3.60 and LD.1.10.
MS.2.3.7 A mechanism for adopting and amending the medical staff bylaws, rules and regulations, and policies; and	MS.1.20 Medical staff bylaws address self governance and accountability to the governing body.	Reformatted and renumbered.
MS.2.3.8 Medical staff representation and participation in any hospital deliberation affecting the discharge of medical staff responsibilities.	MS.1.10 The hospital has an organized, self-governing medical staff that provides oversight of care, treatment, and services provided by practitioners with privileges, provides for a uniform quality of patient care, treatment, and services, and reports to and is accountable to the governing body. MS.1.20 Medical staff bylaws address self governance and accountability to the governing body. MS.1.30 Neither the organized medical staff nor the governing body may unilaterally amend the medical staff bylaws or rules and regulations. MS.4.50 There are mechanisms including a fair hearing and appeal process for addressing adverse decisions regarding reappointment, denial, reduction, suspension or revocation of privileges that may relate to quality of care, treatment, and services issues. MS.1.40 There is a medical staff executive committee.	Medical staff representation in hospital deliberations is implicit in the standard and EPs of MS self-governance, medical staff bylaws requirements as approved by the governing body, the role of the Medical Executive Committee (MEC), and unilateral amendment.
MS.2.4 When necessary, the medical staff bylaws and rules and regulations are revised to reflect the hospital's current practices with respect to medical staff organization and functions.	MS.1.20 Medical staff bylaws address self governance and accountability to the governing body.	No standard or EP specifically requires amendment of bylaws although this is implicit in MS.1.10.
MS.2.4.1 The medical staff bylaws, rules and regulations, and policies and the governing body's bylaws do not conflict.	MS.1.20 Medical staff bylaws address self governance and accountability to the governing body.	Addressed in MS.1.20, EP 7.
MS.2.4.2 If significant changes are made in the medical staff bylaws, rules and regulations, or policies, medical staff members and other individuals who have delineated clinical privileges are provided with revised texts of the written materials.	Deleted.	Administrative requirement; also addressed in MEC at MS.1.40 and LD.3.60.

Crosswalks of Standards

Previous Standards	Current Standards	Comments
MS.2.5 *In hospitals participating in professional graduate education programs, the rules and regulations and policies of the medical staff specify the process for supervision of participants in the program in carrying out their patient care responsibilities, in accordance with MS.6.9.*	**MS.2.30** In hospitals participating in a professional graduate education program(s), the organized medical staff has a defined process for supervision by a licensed independent practitioner with appropriate clinical privileges of each member in the program in carrying out his or her patient care responsibilities.	Reformatted and renumbered; standard is now scorable.
MS.2.6 The medical staff implements a process to identify and manage matters of individual physician health that is separate from the medical staff disciplinary function.	**MS.4.80** The medical staff implements a process to identify and manage matters of individual health for licensed independent practitioners. This identification process is separate from actions taken for disciplinary purposes.	Physician health expanded to all licensed independent practitioner health.
MS.3 *The medical staff is organized to accomplish its functions.*		This standard was not scorable and has been deleted.
MS.3.1 There is an executive committee of the medical staff.	**MS.1.40** There is a medical staff executive committee.	Reformatted and renumbered.
MS.3.1.1 The executive committee's function, size, and composition and the method of selecting its members are defined in the medical staff bylaws.	**MS.1.20** Medical staff bylaws address self governance and accountability to the governing body.	Addressed in **MS.1.20**, EP 10.
MS.3.1.2 The chief executive officer of the hospital or his or her designee attends each executive committee meeting on an ex-officio basis, with or without vote.	**MS.1.40** There is a medical staff executive committee.	Reformatted and renumbered.
MS.3.1.3 No medical staff member actively practicing in the hospital is ineligible for membership on the executive committee solely because of his or her professional discipline or specialty.	**MS.1.40** There is a medical staff executive committee.	Reformatted and renumbered.
MS.3.1.4 A majority of voting executive committee members are fully licensed physician members of the medical staff actively practicing in the hospital.	**MS.1.40** There is a medical staff executive committee.	Addressed in **MS.1.40**, EP 4.
MS.3.1.5 The executive committee is empowered to act for the medical staff in the intervals between medical staff meetings.	**MS.1.40** There is a medical staff executive committee.	Addressed in **MS.1.40**, EP 5.
MS.3.1.6 The executive committee is responsible for making medical staff recommendations directly to the governing body for its approval.	**MS.1.40** There is a medical staff executive committee.	Reformatted and renumbered.
MS.3.1.6.1.1 The medical staff's structure;	**MS.1.40** There is a medical staff executive committee.	Addressed in **MS.1.40**, EP 8.
MS.3.1.6.1.2 The mechanism used to review credentials and to delineate individual clinical privileges;	**MS.1.40** There is a medical staff executive committee.	Addressed in **MS.1.40**, EP 9.
MS.3.1.6.1.3 Recommendations of individuals for medical staff membership;	**MS.1.40** There is a medical staff executive committee.	Addressed in **MS.1.40**, EP 9.
MS.3.1.6.1.4 Recommendations for delineated clinical privileges for each eligible individual;	**MS.1.40** There is a medical staff executive committee.	Addressed in **MS.1.40**, EP 9.
MS.3.1.6.1.5 The participation of the medical staff in organization performance improvement activities;	**MS.3.10** The organized medical staff has a leadership role in hospital performance improvement activities to improve quality of care, treatment, and services and patient safety. **MS.3.20** The organized medical staff participates in the measurement, assessment, and improvement of other processes.	Reformatted and renumbered.
MS.3.1.6.1.6 The mechanism by which medical staff membership may be terminated; and	**MS.1.40** There is a medical staff executive committee.	Addressed in **MS.1.40**, EP 6.

CW – 37

Previous Standards	Current Standards	Comments
MS.3.1.6.1.7 The mechanism for fair-hearing procedures.	MS.4.50 There are mechanisms including a fair hearing and appeal process for addressing adverse decisions regarding reappointment, denial, reduction, suspension, or revocation of privileges that may relate to quality of care, treatment, and services issues.	Reformatted and renumbered.
MS.3.1.7 The executive committee receives and acts on reports and recommendations from medical staff committees, clinical departments, and assigned activity groups.	MS.1.40 There is a medical staff executive committee.	Addressed in **MS.1.40**, EP 12.
MS.4 *When medical staff clinical departments exist:* MS.4.1 *Each department has effective leadership.* MS.4.1.1 The director of each department is certified by an appropriate specialty board, or affirmatively establishes comparable competence, through the credentialing process. MS.4.2 Medical staff department directors' responsibilities are specified in the medical staff bylaws and rules and regulations. MS.4.2.1 *Each department director is responsible for the following:* MS.4.2.1.1 All clinically related activities of the department; MS.4.2.1.2 All administratively related activities of the department, unless otherwise provided for by the hospital; MS.4.2.1.3 Continuing surveillance of the professional performance of all individuals in the department who have delineated clinical privileges; MS.4.2.1.4 Recommending to the medical staff the criteria for clinical privileges that are relevant to the care provided in the department; MS.4.2.1.5 *Recommending clinical privileges for each member of the department;*	MS.1.20 Medical staff bylaws address self governance and accountability to the governing body. MS.4.20 There is a process for granting, renewing or revising setting-specific clinical privileges. LD.2.20 Each organizational program, service, site, or department has effective leadership.	Departmental requirements have been reduced to two EPs within the MS chapter. The majority of scored departmental standards have been deleted or collapsed into one EP (**MS.1.20**, EP 8), stating that the medical staff define the role and responsibilities of the department chair in the medical staff bylaws. An additional EP (**MS.4.20**, EP 8) requires that the department chairperson participate in the evaluation of practitioners at the time privileges are granted and renewed.
MS.4.2.1.6 Assessing and recommending to the relevant hospital authority off-site sources for needed patient care services not provided by the department or the organization.	LD.3.30 A hospital demonstrates a commitment to its community by providing essential services in a timely manner. LD.3.50 Services provided by consultation, contractual arrangements, or other agreements are provided safely and effectively.	Reformatted and renumbered.
MS.4.2.1.7 *the integration of the department or service into the primary functions of the organization; (LD.2.1)* MS.4.2.1.8 *the coordination and integration of interdepartmental and intradepartmental services; (LD.2.2)* MS.4.2.1.9 *the development and implementation of policies and procedures that guide and support the provision of services; (LD.2.3)* MS.4.2.1.10 *the recommendations for a sufficient number of qualified and competent persons to provide care or service; (LD.2.4)*		Not scorable in 2003; requirements appear in **LD.2.20, LD.3.70, LD.3.80, LD.3.90,** and **LD.4.10**. Requirements are also addressed in **PI.1.10, HR.1.10, HR.1.20, HR.2.10,** and **HR.2.30**.

Crosswalks of Standards

Previous Standards	Current Standards	Comments
MS.4.2.1.11 *the determination of the qualifications and competence of department or service personnel who are not licensed independent practitioners and who provide patient care services;* **(LD.2.5)**		
MS.4.2.1.12 *the continuous assessment and improvement of the quality of care and services provided;* **(LD.2.6)**		
MS.4.2.1.13 *the maintenance of quality control programs, as appropriate;* **(LD.2.7)**		
MS.4.2.1.14 *the orientation and continuing education of all persons in the department or service; and* **(LD.2.8)**		
MS.4.2.1.15 *recommendations for space and other resources needed by the department or service.* **(LD.2.9)**		
MS.5 The organization establishes mechanisms for hospital-specific appointment and reappointment of medical staff members and for granting and renewing or revising hospital-specific clinical privileges.	**MS.4.10** The organized medical staff has a credentialing process that is defined in the medical staff bylaws. **MS.4.20** There is a process for granting, renewing, or revising setting-specific clinical privileges. **MS.4.30** An organized medical staff may use an expedited process for appointing to the medical staff and when granting privileges when criteria for that process are met. **MS.4.40** At the time of renewal of privileges, the organized medical staff evaluates individuals for their continued ability to provide quality care, treatment, and services for the privileges requested as defined in the medical staff bylaws.	Reformatted and renumbered.
MS.5.1 The governing body appoints and reappoints to the medical staff and grants initial, renewed, or revised clinical privileges, based on medical staff recommendations, in accordance with the bylaws, rules and regulations, and policies of the medical staff and of the hospital.	**MS.1.20** Medical staff bylaws address self governance and accountability to the governing body. **MS.4.10** The organized medical staff has a credentialing process that is defined in the medical staff bylaws. **MS.4.20** There is a process for granting, renewing, or revising setting-specific clinical privileges. **MS.4.30** An organized medical staff may use an expedited process for appointing to the medical staff and when granting privileges when criteria for that process are met.	Addressed in **MS.1.20**, EPs 3, 4, 13–17, and 19–21; **MS.4.20**, EP 5; and **MS.4.30**, EP 2.
MS.5.1.1 The governing body, pursuant to its bylaws, may elect to delegate the authority to render initial appointment, reappointment, and renewal or modification of clinical privileges decisions to a committee of the governing body.	**MS.4.30** An organized medical staff may use an expedited process for appointing to the medical staff and when granting privileges when criteria for that process are met.	Reformatted and renumbered.
MS.5.1.2 Each applicant for medical staff membership is oriented to these bylaws, rules and regulations, and policies and agrees in writing that his or her activities as a medical staff member will be bound by them.		Deleted; administrative requirement. Also covered under the LD communication provision in **LD.3.60**.

Previous Standards	Current Standards	Comments
MS.5.1.3 Individuals in administrative positions who desire medical staff membership or clinical privileges are subject to the same procedures as all other applicants for membership or privileges.		Deleted; implicit in requirement that all individuals desiring membership or privileges must be "processed" through medical staff mechanisms. All members receiving privileges are to be bound by the same principles.
MS.5.2 There are mechanisms, including a fair hearing and appeal process, for addressing adverse decisions for existing medical staff members and other individuals holding clinical privileges for renewal, revocation, or revision of clinical privileges.	MS.4.50 There are mechanisms including a fair hearing and appeal process for addressing adverse decisions regarding reappointment, denial, reduction, suspension, or revocation of privileges that may relate to quality of care, treatment, and services issues.	Reformatted and renumbered.
MS.5.2.1 *These mechanisms may differ for medical staff members and other individuals holding clinical privileges.*	MS.4.50 There are mechanisms including a fair hearing and appeal process for addressing adverse decisions regarding reappointment, denial, reduction, suspension, or revocation of privileges that may relate to quality of care, treatment, and services issues.	Reformatted and renumbered; standard is now scorable.
MS.5.3 *The mechanisms for appointment or reappointment and initial granting and renewal or revision of clinical privileges are*		This standard was not scorable and has been deleted.
MS.5.3.1 approved and implemented by the medical staff and governing body;	MS.1.20 Medical staff bylaws address self governance and accountability to the governing body.	Addressed in **MS.1.20**, EPs 18, 19, 20.
MS.5.3.2 fully documented in the medical staff bylaws, rules and regulations, and policies; and	MS.1.20 Medical staff bylaws address self governance and accountability to the governing body.	Reformatted and renumbered.
MS.5.3.3 *described to each applicant.*		Deleted; now addressed in **LD.3.60**.
MS.5.4 The mechanisms provide for professional criteria that are specified in the medical staff bylaws and uniformly applied to all applicants for medical staff membership, medical staff members, or applicants for delineated clinical privileges. These criteria constitute the basis for granting initial or continuing medical staff membership and for granting initial, renewed, or revised clinical privileges.	MS.4.10 The organized medical staff has a credentialing process that is defined in the medical staff bylaws. MS.4.20 There is a process for granting, renewing, or revising setting-specific clinical privileges. MS.4.40 At the time of renewal of privileges, the organized medical staff evaluates individuals for their continued ability to provide quality care, treatment, and services for the privileges requested as defined in the medical staff bylaws.	Reformatted and renumbered.
MS.5.4.1 Each clinical department makes recommendations to the medical staff regarding professional criteria for clinical privileges.	MS.1.40 There is a medical staff executive committee. MS.4.20 There is a process for granting, renewing or revising setting-specific clinical privileges.	Addressed in **MS.1.40**, EP 12 and **MS.4.20**, EP 8. The department concepts have been greatly reduced and the exact language of this standard has been deleted, but **MS.1.40**, EP 12 states that the MEC reviews and acts on reports of medical staff committees and departments. EP 8 of **MS.4.20** requires that the department chairperson participate in the evaluation of practitioners.
MS.5.4.2 The professional criteria are designed to assure the medical staff and governing body that patients will receive quality care.		Deleted as a specific requirement. The entire chapter is designed to ensure quality care and oversight of practitioners by the MS. Implicit in EPs, and directly addressed in introduction to Credentialing and Privileging.

Crosswalks of Standards

Previous Standards	Current Standards	Comments
MS.5.4.3 The professional criteria at least pertain to evidence of current licensure, relevant training or experience, current competence, and ability to perform the privileges requested.	**MS.4.10** The organized medical staff has a credentialing process that is defined in the medical staff bylaws. **MS.4.20** There is a process for granting, renewing, or revising setting-specific clinical privileges. **MS.4.30** An organized medical staff may use an expedited process for appointing to the medical staff and when granting privileges when criteria for that process are met. **MS.4.40** At the time of renewal of privileges, the organized medical staff evaluates individuals for their continued ability to provide quality care, treatment, and services for the privileges requested as defined in the medical staff bylaws.	Reformatted and renumbered.
MS.5.4.3.1 For an applicant for initial appointment to the medical staff and for initial granting of clinical privileges, the hospital verifies information about the applicant's licensure, specific training, experience, and current competence provided by the applicant with information from the primary source(s) whenever feasible.	**MS.4.10** The organized medical staff has a credentialing process that is defined in the medical staff bylaws.	Addressed in **MS.4.10**, EP 4.
MS.5.4.3.1.1 Action on an individual's application for appointment or initial clinical privileges is withheld until the information is available and verified.	**MS.4.10** The organized medical staff has a credentialing process that is defined in the medical staff bylaws. **MS.4.20** There is a process for granting, renewing, or revising setting-specific clinical privileges. **MS.4.30** An organized medical staff may use an expedited process for appointing to the medical staff and when granting privileges when criteria for that process are met. **MS.4.40** At the time of renewal of privileges, the organized medical staff evaluates individuals for their continued ability to provide quality care, treatment, and services for the privileges requested as defined in the medical staff bylaws.	Implicit in standards and EPs that privileges may not be granted until information is verified.
MS.5.4.3.2 *The hospital is also encouraged to consider additional information concerning the applicant from other sources, including the Federation of State Medical Boards Physician Disciplinary Data Bank. These databases and other sources may provide the hospital with information that is new or that may flag an inconsistency when compared with the individual's application.*		Deleted; this standard was previously not scorable.
MS.5.4.4 Decisions on reappointments or on revocation, revision, or renewal of clinical privileges must consider criteria that are directly related to the quality of care.	**MS.4.20** There is a process for granting, renewing, or revising setting-specific clinical privileges.	Addressed in **MS.4.20**, EP 14.

Previous Standards	Current Standards	Comments
MS.5.4.4.1 Such decisions are subject to a fair hearing and appeal process.	MS.1.20 Medical staff bylaws address self governance and accountability to the governing body. MS.4.50 There are mechanisms including a fair hearing and appeal process for addressing adverse decisions regarding reappointment, denial, reduction, suspension or revocation of privileges that may relate to quality of care, treatment, and services issues.	Addressed in MS.1.20, EP 17.
MS.5.4.5 Decisions on appointments or on granting of clinical privileges must consider criteria that are directly related to the quality of care.	MS.4.20 There is a process for granting, renewing, or revising setting-specific clinical privileges.	Addressed in MS.4.20, EP 14.
MS.5.5 *The medical staff bylaws, rules and regulations, or policies define the information to be provided by each applicant for appointment or reappointment to the medical staff and initial, renewed, or revised clinical privileges, including at least*		Not scorable; lead-in statement deleted.
MS.5.5.1 *previously successful or currently pending challenges to any licensure or registration (state or district, Drug Enforcement Administration) or the voluntary relinquishment of such licensure or registration;*	MS.4.20 There is a process for granting, renewing, or revising setting-specific clinical privileges. MS.4.30 An organized medical staff may use an expedited process for appointing to the medical staff and when granting privileges when criteria for that process are met.	Addressed in MS.4.20, EP 6 and MS.4.30, EP 1.
MS.5.5.2 *voluntary or involuntary termination of medical staff membership or voluntary or involuntary limitation, reduction, or loss of clinical privileges at another hospital; and*	MS.4.20 There is a process for granting, renewing, or revising setting-specific clinical privileges. MS.4.30 An organized medical staff may use an expedited process for appointing to the medical staff and when granting privileges when criteria for that process are met.	Reformatted and renumbered.
MS.5.5.3 *involvement in a professional liability action under circumstances specified in the medical staff bylaws, rules and regulations, and policies.*	MS.4.20 There is a process for granting, renewing, or revising setting-specific clinical privileges. MS.4.30 An organized medical staff may use an expedited process for appointing to the medical staff and when granting privileges when criteria for that process are met.	Reformatted and renumbered.
MS.5.5.3.1 At a minimum, final judgments or settlements involving the individual are reported.	MS.4.20 There is a process for granting, renewing, or revising setting-specific clinical privileges. MS.4.30 An organized medical staff may use an expedited process for appointing to the medical staff and when granting privileges when criteria for that process are met.	Reformatted and renumbered.
MS.5.6 *Appointment or reappointment to the medical staff and the initial granting and renewal or revision of clinical privileges are also based on information regarding the applicant's competence.*	MS.4.20 There is a process for granting, renewing, or revising setting-specific clinical privileges. MS.4.30 An organized medical staff may use an expedited process for appointing to the medical staff and when granting privileges when criteria for that process are met.	Reformatted and renumbered; standards are now scorable.

Crosswalks of Standards

Previous Standards	Current Standards	Comments
MS.5.7 Deliberations by the medical staff in developing recommendations for appointment to or termination from the medical staff and for the initial granting, revision, or revocation of clinical privileges include information provided by a peer(s) of the applicant.	MS.4.70 Peer recommendations from peers in the same professional discipline as the applicant are used as part of the basis for the initial granting of privileges. Peer recommendations are used to recommend individuals for the renewal of clinical privileges when insufficient peer review data are available.	Reformatted and renumbered.
MS.5.8 *A structured procedure, as defined by medical staff bylaws, rules and regulations, and medical staff policies, is used for the expeditious processing of complete applications for appointment, reappointment, and initial, renewed, or revised clinical privileges.*	MS.1.20 Medical staff bylaws address self governance and accountability to the governing body. MS.4.20 There is a process for granting, renewing or revising setting-specific clinical privileges. MS.4.40 At the time of renewal of privileges, the organized medical staff evaluates individuals for their continued ability to provide quality care, treatment, and services for the privileges requested as defined in the medical staff bylaws.	Addressed in **MS.1.20**, EPs 19 and 20; requirements are now scorable.
MS.5.8.1 A separate record is maintained for each individual requesting medical staff membership or clinical privileges.		Deleted; administrative requirement.
MS.5.8.2 Complete applications are acted on within a reasonable period of time, as specified in the medical staff bylaws.	MS.4.20 There is a process for granting, renewing, or revising setting-specific clinical privileges.	Addressed in **MS.4.20**, EP 12.
MS.5.9 Gender, race, creed, or national origin are not used in making decisions regarding the granting or denying of medical staff membership or clinical privileges.		Deleted; addressed in **LD.1.30** (law and regulation).
MS.5.10 Each applicant		Not scored; lead-in statement deleted.
MS.5.10.1 consents to the inspection of records and documents pertinent to his or her licensure, specific training, experience, current competence, and ability to perform the privileges requested, and, if requested, appears for an interview;		Deleted.
MS.5.10.1.1 The bylaws, rules and regulations, and policies of the medical staff indicate that the applicant for reappointment or renewal of clinical privileges is required to submit any reasonable evidence of current ability to perform privileges that may be requested.	MS.4.20 There is a process for granting, renewing, or revising setting-specific clinical privileges. MS.4.30 An organized medical staff may use an expedited process for appointing to the medical staff and when granting privileges when criteria for that process are met. MS.4.40 At the time of renewal of privileges, the organized medical staff evaluates individuals for their continued ability to provide quality care, treatment, and services for the privileges requested as defined in the medical staff bylaws.	Reformatted and renumbered.
MS.5.10.2 [Each applicant] pledges to provide for continuous care for his or her patients; and	MS.2.10 The organized medical staff oversees the quality of patient care, treatment, and services provided by practitioners privileged through the medical staff process.	Addressed in **MS.2.10**, EP 1.
MS.5.10.3 *[Each applicant] acknowledges any provisions in the medical staff bylaws for release and immunity from civil liability.*		Deleted.

Previous Standards	Current Standards	Comments
MS.5.11 Appointment or reappointment to the medical staff and the granting, renewal, or revision of clinical privileges are made for a period of no more than two years.	MS.4.20 There is a process for granting, renewing or revising setting-specific clinical privileges.	Addressed in MS.4.20, EP 4.
MS.5.12 Appraisal for reappointment to the medical staff or renewal or revision of clinical privileges is based on ongoing monitoring of information concerning the individual's		Not scored; lead-in statement deleted.
MS.5.12.1 professional performance;	MS.4.20 There is a process for granting, renewing, or revising setting-specific clinical privileges. MS.4.40 At the time of renewal of privileges, the organized medical staff evaluates individuals for their continued ability to provide quality care, treatment, and services for the privileges requested as defined in the medical staff bylaws.	Addressed in MS.4.20, EP 7 and MS.4.40, EP 4.
MS.5.12.2 judgment; and	MS.4.20 There is a process for granting, renewing, or revising setting-specific clinical privileges.	Addressed in MS.4.20, EP 7.
MS.5.12.3 clinical or technical skills.	MS.4.20 There is a process for granting, renewing, or revising setting-specific clinical privileges.	Addressed in MS.4.20, EP 7.
MS.5.13 Departmental or major clinical service recommendations are part of the basis for developing recommendations for continued membership on the medical staff or for delineating individual clinical privileges.	MS.4.40 At the time of renewal of privileges, the organized medical staff evaluates individuals for their continued ability to provide quality care, treatment, and services for the privileges requested as defined in the medical staff bylaws.	Addressed in MS.4.20, EP 8.
MS.5.14 All individuals who are permitted by law and by the hospital to provide patient care services independently in the hospital have delineated clinical privileges, whether or not they are medical staff members.	MS.4.20 There is a process for granting, renewing, or revising setting-specific clinical privileges.	Addressed in MS.4.20, EPs 1, 2, 3, 4, and 13.
MS.5.14.1 The delineation of an individual's clinical privileges includes the limitations, if any, on an individual's privileges to admit and treat patients or direct the course of treatment for the conditions for which the patients were admitted.	MS.4.20 There is a process for granting, renewing, or revising setting-specific clinical privileges. MS.4.40 At the time of renewal of privileges, the organized medical staff evaluates individuals for their continued ability to provide quality care, treatment, and services for the privileges requested as defined in the medical staff bylaws.	Implicit in the EPs.
MS.5.14.2 There is a mechanism designed to ensure that all individuals with clinical privileges only provide services within the scope of privileges granted.	MS.4.40 At the time of renewal of privileges, the organized medical staff evaluates individuals for their continued ability to provide quality care, treatment, and services for the privileges requested as defined in the medical staff bylaws.	Addressed in MS.4.40, EP 5.
MS.5.14.3 When physicians or other individuals eligible for delineated clinical privileges are engaged by the hospital to provide patient care services pursuant to a contract, their clinical privileges to admit or treat patients are defined through medical staff mechanisms.	MS.4.20 There is a process for granting, renewing, or revising setting-specific clinical privileges. MS.4.40 At the time of renewal of privileges, the organized medical staff evaluates individuals for their continued ability to provide quality care, treatment, and services for the privileges requested as defined in the medical staff bylaws.	All medical staff processes apply to contracted staff.

Crosswalks of Standards

Previous Standards	Current Standards	Comments
MS.5.14.4 The chief executive officer or his or her designee may grant temporary clinical privileges, when appropriate.	**MS.4.100** Under certain circumstances, temporary clinical privileges may be granted for limited period of time.	Addressed in **MS.4.100**, EP 4.
MS.5.14.4.1 Emergency privileges may be granted when the emergency management plan has been activated, and the organization is unable to handle the immediate patient needs. (See standard **EC.1.4**)	**MS.4.110** Disaster privileges may be granted when the emergency management plan has been activated and the hospital is unable to handle the immediate patient needs (see standard **EC.4.10**).	Reformatted and renumbered.
MS.5.15 Whatever mechanism for granting and renewal or revision of clinical privileges is used, evidence indicates that the clinical privileges are hospital specific and based on the individual's demonstrated current competence.	Deleted as a specific requirement.	Addressed in the introduction to Credentialing, Privileging, and Appointment. Implicit in standards and EPs.
MS.5.15.1 *Privileges are related to*		Not scored; lead-in statement deleted.
MS.5.15.1.1 *an individual's documented experience in categories of treatment areas or procedures;*	**MS.4.20** There is a process for granting, renewing, or revising setting-specific clinical privileges. **MS.4.30** An organized medical staff may use an expedited process for appointing to the medical staff and when granting privileges when criteria for that process are met. **MS.3.10** The organized medical staff has a leadership role in hospital performance improvement activities to improve quality of care, treatment, and services and patient safety.	Previous standard not scorable; specific language excluded but concept is implicit in standards and EPs.
MS.5.15.1.2 *the results of treatment; and*	**MS.4.20** There is a process for granting, renewing, or revising setting-specific clinical privileges. **MS.4.30** An organized medical staff may use an expedited process for appointing to the medical staff and when granting privileges when criteria for that process are met. **MS.3.10** The organized medical staff has a leadership role in hospital performance improvement activities to improve quality of care, treatment, and services and patient safety.	Previous standard not scorable; specific language excluded but concept is implicit in standards and EPs.
MS.5.15.1.3 *the conclusions drawn from organization performance improvement activities when available.*	**MS.3.10** The organized medical staff has a leadership role in hospital performance improvement activities to improve quality of care, treatment, and services and patient safety.	Previous standard not scorable; specific language excluded but concept is implicit in standards and EPs.
MS.5.15.2 Board certification is an excellent benchmark and is considered when delineating clinical privileges.		Deleted; not scorable.
MS.5.15.3 When privilege delineation is based primarily on experience, the individual's credentials record reflects the specific experience and successful results that form the basis for the granting of privileges.	**MS.4.20** There is a process for granting, renewing, or revising setting-specific clinical privileges.	Addressed in **MS.4.20**, EPs 3, 6, and 7.
MS.5.15.4 When the medical staff uses a system involving classification or categorization of privileges, the scope of each level of privileges is well defined, and the standards to be met by the applicant are stated clearly for each category.	**MS.4.20** There is a process for granting, renewing, or revising setting-specific clinical privileges. **MS.4.40** At the time of renewal of privileges, the organized medical staff evaluates individuals for their continued ability to provide quality care, treatment, and services for the privileges requested as defined in the medical staff bylaws.	Implicit in credentialing and privileging standards.

Previous Standards	Current Standards	Comments
MS.5.15.5 When medical staff clinical departments exist, all licensed independent practitioners are assigned to at least one clinical department and are granted clinical privileges that are relevant to the care provided in that department.		Deleted.
M.S.5.15.5.1 There is a satisfactory method to coordinate appraisal for granting or renewal or revision of clinical privileges when an individual currently holding clinical privileges or applying for clinical privileges requests privileges that are relevant to the care provided in more than one department or clinical specialty area.		Deleted.
MS.5.15.6 The exercise of clinical privileges within any department is subject to the rules and regulations of that department and to the authority of the department's director.		Deleted.
MS.5.15.7 When there are no medical staff clinical departments, all individuals with clinical privileges have their privileges recommended and the quality of their care reviewed through designated medical staff mechanisms, described in the medical staff or governing body bylaws and rules and regulations.	**MS.4.20** There is a process for granting, renewing, or revising setting-specific clinical privileges. **MS.4.40** At the time of renewal of privileges, the organized medical staff evaluates individuals for their continued ability to provide quality care, treatment, and services for the privileges requested as defined in the medical staff bylaws.	Reformatted and renumbered; standards are now scorable.
MS.5.16 Practitioners who diagnose or treat patients via telemedicine link are subject to the credentialing and privileging processes of the organization that receives the telemedicine service.	**MS.4.120** Licensed independent practitioners who are responsible for the care, treatment, and services of the patient via telemedicine link are subject to the credentialing and privileging processes of the originating site.	Reformatted and renumbered.
MS.5.16.1 The medical staff recommends the clinical services to be provided by telemedicine.	**MS.4.130** The medical staffs at both the originating and distant sites recommend the clinical services to be provided by licensed independent practitioners through a telemedical link at their respective sites.	Reformatted and renumbered.
MS.6 Individuals who admit patients are granted specific privileges to do so.	**MS.4.20** There is a process for granting, renewing, or revising setting-specific clinical privileges. **MS.4.30** An organized medical staff may use an expedited process for appointing to the medical staff and when granting privileges when criteria for that process are met. **MS.2.10** The organized medical staff oversees the quality of patient care, treatment, and services provided by practitioners privileged through the medical staff process.	Addressed in **MS.2.10**, EP 1.
MS.6.1 Individuals are granted the privilege to admit patients to inpatient services in accordance with state law and criteria for standards of medical care established by the medical staff.	**MS.4.20** There is a process for granting, renewing, or revising setting-specific clinical privileges. **MS.4.40** At the time of renewal of privileges, the organized medical staff evaluates individuals for their continued ability to provide quality care, treatment, and services for the privileges requested as defined in the medical staff bylaws.	Addressed in **MS.4.20** EPs 1 and 2; **MS.4.40**, EPs 1 and 2.

Crosswalks of Standards

Previous Standards	Current Standards	Comments
MS.6.2 A patient admitted for inpatient care has a medical history taken and an appropriate physical examination performed by a qualified physician.	**MS.2.10** The organized medical staff oversees the quality of patient care, treatment, and services provided by practitioners privileged through the medical staff process. **MS.4.20** There is a process for granting, renewing, or revising setting-specific clinical privileges.	Reformatted and renumbered.
MS.6.2.1 Qualified oral and maxillofacial surgeons may perform the medical history and physical examination, if they have such privileges, in order to assess the medical, surgical, and anesthetic risks of the proposed operative and other procedure(s).	**MS.2.10** The organized medical staff oversees the quality of patient care, treatment, and services provided by practitioners privileged through the medical staff process.	Addressed in **MS.2.10**, EP 8.
MS.6.2.2 Other licensed independent practitioners who are permitted to provide patient care services independently may perform all or part of the medical history and physical examination, if granted such privileges.	**MS.2.10** The organized medical staff oversees the quality of patient care, treatment, and services provided by practitioners privileged through the medical staff process.	Addressed in **MS.2.10**, EP 8.
MS.6.2.2.1 The findings, conclusions, and assessment of risk are confirmed or endorsed by a qualified physician prior to major high-risk (as defined by the medical staff) diagnostic or therapeutic interventions.	**MS.2.10** The organized medical staff oversees the quality of patient care, treatment, and services provided by practitioners privileged through the medical staff process.	Addressed in **MS.2.10**, EP 10.
MS.6.2.2.2 Dentists are responsible for the part of their patients' history and physical examination that relates to dentistry.	**MS.2.10** The organized medical staff oversees the quality of patient care, treatment, and services provided by practitioners privileged through the medical staff process.	Addressed in **MS.2.10**, EP 8.
MS.6.2.2.3 Podiatrists are responsible for the part of their patients' history and physical examination that relates to podiatry.	**MS.2.10** The organized medical staff oversees the quality of patient care, treatment, and services provided by practitioners privileged through the medical staff process.	Addressed in **MS.2.10**, EP 8.
MS.6.3 The medical staff determines those nonpatient services (for example, ambulatory surgery), if any, for which a patient must have a medical history taken and appropriate physical examination performed by a qualified physician who has such privileges, except as provided for in **MS.6.2.1** through **MS.6.2.2.3**.	**MS.2.10** The organized medical staff oversees the quality of patient care, treatment, and services provided by practitioners privileged through the medical staff process.	Addressed in **MS.2.10**, EP 11.
MS.6.4 Individuals provide treatment and perform operative and other procedure(s) within those areas of competence indicated by the scope of their delineated clinical privileges.	**MS.4.20** There is a process for granting, renewing, or revising setting-specific clinical privileges. **MS.4.40** At the time of renewal of privileges, the organized medical staff evaluates individuals for their continued ability to provide quality care, treatment, and services for the privileges requested as defined in the medical staff bylaws.	Reformatted and renumbered.
MS.6.5 The management of each patient's care is the responsibility of a qualified licensed independent practitioner with appropriate clinical privileges.	**MS.2.20** The management and coordination of each patient's care, treatment, and services is the responsibility of a practitioner with appropriate privileges.	Addressed in **MS.2.20**, EP 1.
MS.6.5.1 Management of a patient's general medical condition is the responsibility of a qualified physician member of the medical staff.	**MS.2.20** The management and coordination of each patient's care, treatment, and services is the responsibility of a practitioner with appropriate privileges.	Reformatted and renumbered.

CW

CW – 47

Previous Standards	Current Standards	Comments
MS.6.5.2 The medical staff, through its designated mechanism, determines the circumstances under which consultation or management by a physician or other qualified licensed independent practitioner is required.	**MS.2.20** The management and coordination of each patient's care, treatment, and services is the responsibility of a practitioner with appropriate privileges.	Addressed in **MS.2.20**, EP 4.
MS.6.6 When a hospital that provides psychiatric or substance-abuse services determines that multidisciplinary treatment plans are appropriate, written policies address multidisciplinary treatment plans. **MS.6.6.1** The written policies provide for appropriate physician involvement in and approval of the multidisciplinary treatment plan.	**MS.2.20** The management and coordination of each patient's care, treatment, and services is the responsibility of a practitioner with appropriate privileges.	No longer a specific reference to substance abuse programs and multidisciplinary treatment plan. EPs are general enough to address this concern.
MS.6.7 In hospitals that do not primarily provide psychiatric or substance-abuse services, the medical staff's role in the care or appropriate referral of patients who are emotionally ill, who become emotionally ill while in the hospital, or who suffer the results of alcoholism or drug abuse is clearly defined in a written plan.		Moved to **LD.3.140**.
MS.6.8 *There is a mechanism designed to ensure that the same level of quality of patient care is provided by all individuals with delineated clinical privileges, within medical staff departments, across departments, and between members and nonmembers of the medical staff who have delineated clinical privileges.*	**MS.1.10** The hospital has an organized, self-governing medical staff that provides oversight of care, treatment, and services provided by practitioners with privileges, provides for a uniform quality of patient care, treatment, and services, and reports to and is accountable to the governing body.	Reformatted and renumbered; standard is now scorable.
MS.6.9 In hospitals participating in a professional graduate education program(s), the medical staff has a defined process for supervision by a licensed independent practitioner with appropriate clinical privileges of each participant in the program(s) in carrying out patient care responsibilities.	**MS.2.30** In hospitals participating in a professional graduate education program(s), the organized medical staff has a defined process for supervision by a licensed independent practitioner with appropriate clinical privileges of each member in the program in carrying out his or her patient care responsibilities.	Reformatted and renumbered.
MS.6.9.1 There is a mechanism for effective communication between the committee(s) responsible for professional graduate education and the medical staff and governing body.	**MS.2.30** In hospitals participating in a professional graduate education program(s), the organized medical staff has a defined process for supervision by a licensed independent practitioner with appropriate clinical privileges of each member in the program in carrying out his or her patient care responsibilities.	Reformatted and renumbered.
MS.7 All individuals with delineated clinical privileges participate in continuing education.	**MS.5.10** All licensed independent practitioners and other practitioners privileged through the medical staff process participate in continuing education.	Reformatted and renumbered.
MS.7.1 Hospital-sponsored educational activities are offered.	**MS.5.10** All licensed independent practitioners and other practitioners privileged through the medical staff process participate in continuing education.	Reformatted and renumbered.
MS.7.1.1.1 the type and nature of care offered by the hospital; and	**MS.5.10** All licensed independent practitioners and other practitioners privileged through the medical staff process participate in continuing education.	Reformatted and renumbered.
MS.7.1.1.2 the findings of performance improvement activities.	**MS.5.10** All licensed independent practitioners and other practitioners privileged through the medical staff process participate in continuing education.	Reformatted and renumbered.

Crosswalks of Standards

Previous Standards	Current Standards	Comments
MS.7.2 Each individual's participation in continuing education is documented; and	**MS.5.10** All licensed independent practitioners and other practitioners privileged through the medical staff process participate in continuing education.	Reformatted and renumbered; standard is now scorable.
MS.7.2.1 considered in decisions about reappointment to the medical staff or renewal or revision of individual clinical privileges.	**MS.5.10** All licensed independent practitioners and other practitioners privileged through the medical staff process participate in continuing education.	Reformatted and renumbered.
MS.8 *The medical staff has a leadership role in organization performance improvement activities designed to*	**MS.3.10** The organized medical staff has a leadership role in hospital performance improvement activities to improve quality of care, treatment, and services and patient safety.	Reformatted and renumbered; standard is now scorable.
MS.8.1 ensure that when the performance of a process is dependent primarily on the activities of one or more individuals with clinical privileges (for example, on what surgeons as a component of the medical staff do), the medical staff provides leadership for the process measurement, assessment, and improvement. These processes include, though are not limited to, those within the:	**MS.3.10** The organized medical staff has a leadership role in hospital performance improvement activities to improve quality of care, treatment, and services and patient safety.	Reformatted and renumbered.
MS.8.1.1 Medical assessment and treatment of patients;	**MS.3.10** The organized medical staff has a leadership role in hospital performance improvement activities to improve quality of care, treatment, and services and patient safety.	Reformatted and renumbered.
MS.8.1.2 Use of medications; (PI.3.1.1)	**MS.3.10** The organized medical staff has a leadership role in hospital performance improvement activities to improve quality of care, treatment, and services and patient safety.	Reformatted and renumbered.
MS.8.1.3 Use of blood and blood components; (PI.3.1.1)	**MS.3.10** The organized medical staff has a leadership role in hospital performance improvement activities to improve quality of care, treatment, and services and patient safety.	Reformatted and renumbered.
MS.8.1.4 Use of operative and other procedure(s); (PI.3.1.1)	**MS.3.10** The organized medical staff has a leadership role in hospital performance improvement activities to improve quality of care, treatment, and services and patient safety.	Reformatted and renumbered.
MS.8.1.5 Efficiency of clinical practice patterns; and	**MS.3.10** The organized medical staff has a leadership role in hospital performance improvement activities to improve quality of care, treatment, and services and patient safety.	Reformatted and renumbered.
MS.8.1.6 Significant departures from established patterns of clinical practice.	**MS.3.10** The organized medical staff has a leadership role in hospital performance improvement activities to improve quality of care, treatment, and services and patient safety.	Reformatted and renumbered.
MS.8.2 *ensure that the medical staff participates in the measurement, assessment, and improvement of other patient care processes. The processes include, though are not limited to, those related to:*		Addressed in **MS.3.20**.
MS.8.2.1 Education of patients and families;	**MS.3.20** The organized medical staff participates in the measurement, assessment, and improvement of other processes.	Reformatted and renumbered.
MS.8.2.2 Coordination of care with other practitioners and hospital personnel, as relevant to the care of an individual patient; and	**MS.3.20** The organized medical staff participates in the measurement, assessment, and improvement of other processes.	Reformatted and renumbered.

Previous Standards	Current Standards	Comments
MS.8.2.3 Accurate, timely, and legible completion of patients' medical records. (IM.7.10)	**MS.3.20** The organized medical staff participates in the measurement, assessment, and improvement of other processes.	Reformatted and renumbered.
MS.8.3 ensure that when the findings of the assessment process are relevant to an individual's performance, the medical staff is responsible for determining their use in peer review or the ongoing evaluations of a licensed independent practitioner's competence, in accordance with the standards on renewing or revising clinical privileges delineated in this chapter;	**MS.3.20** The organized medical staff participates in the measurement, assessment, and improvement of other processes.	Reformatted and renumbered.
MS.8.4 ensure that the findings, conclusions, recommendations, and actions taken to improve organization performance are communicated to appropriate medical staff members; and	**MS.3.20** The organized medical staff participates in the measurement, assessment, and improvement of other processes.	Reformatted and renumbered.
MS.8.5 ensure that the medical staff, with other appropriate hospital staff, develops and uses criteria that identify deaths in which an autopsy should be performed.	**MS.3.10** The organized medical staff has a leadership role in hospital performance improvement activities to improve quality of care, treatment, and services and patient safety.	Reformatted and renumbered.
MS.8.5.1 *The medical staff attempts to secure autopsies in all deaths that meet the criteria.*	**MS.3.10** The organized medical staff has a leadership role in hospital performance improvement activities to improve quality of care, treatment, and services and patient safety.	Reformatted and renumbered; standard is now scorable.
MS.8.5.2 The mechanism for documenting permission to perform an autopsy is defined.	**MS.3.10** The organized medical staff has a leadership role in hospital performance improvement activities to improve quality of care, treatment, and services and patient safety.	Reformatted and renumbered.
MS.8.5.3 There is a system for notifying the medical staff, and specifically the attending practitioner, when an autopsy is being performed.	**MS.3.10** The organized medical staff has a leadership role in hospital performance improvement activities to improve quality of care, treatment, and services and patient safety.	Reformatted and renumbered.

Crosswalk of Previous Nursing Standards for Hospitals to Current Nursing Standards for Hospitals

This crosswalk is designed to show where the previous Nursing (NR) standards requirements appear in the reformatted NR standards. The left column (Previous Standards) lists consecutively each previous NR standard. The middle column, Current Standards, indicates the NR standards with revised numbers. The right column, Comments, identifies what changes have occurred between the previous standards and the current standards.

Previous Standards	Current Standards	Comments
NR.1 Nursing services are directed by a nurse executive who is a registered nurse qualified by advanced education and management experience.	**NR.1.10** A nurse executive directs the hospital's nursing services. **NR.2.10** The nurse executive is a registered nurse qualified by advanced education and management experience.	Reformatted and renumbered.
NR.2 The nurse executive has the authority and responsibility for establishing standards of nursing practice.	**NR.3.10** The nurse executive establishes nursing policies and procedures, nursing standards of patient care, treatment, and services and standards of nursing practice.	Reformatted and renumbered.
NR.3 Nursing policies and procedures, nursing standards of patient care, and standards of nursing practice are approved by the nurse executive or a designee(s).	**NR.1.10** Element of Performance 3 The nurse executive or a designee(s) approves nursing policies and procedures, nursing standards of patient care, treatment, and services, and standards of nursing practice before implementation.	Reformatted and renumbered.
NR.4 The nurse executive and other nursing leaders participate with leaders from the governing body, management, medical staff, and clinical areas in planning, promoting, and conducting organizationwide performance improvement activities.	**NR.1.10** Element of Performance 1 An identified nurse leader at the executive level coordinates the following functions: • Participating with governing body, management, medical staff, and clinical leaders in the hospital's decision-making structures and processes • Implementing an effective, ongoing program to measure, assess, and improve the quality of nursing care, treatment, and services delivered to patients	Reformatted and renumbered.

Glossary

abuse   Intentional maltreatment of an individual which may cause injury, either physical or psychological. *See also* neglect.

   mental abuse   Includes humiliation, harassment, and threats of punishment or deprivation.

   physical abuse   Includes hitting, slapping, pinching, or kicking. Also includes controlling behavior through corporal punishment.

   sexual abuse   Includes sexual harassment, sexual coercion, and sexual assault.

accountability   *See* information management.

accreditation   Determination by the Joint Commission's accrediting body that an eligible health care organization complies with applicable Joint Commission standards. *See also* accreditation decisions.

accreditation cycle   A period of accreditation at the conclusion of which, accreditation expires unless a full survey is performed.

accreditation decisions   Categories of accreditation that an organization can achieve based on a Joint Commission full survey. These decision categories are

- **Accredited**   The organization is in compliance with all standards at the time of the on-site survey or has successfully addressed all requirements for improvement in an Evidence of Standards Compliance (*see* definition) within 90 days following the survey (45 days beginning July 1, 2005).

- **Provisional Accreditation**   The organization fails to successfully address all requirements for improvement in an ESC within 90 days following the survey (45 days beginning July 1, 2005).

- **Conditional Accreditation**   The organization is not in substantial compliance with the standards, as usually evidenced by a count of the number of standards identified as not compliant at the time of survey which is between two and three standard deviations above the mean number of noncompliant standards for organizations in that accreditation program. The organization must remedy identified problem areas through preparation and submission of an ESC and subsequently undergo an on-site, follow-up survey.

- **Preliminary Denial of Accreditation**   There is justification to deny accreditation to the organization as usually evidenced by a count of the number of non-compliant standards at the time of survey which is at least three standard deviations above the mean number of standards identified as not compliant for organizations in that accreditation program. The decision is subject to appeal prior to the determination to deny accreditation; the appeal process may also result in a decision other than Denial of Accreditation.

- **Denial of Accreditation**   The organization has been denied accreditation. All review and

GL – 1

appeal opportunities have been exhausted.

- **Preliminary Accreditation** The organization demonstrates compliance with selected standards in the first of two surveys conducted under the Early Survey Policy Option 1 (*see* definition).

accreditation process A continuous process whereby health care organizations are required to demonstrate to the Joint Commission that they are providing safe, high quality of care, as determined by compliance with Joint Commission standards, National Patient Safety Goals recommendations, and performance measurement requirements. Key components of this process are an on-site evaluation of an organization by Joint Commission surveyors, a Periodic Performance Review, and quarterly submission of performance measurement data to the Joint Commission, as applicable.

accreditation report A report of an organization's survey findings; the report includes organization strengths, requirements for improvement (*see* definition) and supplemental findings (*see* definition), as appropriate.

accreditation survey findings Findings from an on-site evaluation conducted by Joint Commission's surveyors that results in an organization's accreditation decision.

activity services Structured activities designed to help an individual develop or maintain creative, physical, and social skills through participation in recreation, art, dance, drama, social, or other activities.

administration 1. The fiscal and general management of an organization, as distinct from the direct provision of services. 2. *See* medication management/administration.

administrative/financial measures Measures that address the organizational structure for coordinating and integrating services, functions, or activities across operational components, including financial management (for example, financial stability, utilization/length of stay, credentialing).

admitting privileges Authority issued to admit individuals to a health care organization. Individuals with admitting privileges may practice only within the scope of the clinical privileges granted by the organization's governing body.

advance directive A document or documentation allowing a person to give directions about future medical care or to designate another person(s) to make medical decisions if the individual loses decision-making capacity. Advance directives may include living wills, durable powers of attorney, do-not-resuscitate (DNRs) orders, right to die, or similar documents listed in the Patient Self-Determination Act which express the patient's preferences.

advanced practice nurse A registered nurse who has gained additional knowledge and skills through successful completion of an organized program of nursing education that prepares nurses for advanced practice roles and has been certified by the Board of nursing to engage in the practice of advanced practice nursing.

adverse drug event A patient injury resulting from a medication, either because of a pharmacological reaction to a normal dose, or because of a preventable adverse reaction to a drug resulting from an error.

adverse drug reaction (ADR) Unintended, undesirable, or unexpected effects of prescribed medications or of medication errors that require discontinuing a medication or modifying the dose; require initial or prolonged hospitalization; result in disability; require treatment with a prescription medication; result in cognitive deterioration or impairment; are life threatening; result in death; or result in congenital anomalies.

advocate A person who represents the rights and interests of another individual as though they were the person's own, in order to realize the rights to which the individual is entitled, obtain needed services, and remove barriers to meeting the individual's needs. *See also* surrogate decision maker.

ambulatory health care All types of health services provided to individuals on an outpatient basis. Ambulatory care services are provided in many settings ranging from freestanding ambulatory surgical facilities to cardiac catheterization centers.

ambulatory health care occupancy *See* occupancy.

analyzing *See* information management.

anesthesia and sedation The administration to an individual, in any setting, for any purpose, by any route, medication to induce a partial or total loss of sensation for the purpose of conducting an operative or other procedure. Definitions of four levels of sedation and anesthesia include the following:

minimal sedation (anxiolysis) A drug-induced state during which patients respond normally to verbal commands. Although cognitive function and coordination may be impaired, ventilatory and cardiovascular functions are unaffected.

moderate sedation/analgesia ("conscious sedation") A drug-induced depression of consciousness during which patients respond purposefully to verbal commands, either alone or accompanied by light tactile stimulation. Reflex withdrawal from a painful stimulus is *not* considered a purposeful response. No interventions are required to maintain a patent airway, and spontaneous ventilation is adequate. Cardiovascular function is usually maintained.

deep sedation/analgesia A drug-induced depression of consciousness during which patients cannot be easily aroused, but respond purposefully following repeated or painful stimulation. The ability to independently maintain ventilatory function may be impaired. Patients may require assistance in maintaining a patent airway and spontaneous ventilation may be inadequate. Cardiovascular function is usually maintained.

anesthesia Consists of general anesthesia and spinal or major regional anesthesia. It does *not* include local anesthesia. General anesthesia is a drug-induced loss of consciousness during which patients are not arousable, even by painful stimulation. The ability to independently maintain ventilatory function is often impaired. Patients often require assistance in maintaining a patent airway, and positive pressure ventilation may be required because of depressed spontaneous ventilation or drug-induced depression of neuromuscular function. Cardiovascular function may be impaired.

anesthetic gases Any gas delivered throughout the respiratory system as a component of general anesthesia or sedation. This may include inhalation anesthetics distributed in liquid form that when vaporized produce an anesthetic gas (for example, isoflurane, sevoflurane) or nonliquid compresssed gases (for example, nitrous oxide). Oxygen is not included in this definition.

anesthetizing location Any area used for the administration of anesthetic agents.

appeal process The process afforded to an organization that receives a Preliminary Denial of Accreditation (*see* definition), which includes the organization having a right to make a presentation to a Review Hearing Panel (*see* definition) before the Accreditation Committee takes final action to deny accreditation.

assessment 1. For purposes of patient assessment, the process established by an organization for obtaining appropriate and necessary information about each individual seeking entry into a health care setting or service. The information is used to match an individual's need with the appropriate setting, care level, and intervention. 2. For purposes of performance improvement, the systematic collection and review of patient-specific data.

auditability *See* information management.

authenticate To verify that an entry is complete, accurate, and final.

authentication *See* information management.

aversive procedures Procedures in which the patient is exposed to an unpleasant or noxious stimulus (the aversion) while engaging in the target behavior, the goal being to create an association of the aversion to the target behavior. Positive punishment is considered to be a type of aversive procedure. Positive punishment is a procedure in which target behavior is followed by the presentation of an unpleasant or noxious stimulus to decrease probability that the behavior will occur again, for example, spraying water mist in the individual's face. Negative punishment is not an aversive procedure. Negative punishment is a procedure in which the target behavior is followed by the removal of a desirable stimulus to decrease probability behavior will occur again, for example, turning off the television.

behavior management and treatment The use of basic behavioral or learning-based techniques designed to help the patient develop socially appropriate and safe replacement behavior. Characteristics of a behavior management and treatment program are that all the direct care staff are trained in the application of the program; it is a written, planned program; it is applied at all times the patient is under the supervision of direct care staff; it is individualized; and it is distinct from routine interactions with the patient.

behavioral health A broad array of mental health, chemical dependency, habilitation, and rehabilitation services provided in settings such as inpatient, residential, and outpatient.

best practices Clinical, scientific, or professional practices that are recognized by a majority of professionals in a particular field. These practices are typically evidence based and consensus-driven.

biologicals Medicines made from living organisms and their products, including serums, vaccines, antigens, and antitoxins.

blood component A fraction of separated whole blood, for example, red blood cell, plasma, platelets, and granulocytes.

blood derivative A pooled blood product, such as albumin, gamma globulin, or Rh immune globulin whose use is considered significantly lower in risk than that of blood or blood components.

blood transfusion services Services relating to transfusing and infusing individuals with blood, blood components, or blood derivatives.

blood usage measurement An activity that entails measuring, assessing, and improving the ordering, distributing, handling, dispensing, administering, and monitoring of blood and blood components.

business occupancy *See* occupancy.

bylaws A governance framework that establishes the roles and responsibilities of a body and its members.

capture *See* information management.

care plan A written plan, based on data gathered during assessment, that identifies care needs, describes the strategy for providing services to meet those needs, documents treatment goals and objectives, outlines the criteria for terminating specified interventions, and documents the progress in meeting goals and objectives. The format of the plan in some organizations may be guided by patient-specific policies and procedures, protocols, practice guidelines, clinical paths, care maps, or a combination thereof. The care plan may include care, treatment, habilitation, and rehabilitation.

care planning (or planning of care) Individualized planning and provision of services that addresses the needs, safety, and well-being of the patient. The plan, which formulates strategies, goals, and objectives, may include narratives, policies and procedures, protocols, practice guidelines, clinical paths, care maps, or a combination of these.

chemical restraint *See* restraint.

CLIA '88 The Clinical Laboratory Improvement Amendments of 1988.

clinical laboratory A facility that is equipped to examine material derived from the human body to provide information for use in the diagnosis, prevention, or treatment of disease; also called medical laboratory.

clinical privileges Authorization granted by the appropriate authority (for example, the governing body) to a practitioner to provide specific care, treatment, and services in an organization within well-defined limits, based on the following factors, as applicable: license, education, training, experience, competence, health status, and judgment.

clinical respiratory services The provision of health care services by respiratory care practitioners or respiratory therapists to individuals in their place of residence, associated with provision of home medical equipment services. This includes, but is not limited to, performing assessments and testing, administration of treatment, provision of education, and/or monitoring of the patient's respiratory status.

clinical service groups Groups of patients in distinct, clinical populations for which data are collected. Tracer patients are selected according to clinical service groups.

community The individuals, families, groups, agencies, facilities, or institutions within the geographic area served by a health care organization.

competence or competency A determination of an individual's skills, knowledge, and capability to meet defined expectations.

complex organization An organization that provides or provides for more than one level of care (for example, acute, subacute, chronic) and type (for example, pediatric, dental, behavioral health) of health care service, usually in more than one type of setting (for example, hospital, behavioral, home). An example is an organization that provides acute care, long term care, and home care services.

complex organization survey A Joint Commission survey in which standards from more than one accreditation manual are used in assessing compliance. This type of survey may include using specialist surveyors appropriate to the standards selected for survey.

compliance with a standard (*see definition*) Meeting the requirements of a standard through compliance with its element(s) of performance.

component A health care delivery entity (for example, service, program, related entity) that meets survey eligibility criteria under one of the Joint Commission accreditation programs. Multiple components comprise a complex organization.

confidentiality An individual's right, within the law, to personal and informational privacy, including his or her health care records. *See also* information management.

consultation 1. Provision of professional advice or services. 2. For purposes of Joint Commission accreditation, advice that is given to staff members of surveyed organizations relating to compliance with standards that are the subject of the survey.

consultation report 1. A written opinion by a consultant that reflects, when appropriate, an examination of the individual and the individual's medical record(s). 2. Information given verbally by a consultant to a care provider that reflects, when appropriate, an examination of the individual. The individual's care provider usually documents those opinions in the clinical/case record.

continuing care Care provided over time; in various settings, programs, or services; spanning the illness-to-wellness continuum.

continuing education Education beyond initial professional preparation that is relevant to the type of care delivered in an organization, that provides current knowledge relevant to an individual's field of practice or service responsibilities, and that may be related to findings from performance improvement activities.

continuity The degree to which the care of individuals is coordinated among practitioners, among organizations, and over time.

continuum of care Matching the individual's ongoing needs with the appropriate level and type of care, treatment, and service within an organization or across multiple organizations.

contract A formal agreement for care, treatment, and services with any organization, agency, or individual that specifies the services, personnel, products, or space provided by, to, or on behalf of the organization and specifies the consideration to be expended in exchange. The agreement is approved by the governing body or comparable entity.

contracted services Services provided through a written agreement with another organization, agency, or individual. The agreement specifies the services or personnel to be provided on behalf of the applicant organization and the fees to provide these services or personnel.

control chart A graphic display of data in the order they occur with statistically determined upper and lower limits of expected common-cause variation. A control chart is used to identify special causes of variation, to monitor a process for maintenance, and to determine if process changes have had the desired effect.

control limit In statistics, an expected limit of common-cause variation, sometimes referred to as either an upper or a lower limit. Variation beyond a control limit is evidence that special causes are affecting a process. Control limits are calculated from process data and are not to be confused with engineering specifications or tolerance limits. Control limits are typically plotted on a control chart.

coordination of care The process of coordinating care, treatment, and services provided by a health care organization, including referral to appropriate community resources and liaison with others (such as the individual's physician, other health care organizations, or community services involved in care, treatment, and services) to meet the ongoing identified needs of individuals, to ensure implementation of the plan of care, and to avoid unnecessary duplication of services.

credentialing The process of obtaining, verifying, and assessing the qualifications of a health care practitioner to provide patient care services in or for a health care organization.

credentials Documented evidence of licensure, education, training, experience, or other qualifications.

criteria 1. Expected level(s) of achievement, or specifications against which performance or quality may be compared. 2. For purposes of eligibility for a Joint Commission survey, the conditions necessary for health care organizations and networks to be surveyed for accreditation by the Joint Commission.

critical access hospital A hospital that offers limited services and is located more than 35 miles from a hospital or another critical access hospital, or is certified by the state as being a necessary provider of health care services to residents in the area.

It maintains no more than 25 beds that could be used for inpatient care. A critical access hospital provides acute inpatient care for a period that does not exceed, on an annual average basis, 96 hours per patient.

data *See* information management.

decentralized laboratory testing *See* point-of-care testing.

decentralized pharmaceutical services *See* pharmaceutical care and services.

deemed status Status conferred by the Centers for Medicare & Medicaid Services (CMS) on a health care provider when that provider is judged or determined to be in compliance with relevant Medicare Conditions of Participation because it has been accredited by a voluntary organization whose standards and survey process are determined by CMS to be equivalent to those of the Medicare program or other federal laws, such as the Clinical Laboratory Improvement Amendments of 1988 (CLIA '88).

delineation of clinical privileges The listing of the specific clinical privileges an organization's staff member is permitted to perform in the organization.

dental services Services provided by a dentist, or a qualified individual under the supervision of a dentist, to improve or maintain the health of an individual's teeth, oral cavity, and associated structures.

dentist An individual who has received the degree of either doctor of dental surgery or doctor of dental medicine and who is licensed to practice dentistry.

dietetic services The delivery of care pertaining to the provision of nutrition and food service to individuals.

disaster *See* emergency.

disaster plan *See* emergency management plan.

discharge The point at which an individual's active involvement with an organization or program is terminated and the organization or program no longer maintains active responsibility for the care of the individual.

discharge planning A formalized process in a health care organization through which the need for a program of continuing and follow-up care is ascertained and, if warranted, initiated for each patient.

disinfection The use of a chemical procedure that eliminates virtually all recognized pathogenic microorganisms but not necessarily all microbial forms (for example, bacterial endospores) on inanimate objects.

dispensing *See* medication management; pharmacy services.

distant site In telemedicine, the site at which the practitioner providing the professional service is located.

drug *See* medication.

drug administration *See* medication management.

drug allergies A state of hypersensitivity induced by exposure to a particular drug antigen resulting in harmful immunologic reactions on subsequent drug exposures, such as a penicillin drug allergy. *See* medication.

drug dispensing *See* medication management.

e-App The electronic version of an organization's application for accreditation.

Early Survey Policy A policy that provides two options to organizations undergoing their first Joint Commission survey. Under both options, the organization undergoes two surveys. Under the first option, the first survey is limited in scope and successful completion results in Preliminary Accreditation (*see* definition). Under the second option, the first survey is a full survey, and successful completion can lead to the organization being Accredited (*see* definition). The second survey in both options is required and will address all standards and a 4-month track record of compliance with the standards.

effectiveness The degree to which care is provided in the correct manner, given the current state of knowledge, to achieve the desired or projected outcome(s) for the individual.

efficacy The degree to which the care of the individual has been shown to accomplish the desired or projected outcome(s).

efficiency The relationship between the outcomes (results of care) and the resources used to deliver care.

electroconvulsive therapy A form of therapy that uses electricity to evoke a convulsive response.

electronic health information *See* information management.

Elements of Performance (EPs) The specific performance expectations and/or structures or processes that must be in place in order for an organization to provide safe, high-quality care, treatment, and services.

emergency **1.** An unexpected or sudden occasion, as in emergency surgery needed to prevent death or serious disability. **2.** A natural or man-made event that significantly disrupts the environment of care (for example, damage to the organization's building(s) and grounds due to severe winds, storms, or earthquakes); that significantly disrupts care and treatment (for example, loss of utilities such as power, water, or telephones due to floods, civil disturbances, accidents, or emergencies in the organization or its community); or that results in sudden, significantly changed or increased demands for the organization's services (for example, bioterrorist attack, building collapse, or plane crash in the organization's community). Some emergencies are called "disasters" or "potential injury creating events" (PICEs).

emergency management plan The organization's written document describing the process it would implement for managing the consequences of natural disasters or other emergencies that could disrupt the organization's ability to provide care, treatment, and services. The plan identifies specific procedures that describe mitigation, preparedness, response, and recovery strategies, actions, and responsibilities. *See also* emergency, mitigation activities, preparedness activities.

encryption *See* information management.

endemic infection *See* infection, endemic.

enteral nutrition *See* nutrition, enteral.

entry The process by which an individual comes into a setting, including screening and/or assessment by the organization or the practitioner in order to determine the capacity of the organization or practitioner to provide the care, treatment, and services required to meet the individual's needs.

environmental tours Activities routinely used by the organization to determine the presence of unsafe conditions and whether the organization's current processes for managing environmental safety risks are being practiced correctly and are effective.

epidemic infection *See* infection, epidemic.

epidemiologically significant infection *See* infection, epidemiologically significant.

equipment management Activities selected and implemented by the organization to assess and control the clinical and physical risks of fixed and portable equipment used for diagnosis, treatment, monitoring, and care.

evidence-based guidelines Guidelines that have been scientifically developed based on current literature and are consensus driven. These are also referred to as National Guidelines or Professional Guidelines.

Evidence of Standards Compliance (ESC) A report submitted by a surveyed organization within 30 days (90 days between January 1, 2004 and June 30, 2005) of its survey, which details the action(s) that it took to bring itself into compliance with a standard or clarifies why the organization believes that was in compliance with the standard for which it received a recommendation. An ESC must address compliance at the element of performance (EP) level and include a measurement of success (MOS) (*see* definition) for all appropriate EP corrections.

failure modes and effect analysis *See* risk assessment, proactive.

family The person(s) who plays a significant role in an individual's life. This may include a person(s) not legally related to the individual. This person(s) is often referred to as a surrogate decision maker if authorized to make care decisions for the individual should he or she lose decision-making capacity. *See also* guardian; surrogate decision maker.

fire safety management Activities selected and implemented by the organization to assess and control the risks of fire, smoke, and other byproducts of combustion that could occur during the organization's provision of care, treatment, and services.

forensic program or service An identified program/service (for example, jail or prison mental health services, court evaluation centers, outpatient probation, parole services, DUI programs or services) that provides diagnosis, evaluation, or services mandated by the legal/corrections system.

formulary A list of medications and associated information related to medication use.

free text *See* information management.

governance The individual(s), group, or agency that has ultimate authority and responsibility for establishing policy, maintaining quality of care, and providing for organization management and planning. Other names for this group include the board, board of trustees, board of governors, and board of commissioners.

guardian A parent, trustee, conservator, committee, or other individual or agency empowered by law to act on behalf of or be responsible for an individual. *See also* family; surrogate decision maker.

hazard vulnerability analysis The identification of potential emergencies and the direct and indirect effects these emergencies may have on the health care organization's operations and the demand for its services.

hazardous condition Any set of circumstances (exclusive of the disease, disorder, or condition for which the patient is undergoing care, treatment, and services) defined by the organization that significantly increases the likelihood of a serious adverse outcome.

hazardous materials and waste Materials whose handling, use, and storage are guided or defined by local, state, or federal regulation (for example, the Occupational Safety and Health Administration's Regulations for Bloodborne Pathogens regarding the disposal of blood and blood-soaked items; the Nuclear Regulatory Commission's regulations for the handling and disposal of radioactive waste), hazardous vapors (for example, gluteraldehyde, ethylene oxide, nitrous oxide), and hazardous energy sources (for example, ionizing or non-ionizing radiation, lasers, microwave, ultrasound). Although the Joint Commission considers infectious waste as falling into this category of materials, federal regulations do not define infectious or medical waste as hazardous waste.

hazardous materials and waste management Activities selected and implemented by the organization to assess and control occupational and environmental hazards of materials and waste that require special handling. *See* hazardous materials and waste.

health care occupancy *See* occupancy.

home care The provision of health care and related services by a licensed home health agency to individuals in their place of residence except when the individual resides in a licensed health care facility, such as a nursing home or hospital.

home health services The provision of any health care services by health care professionals to patients in their place of residence. This includes, but is not limited to, performing assessments, provision of care, treatment, counseling, and/or monitoring of the patient's clinical status by nurses (both intermittent skilled and private duty), occupational therapists, physical therapists, speech-language pathologists, audiologists, social workers, dietitians, dentists, physicians, and other licensed health care professionals in the patient's home. It includes the extension or follow-up of health care services provided by hospital professional staff in the patient's home.

home personal care and/or support services The provision of assistance because of a health-related condition with personal care, activities of daily living, and management of household routine by paraprofessional personnel to individuals in their place of residence. This includes the provision of services by home health aides, personal care aides, home attendants, nursing assistants, companions, and homemakers.

hospice An organized program that consists of services provided and coordinated by an interdisciplinary team to meet the needs of patients who are diagnosed with a terminal illness and have a limited life span. The program specializes in palliative management of pain and other physical symptoms, meeting the psychosocial and spiritual needs of the patient and the patient's family or other primary care person(s), utilization of volunteers and provision of bereavement care to survivors. This includes, but is not limited to, all programs licensed as hospices, and Medicare-certified hospice programs. All services provided by the hospice (for example, pharmacy and home medical equipment services), and care provided in all settings (inpatient, nursing home, and so forth) are included.

hospital A health care organization that has a governing body, an organized medical staff and professional staff, and inpatient facilities and provides medical, nursing, and related services for ill and injured patients 24 hours per day, seven days per week. For licensing purposes, each state has its own definition of a hospital.

housestaff Individuals, licensed as appropriate, who are graduates of medical, dental, osteopathic, or podiatric schools; who are appointed to a hospital's professional graduate training program that is approved by a nationally recognized accrediting body approved by the U.S. Department of Education; and who participate in patient care under the direction of licensed independent practitioners of the pertinent clinical disciplines who have clinical privileges in the hospital and are members of, or are affiliated with, the medical staff.

human subject research The use of individuals in the systematic study, observation, or evaluation of factors on preventing, assessing, treating, and understanding an illness. The term applies to all behavioral and medical experimental research that involves human beings as experimental subjects.

indicator A measure used to determine, over time, an organization's performance of functions, processes, and outcomes.

infection The transmission of a pathogenic microorganism to a host, with subsequent invasion and multiplication, with or without resulting symptoms of disease.

> **endemic infection** The usual level or presence of an agent or disease in a defined population during a defined period.
>
> **epidemic infection** A higher than expected level of infection by a common agent in a defined population during a defined period.
>
> **health care–associated infection** An infection acquired while receiving care, treatment, and services in the health care organization.

infection control program Organized system of services designed to meet the needs of the organization or individual in relation to the surveillance, prevention, and control of infection.

information management Terms applicable to information management functions:

- **accountability** All information is attributable to its source (person or device).

Glossary

- **analyzing** The process that interprets data and transforms it into information.
- **auditability** The ability to do a methodical examination and verification of all information activities such as entering and accessing.
- **authentication** The validation of correctness for both the information itself and the person who is the author or user of information.
- **capture** The process of recording representations of human thought, perceptions, or actions, as well as device-generated data or information that is gathered and/or computed about a patient as part of a health care encounter or about other matters in a health care organization.
- **confidentiality** The safekeeping of data/information so as to restrict access to individuals who have need, reason, and permission for such access.
- **data** Uninterpreted observations or facts.
- **electronic health information** A computerized format of the health care information in paper records that is used for the same range of purposes as paper records, namely to familiarize readers with the patient's status; to document care, treatment, and services; to plan for discharge; to document the need for care, treatment, and services; to assess the quality of care, treatment, and services; to determine reimbursement rates; to justify reimbursement claims; to pursue clinical or epidemiological research; and to measure outcomes of the care, treatment, and service process.
- **encryption** The process of transforming plain text (readable) into cipher text that is unreadable without a special software key.
- **free text** Free-flowing, non-structured type of speaking, writing, or inputting information.
- **integrity** In the context of data security, data integrity means the protection of data from accidental or unauthorized intentional change.
- **interactive text** A more complex version of structured text, as it interactively prompts and provides feedback to the person using it. Typically, it uses a higher level of computer intelligence that interacts with the person who records information.
- **interoperability** Enables authorized users to capture, share, and report information from any system, whether paper-based or electronic-based.
- **knowledge-based information** A collection of stored facts, models, and information that can be used for designing and redesigning processes and for problem solving. In the context of the manual, knowledge-based information is found in the clinical, scientific, and management literature.
- **nonrepudiation** The inability to dispute a document's content or authorship.
- **privacy** An individual's right to limit the disclosure of personal information.
- **processing** The manipulation of data and information by editing and updating.

- **protected health information** Health information that contains information such that an individual person can be identified as the subject of that information.
- **report generation** The process of analyzing, organizing, and presenting recorded information for authentication and inclusion in the patient's health care record or in financial or business records.
- **retrievability** The capability of efficiently finding relevant information.
- **security** The protection of data from intentional or unintentional destruction, modification, or disclosure.
- **structured text** Process that requires authors to put specific information into specific fields with passive guidance by the information system. In paper-based systems, a form encourages a practitioner to fill in fields or boxes. Electronic systems use the same principle for templates or macros, which are guides used to create standardized information documentation. The purpose is to produce data of more consistent quality, make information more usable for decision support, make information more complete and more easily retrievable, and save documentation time.
- **timeliness** The time between the occurrence of an event and the availability of data about the event. Timeliness is related to the use of the data.
- **transmission** The sending of data and information from one location to another.

informed consent Agreement or permission accompanied by full notice about what is being consented to. A patient must be apprised of the nature, risks, and alternatives of a medical procedure or treatment before the physician or other health care professional begins any such course. After receiving this information, the patient then either consents to or refuses such a procedure or treatment.

initial survey An accreditation survey of a health care organization not previously accredited by the Joint Commission, or an accreditation survey of an organization performed without reference to any prior survey findings.

integrity *See* information management.

interactive text *See* information management.

interdisciplinary Communication; discussion; planning; evaluation; and care, treatment, and service activities that occur formally and informally between and among team members who are representatives of multiple disciplines.

interim life safety measures (ILSM) A series of 11 administrative actions intended to temporarily compensate for significant hazards posed by existing National Fire Protection Association 101® 2000 *Life Safety Code®* (*LSC*) deficiencies or construction activities. *See also Life Safety Code®*; fire safety management.

interoperability *See* information management.

intravenous (IV) admixture The preparation of pharmaceutical product which requires the measured addition of a medication to a 50ml or greater bag or bottle of IV fluid (for example, IV, IM, IT, SC, and so forth). It does not include the drawing-up of medications into a syringe for immediate use (that is, reconstitution), or the assembly and activation of an IV system that does not involve the measurement of the additive.

invasive procedure A procedure involving puncture or incision of the skin, or insertion of an instrument or foreign material into the body.

investigational medication A medication or placebo used as part of a research protocol or clinical trial.

Joint Commission on Accreditation of Healthcare Organizations (JCAHO) An independent, not-for-profit organization dedicated to improving the quality of care in organized health care settings. Founded in 1951, its members represent the American College of Physicians-American Society of Internal Medicine, the American College of Surgeons, the American Dental Association, the American Hospital Association, the American Medical Association, the public, and the nursing profession. The Joint Commission engages in issues and activities concerning the advancement of health care safety and quality, including public policy initiatives, standards development, and accreditation and certification programs.

knowledge-based information *See* information management.

laboratory *See* pathology and clinical laboratory services.

leader An individual who sets expectations, develops plans, and implements procedures to assess and improve the quality of the organization's governance, management, clinical, and support functions and processes. The leaders described in the leadership function include at least the leaders of the governing body; the chief executive officer and other senior managers; departmental leaders; the elected and the appointed leaders of the medical staff and the clinical departments and other medical staff members in organizational administrative positions; and the nurse executive and other senior nursing leaders.

licensed independent practitioner Any individual permitted by law and by the organization to provide care and services, without direction or supervision, within the scope of the individual's license and consistent with individually granted clinical privileges.

licensure A legal right that is granted by a government agency in compliance with a statute governing an occupation (such as medicine, nursing, psychiatry, or clinical social work) or the operation of an activity (such as in a long term care or residential treatment center).

***Life Safety Code*® (*LSC*)** A set of standards for the construction and operation of buildings, intended to provide a reasonable degree of safety to life during fires; prepared, published, and periodically revised by the National Fire Protection Association and adopted by the Joint Commission to evaluate health care organizations under its life-safety management program. *See also* interim life safety measures; fire safety management; occupancy.

life support equipment Any device used for the purpose of sustaining life and whose failure to perform its primary function, when used according to manufacturer's instructions and clinical protocol, will lead to patient death in the absence of immediate intervention (examples include ventilators, anesthesia machines, and heart-lung bypass machines).

long term care The health and personal care services provided to chronically ill, aged, physically disabled, or developmentally disabled persons in an institution or in the place of residence. These persons are not in an acute phase of illness, but require convalescent, physical, supportive, and/or restorative services on a long-term basis.

loss of protective reflexes An inability to handle secretions without aspiration or to maintain a patent airway independently.

measure of success (MOS) A numerical or quantifiable measure usually related to an audit that determines if an action was effective and sustained due four months after Evidence of Standards Compliance (*see* definition) approval.

measurement The systematic process of data collection, repeated over time or at a single point in time.

medical equipment Fixed and portable equipment used for the diagnosis, treatment, monitoring, and direct care of individuals. *See also* equipment management.

medical history A component of the medical record consisting of an account of an individual's history, obtained whenever possible from the individual, and including at least the following information: chief complaint, details of the present illness or care needs, relevant past history, and relevant inventory by body systems.

medical record *See* record.

medical record review The process of measuring, assessing, and improving the quality of medical record documentation—that is, the degree to which medical record documentation is accurate, complete, and performed in a timely manner. This process is carried out with the cooperation of relevant departments or services.

medical staff Individuals who are subject to the bylaws and rules and regulations of the organized medical staff. *See also* organized medical staff.

medical staff bylaws Regulations and/or rules adopted by the organized medical staff and the governing body of an organization for internal governance, defining rights and obligations of various officers, persons, or groups within the organized medical staff's structure.

medical staff executive committee A group of medical staff members, a majority of whom are licensed physician members of the medical staff practicing in the organization, selected by the medical staff or appointed in accordance with governing body bylaws. This group is responsible for making specific recommendations directly to the organization's governing body for approval, as well as receiving and acting on reports and recommendations from medical staff committees, clinical departments or services, and assigned activity groups. The medical staff as a whole may serve as the executive committee. In smaller, less complex hospitals where the entire medical staff functions as the executive committee, it is often designated as the committee of the whole.

Medicare Provider Analysis and Review (MedPar) Data Data which are collected by the Centers for Medicare & Medicaid Services (CMS) from hospitals in order for hospitals to receive reimbursement for performed services and procedures.

medication Any prescription medications; sample medications; herbal remedies; vitamins; nutriceuticals; over-the-counter drugs; vaccines; diagnostic and contrast agents used on or administered to persons to diagnose, treat, or prevent disease or other abnormal conditions; radioactive medications; respiratory therapy treatments; parenteral nutrition; blood derivatives; intravenous solutions (plain, with electrolytes and/or drugs); and any product designated by the Food and Drug Administration (FDA) as a drug. This definition of medication does not include enteral nutrition solutions (which are considered food products), oxygen, and other medical gases.

medication error Any preventable event that may cause inappropriate medication use or jeopardize patient safety. *See also* adverse drug reaction; sentinel event.

medication history A delineation of the drugs used by an individual (both past and present), including prescribed and unprescribed drugs and alcohol, along with any unusual reactions to those drugs. *See* medication.

medication management The process an organization uses to provide medication therapy to individuals served by the organization. The steps in the medication management process include the following:

- **selection** Safe and appropriate selection of medications available for prescribing, storage, and/or use in the organization.
- **procurement** The task of obtaining selected medications from a source outside the organization. It does not include obtaining a medication from the organization's own pharmacy, which is considered as part of the ordering and dispensing processes.
- **storage** The task of appropriately maintaining a supply of medications on the organization's premises.
- **prescribing or ordering** Synonymous terms for when a licensed independent practitioner transmits a legal order or prescription to the organization directing the preparing, dispensing, and administering of a specific medication to a specific patient. It does not include requisitions for medication supplies.
- **transcribing** The process by which an order from a licensed independent practitioner is documented either in writing or electronically.
- **preparing** The compounding, manipulation, or other activity needed to get a medication ready for administration exactly as ordered by the licensed independent practitioner.
- **dispensing** Providing, furnishing, or otherwise making available a supply of medications to the individual for whom it was ordered or their representative by a licensed pharmacy according to a specific prescription or medication order, or by a licensed independent practitioner authorized by

law to dispense. Dispensing does not involve providing an individual a dose of medication previously dispensed by the pharmacy.

- **administration** The provision of a prescribed and prepared dose of an identified medication to the individual for whom it was ordered to achieve its pharmacological effect. This includes directly introducing the medication into or onto the individual's body.
- **self-administration** Independent use by a patient of a medication, including medications that may be held by the organization for independent use by the patient.
- **monitoring** The ongoing evaluation of an individual to whom a medication was administered, to ascertain the effectiveness and efficacy of the medication therapy and prevent the occurrence of any serious adverse outcomes.

medication-management measurement The measurement, assessment, and improvement of the prescribing or ordering, preparing and dispensing, administering, and monitoring of medications.

mental abuse *See* abuse.

minimum data set An agreed-on and accepted set of terms and definitions constituting a core of data; a collection of related data items.

mission statement A written expression that sets forth the purpose of an organization or one of its components. The generation of a mission statement usually precedes the formation of goals and objectives.

mitigation activities Those activities an organization undertakes in attempting to lessen the severity and impact of a potential emergency. *See* emergency.

multidisciplinary team A group of clinical staff members composed of representatives of a range of professions, disciplines, or service areas.

near miss Used to describe any process variation which did not affect an outcome, but for which a recurrence carries a significant chance of a serious adverse outcome. Such a "near miss" falls within the scope of the definition of a sentinel event, but outside the scope of those sentinel events that are subject to review by the Joint Commission under its Sentinel Event Policy.

neglect The absence of minimal services or resources to meet basic needs. Neglect includes withholding or inadequately providing food and hydration (without physician, patient, or surrogate approval), clothing, medical care, and good hygiene. It may also include placing the individual in unsafe or unsupervised conditions. *See also* abuse.

network An entity offering comprehensive or specialty services that provides, or provides for, integrated health care services to a defined population of individuals. Networks are characterized by a centralized structure that coordinates and integrates services provided by components and practitioners participating in the network.

nonrepudiation *See* information management.

nurse executive A registered professional nurse who is responsible for the full-time, direct supervision of nursing services and who is currently licensed by the state in which he or she practices. Attributes of this position may be further defined in regulatory statutes.

nursing The health profession dealing with nursing care and services as (1) defined by the Code of Ethics for Nurses with Interpretive Statements, Nursing's Social Policy Statement, Nurses' Bill of Rights, Scope and Standards of Nursing Practice of the American Nurses Association and specialty nursing organizations; and (2) defined by relevant state, commonwealth, or territory nurse practice acts and other applicable laws and regulations.

nursing care Professional processes of assessment, diagnosis, planning, implementation, and evaluation based on the art and science of nursing to promote health, its recovery, or a peaceful and dignified death. This includes, but is not limited to, assisting individuals, families, communities, and/or populations in understanding health needs and carrying out therapeutic plans and activities.

nursing home A nonhospital health care organization with inpatient beds and an organized professional staff that provides continuous nursing and other health-related, psychosocial, and personal services to patients who are not in an acute phase of illness, but who require continued care on an inpatient basis.

nursing services One or more defined units or departments within a health care organization with accountability for the delivery of quality nursing care to individuals, families, communities, and/or populations. Personnel, fiscal, capital, and intellectual resources focus on patient safety via interdisciplinary collaboration, integrated data and information management, and communication within all planning, implementation, and evaluation activities.

nursing staff Personnel within a health care organization who are accountable for providing and assisting in the provision of nursing care. Such personnel must include Registered Nurses (RNs), and may include others such as Advanced Practice Registered Nurses (APRNs), Licensed Practical or Vocational Nurses (LPNs/LVNs), and nursing assistants or other designated unlicensed assistive personnel.

nutriceuticals Nutritional supplements formulated in a pharmaceutical dosage form and used with the intention of deriving medical or health benefits, including preventing and treating disease. Such products may range from isolated nutrients, dietary supplements, and diets to genetically engineered "designer" foods, herbal products, and processed foods such as cereals, soups, and beverages.

nutrition The sum of the processes by which one takes in and uses nutrients.

> **enteral nutrition** Nutrition provided via the gastrointestinal tract. Enteral nutrition encompasses both oral (delivered through the mouth) and tube (provided through a tube or catheter that delivers nutrients distal to the mouth) routes.
>
> **parenteral nutrition** Nutrients that are provided intravenously, bypassing the digestive tract, which may contain protein, sugar,

fat, and added vitamins and minerals as needed by the patient. Other terms used are total parenteral nutrition (TPN), partial parenteral nutrition (PPN), and hyperalimentation (HA).

nutrition assessment A comprehensive process for defining an individual's nutrition and hydration status using medical, nutrition, and medication intake histories, physical examination, anthropomorphic measurements, and laboratory data.

nutrition care Interventions and counseling to promote appropriate nutrition and fluid intake, based on nutrition and hydration assessment and information about food, other sources of nutrients, and meal preparation consistent with the individual's cultural background and socioeconomic status. Nutrition therapy, a component of medical treatment, includes enteral and parenteral nutrition. *See also* nutrition.

nutrition screening A process used to indicate the need for a nutritional assessment to determine whether a patient is malnourished or at risk for malnourishment.

occupancy

    ambulatory health care occupancy
An occupancy used to provide services or treatment to four or more patients at the same time that either (1) renders them incapable of providing their own means of self-preservation in an emergency or (2) provides outpatient surgical treatment requiring general anesthesia.

    business occupancy An occupancy used to provide outpatient care, treatment, and services that does not meet the criteria in the ambulatory health care occupancy definition (for example, three or fewer patients at the same time who are either rendered incapable of self-preservation in an emergency or are undergoing general anesthesia).

    health care occupancy An occupancy used for purposes such as medical or other treatment or care of persons suffering from physical or mental illness, disease or infirmity; and for the care of infants, convalescents, or infirm aged persons. Health care occupancies provide sleeping facilities for four or more occupants and are occupied by persons who are mostly incapable of self-preservation because of age, physical or mental disability, or because of security measures not under the occupant's control. Health care occupancies include hospitals, nursing homes, and limited care facilities.

    residential occupancy An occupancy in which sleeping accommodations are provided for normal residential purposes and include all buildings designed to provide sleeping accommodations.

operative and other high risk procedures Surgical or other procedures that put the patient at risk of death or disability. This does not include use of medications that place patients at risk.

oral and maxillofacial surgeon An individual who has successfully completed a postgraduate program in oral and maxillofacial surgery accredited by a nationally recognized accrediting body approved by the

U.S. Department of Education. As determined by the medical staff, the individual is also currently competent to perform a complete history and physical examination in order to assess the medical, surgical, and anesthetic risks of the proposed operative and other procedure(s).

organization's strengths   Areas in which an organization's performance is exemplary, as evidenced by the implementation of innovative approaches to meeting Joint Commission standards. An organization will not be cited for having a strength if the organization has a related noncompliant standard and/or partially compliant element of performance (EP).

originating site   In telemedicine, the site at which the patient is located at the time the service is provided.

organized medical staff   The governance structure of the medical staff, including the medical staff bylaws and rules and regulations to which the medical staff is subject. This structure is approved by the governing body of the organization. *See also* medical staff.

outpatient program   A program that provides services to persons who generally do not need the level of care associated with the more structured environment of an inpatient or a residential program.

parenteral nutrition   *See* nutrition, parenteral.

parenteral product   A sterile pharmaceutical preparation introduced into the body through a route other than the digestive tract, as by subcutaneous, intramuscular, or intravenous injection or infusion.

partial-hospitalization program   A program that provides services to persons who spend only part of a 24-hour period in a behavioral health facility. Partial-hospitalization programs do not provide overnight care.

pathology and clinical laboratory services   The services that provide information on diagnosis, prevention, or treatment of disease or the assessment of health, through the examination of the structural and functional changes in tissues and organs of the body that cause or are caused by disease. It also includes the biological, microbiological, serological, chemical, immunohematological, hematological, or other examination of materials derived from the human body.

patient   An individual who receives care, treatment, and services. For hospice providers, the patient and family are considered a single unit of care. Synonyms used by various health care fields include client, resident, customer, patient and family unit, consumer, and health care consumer.

patient tracer   The process of evaluating a patient's total care experience within a health care organization.

performance improvement   The continuous study and adaptation of a health care organization's functions and processes to increase the probability of achieving desired outcomes and to better meet the needs of individuals and other users of services.

performance measurement system   An entity consisting of an automated database(s), that facilitates performance improvement in health care organizations through the collection and dissemination of process and/or outcome measures of performance.

Measurement systems must be able to generate internal comparisons of organization performance over time, and external comparisons of performance among participating organizations at comparable times.

Periodic Performance Review (PPR) An additional requirement of the accreditation process whereby an organization reviews its compliance with all applicable Joint Commission standards, completes and submits to the Joint Commission a plan of action (*see* definition) for any standard not in full compliance, including the identification of a measure of success (MOS) (*see* definition), and engages in a telephone discussion with a member of the Standards Interpretation Group staff to determine the acceptability of the plan of action. The PPR will encourage organizations to be in continuous compliance with Joint Commission standards. At the time of the next full survey, surveyors will validate that the MOS(s) were implemented and effective.

personal care and support services Services provided in an individual's place of residence on a per-visit or per-hour basis to meet the identified needs of patients who have or are at risk of an injury, an illness, or a disabling condition and who require assistance in personal care, activities of daily living, or the administration of treatments. These services may include, but are not limited to, those provided by home health aides, personal care aides, or home attendants. These services may be provided directly or through contract with another organization or individual.

pharmaceutical care and services Services provided directly or through written contract with another organization that include procuring, preparing, dispensing, and/or distributing pharmaceutical products and the ongoing monitoring of the recipient to identify, prevent, and resolve medication-related problems.

pharmaceutical equivalence The degree to which two formulations of the same medication are identical in strength, concentration, and dosage form.

pharmacist An individual who has a degree in pharmacy and is licensed and registered to prepare, preserve, compound, and dispense drugs and chemicals.

pharmacy A licensed location where drugs are stored and dispensed.

pharmacy services The provision of pharmaceutical care and services involving the preparation and dispensing of medications, and medication-related devices and supplies by a licensed pharmacy, with or without the provision of clinical or consultant pharmacist services.

physical abuse *See* abuse.

physical restraint *See* restraint.

physician A doctor of medicine or doctor of osteopathy who, by virtue of education, training, and demonstrated competence, is granted clinical privileges by the organization to perform a specific diagnostic or therapeutic procedure(s) and who is fully licensed to practice medicine.

physician assistant An individual who practices medicine with supervision by licensed physicians, providing patients with services ranging from primary medicine to specialized surgical care. The scope of practice is determined by state law, the supervising physician's delegation of responsibilities, the individual's education and experience, and the specialty and setting in which the individual works.

physician licensure The process by which a legal jurisdiction, such as a state, grants permission to a physician to practice medicine after finding that he or she has met acceptable qualification standards. Licensure also involves ongoing regulation of physicians by the legal jurisdiction, including the authority to revoke or otherwise restrict a physician's license to practice.

plan A detailed method, formulated beforehand, that identifies needs, lists strategies to meet those needs, and sets goals and objectives. The format of the plan may include narratives, policies and procedures, protocols, practice guidelines, clinical paths, care maps, or a combination of these.

plan for improvement For purposes of Joint Commission accreditation, an organization's written statement that details the procedures to be taken and time frames to correct existing *Life Safety Code®* deficiencies. *See also* Statement of Conditions™ (SOC); interim life safety measures; *Life Safety Code®*.

plan of action A plan detailing the action(s) that an organization will take in order to come into compliance with a Joint Commission standard. A plan of action must be completed for each element of performance (EP) (*see* definition) associated with a noncompliant standard. A measure of success (MOS) (*see* definition) must also be included in the plan of action as indicated in the accreditation manual.

podiatrist An individual who has received the degree of doctor of podiatry medicine and who is licensed to practice podiatry.

point-of-care testing Analytical testing performed at sites outside the traditional laboratory environment, usually at or near where care is delivered to individuals. Testing may range from simple waived procedures, such as fecal occult blood, to more sophisticated chemical analyzers. The testing may be under the control of the main laboratory the direction of another specialized laboratory (such as for arterial blood gas), or under the nursing service. Testing may be categorized as waived, moderate, or high complexity under CLIA '88. Also called alternate site testing, decentralized laboratory testing, and distributed site testing.

policies and procedures The formal, approved description of how a governance, management, or clinical care process is defined, organized, and carried out.

practice guidelines Tools that describe processes found by clinical trials or by consensus opinion of experts to be the most effective in evaluating and/or treating a patient who has a specific symptom, condition, or diagnosis, or describe a specific procedure. Synonyms include practice parameter, protocol, preferred practice pattern, and guideline.

practitioner Any individual who is qualified to practice a health care profession (for example, a physician or nurse) and is engaged in the provision of care and services. Practitioners are often required to be licensed as defined by law.

Preliminary Denial of Accreditation
See accreditation decisions.

preparedness activities Those activities an organization undertakes to build capacity and identify resources that may be used if an emergency occurs. *See* emergency.

prescribing or ordering *See* medication management.

primary source The original source of a specific credential that can verify the accuracy of a qualification reported by an individual health care practitioner. Examples include medical school, graduate medical education program, and state medical board.

priority focus areas Processes, systems, or structures in a health care organization that significantly impact the quality and safety of care. The priority focus areas are

- Assessment and Care/Services
- Communication
- Credentialed Practitioners
- Equipment Use
- Infection Control
- Information Management
- Medication Management
- Organizational Structure
- Orientation and Training
- Patient Safety
- Physical Environment
- Quality Improvement Expertise and Activity
- Rights and Ethics
- Staffing

primary priority focus area
Every standard is linked to one or more priority focus areas. When a surveyor has findings under a standard, he/she determines which of the linked priority focus areas is most related to the specific finding and this becomes the *primary* priority focus area. For example, a finding under standard HR.1.10 may be assigned a primary priority focus area of Staffing. The organization's accreditation report is organized by priority focus area.

secondary priority focus areas
The additional priority focus areas that are also related to a specific finding, in addition to the primary priority focus area. For example, a finding under standard HR.1.10 may be assigned a secondary priority focus area of Orientation and Training. The organization's accreditation report also lists the secondary priority focus area(s).

priority focus process (PFP) The process for standardizing the priorities for sampling during an organization's survey based on information collected about the organization prior to survey. The process also helps to focus the survey on areas that are critical to that organization's patient safety and quality of care processes. Examples of such information may include, but not be limited to, data from the organization's e-App (*see* definition); the organization's plan of action prepared as part of the Periodic Performance Review (*see* definition) process; complaint and sentinel event information; data collected from external sources, such as Med-Par (*see* definition) data; performance measurement data; and previous survey results.

priority focus tool (PFT) An automated tool that supports the priority focus process through the use of algorithms, or sets of rules, to transform a health care organization's data into information that guides the survey process.

privacy *See* information management.

privileging The process whereby a specific scope and content of patient care services (that is, clinical privileges) are authorized for a health care practitioner by a health care organization, based on evaluation of the individual's credentials and performance. *See* licensed independent practitioner.

processing *See* information management.

program An organized system of services designed to address the needs of the organization or individual.

protected health information *See* information management.

protective services A range of sociolegal, assistive, and remedial services that facilitate the exercise of individual rights and provide certain supportive and surrogate mechanisms. Such mechanisms are designed to help developmentally disabled individuals reach the maximum independence possible, yet protect them from exploitation, neglect, or abuse. Depending on the nature and extent of individual needs, protective services may range from counseling to full guardianship.

provisional accreditation *See* accreditation decisions.

psychiatrist A physician who specializes in assessing and treating persons having psychiatric disorders; is certified by the American Board of Psychiatry and Neurology or has the documented equivalent in education, training, or experience; and is fully licensed to practice medicine in the state in which he or she practices.

psychoactive *See* psychotropic/psychopharmacologic medication.

psychotropic/psychopharmacologic medication Any medication whose intended purpose is to alter perception, mental status, or behavior. These include, but are not limited to, those drugs that produce drug dependence. Some examples of drug classes that are considered psychotropic/psychopharmacologic medications include, but are not limited to, hypnotics, antipsychotics, long- and short-acting benzodiazepines, sedatives/anxiolytics, and antidepressants.

Public Information Policy A Joint Commission policy governing the disclosure of specific information about the performance of a health care organization or network, as well as accreditation-related information that will remain confidential. This policy covers the Joint Commission's performance reports, information publicly disclosed on request, complaint information, aggregate performance data, data released to government agencies, and the Joint Commission's right to clarify information an accredited organization releases about its accreditation status.

qualified individual An individual or staff member who is qualified to provide care, treatment, and services by virtue of the following: education, training, experience, competence, registration, certification, or applicable licensure, law or regulation. Examples of qualified individuals can include the following: activities coordinator, administrator, audiologist, child psychiatrist, clinical chaplain, creative arts therapist, dietetic services supervisor, dietitian, registered dietitian, health information administrator, health information technician, licensed practical nurse (LPN), medical radiation physician, medical technologist, music therapist, occupational therapist, occupational therapy assistant, physiatrist, physical therapist assistant, physical therapist, psychiatric nurse, psychologist, radiologic technologist, recreational therapist, recreational therapist assistant or technician, respiratory care technician, respiratory therapist, respiratory therapy technician, social work assistant, social worker, and speech-language pathologist.

qualified individual, infection control An individual who is qualified to participate in one or all of the mechanisms outlined in the standards by virtue of one or more of the following: education, training, certification or licensure, or experience. Certification by the Certification Board for infection control is often a requirement for infection control practitioners.

quality control A process that consists of measuring performance, comparing performance against goals, and acting on the differences when performance falls short of defined goals.

quality of care The degree to which health services for individuals and populations increase the likelihood of desired health outcomes and are consistent with current professional knowledge. Dimensions of performance include the following: patient perspective issues; safety of the care environment; and accessibility, appropriateness, continuity, effectiveness, efficacy, efficiency, and timeliness of care.

Quality Report A report that is available to the public that provides information about an organization's accreditation decision and the effective date for the decision, any special quality awards the organization received, the accreditation services included in the organization's accreditation award, any disease-specific care certification(s) and the effective date of each certification received by the organization, the implementation of National Patient Safety Goals by the organization, the organization's performance against National Quality Goals and the organization's performance in relation to Patient Experience of Care measures.

range orders Orders in which the dose or dosing interval varies over a prescribed range, depending on the situation or individual's status.

rationale for a standard Background, justification, or additional information about a standard. A rationale is *not* scored. Not every standard has a rationale.

reassessment Ongoing data collection, which begins on initial assessment, comparing the most recent data with the data collected at earlier assessments.

record 1. The account compiled by physicians and other health care professionals of a variety of patient health information, such as assessment findings, treatment details, and progress notes. 2. (data source) Data obtained from the records or documentation maintained on a patient in any health care setting (for example, hospital, home care, long term care, practitioner office). Includes automated and paper medical record systems.

referral The sending of an individual (1) from one clinician to another clinician or specialist, (2) from one setting or service to another, or (3) by one physician (the referring physician) to another physician(s) or other resource, either for consultation or care.

registered nurse An individual who is qualified by an approved postsecondary program or baccalaureate or higher degree in nursing and licensed by the state, commonwealth, or territory to practice professional nursing.

report generation See information management.

reprocessing All operations performed to render a contaminated reusable or single-use device patient-ready. The steps may include cleaning and disinfection/sterilization. The manufacturer of reusable devices and single use devices that are marketed as non-sterile should provide validated reprocessing instructions in the labeling.

requirement for improvement A recommendation which was not sufficiently addressed in an organization's Evidence of Standards Compliance (see definition), and needs to be addressed in order for the organization to retain its accreditation decision. Failure to address a requirement for improvement (see definition) after two opportunities will result in a recommendation to place the organization in Conditional Accreditation (see definition).

residential occupancy See occupancy.

residential program A program that provides services to individuals who need a less structured environment than that of an inpatient program and who are capable of self-preservation in the event of an internal disaster. See also inpatient services; outpatient program.

respiratory care services Delivery of care to provide ventilatory support and associated services for individuals.

restraint Any method (chemical or physical) of restricting a patient's freedom of movement, including seclusion, physical activity, or normal access to his or her body that (1) is not a usual and customary part of a medical diagnostic or treatment procedure to which the patient or his or her legal representative has consented; (2) is not indicated to treat the patient's medical condition or symptoms; or (3) does not promote the patient's independent functioning.

  chemical restraint The inappropriate use of a sedating psychotropic drug to manage or control behavior.

  physical restraint Any method of physically restricting a person's freedom of movement, physical activity, or normal access to his or her body.

retrievability See information management.

Review Hearing Panel A panel of three individuals, including one member of the Joint Commission Accreditation Committee, which hears a presentation on the facts of the case by an organization in Preliminary Denial of Accreditation, should the organization desire such a presentation.

risk assessment, proactive An assessment that examines a process in detail including sequencing of events; assesses actual and potential risk, failure, or points of vulnerability;

and, through a logical process, prioritizes areas for improvement based on the actual or potential patient care impact (criticality).

risk-management activities Clinical and administrative activities that organizations undertake to identify, evaluate, and reduce the risk of injury to patients, staff, and visitors and the risk of loss to the organization itself.

root cause analysis A process for identifying the basic or causal factor(s) that underlie variation in performance, including the occurrence or possible occurrence of a sentinel event.

run chart A display of data in which data points are plotted as they occur over time (for example, observed weights over time) to detect trends or other patterns and variation occurring over time. Run charts, as opposed to tabular frequency displays, are capable of time-order analytic studies.

safety The degree to which the risk of an intervention (for example, use of a drug or a procedure) and risk in the care environment are reduced for a patient and other persons, including health care practitioners.

safety management Activities selected and implemented by the organization to assess and control the impact of environmental risk, and to improve general environmental safety.

scope of care or services The activities performed by governance, managerial, clinical, or support staff.

secure In locked containers, in a locked room, or under constant surveillance.

security *See* information management.

security management A component of an organization's management of the environment of care program that maintains and improves the general security of the care environment.

self-admimistration *See* medication management, administration.

sentinel event An unexpected occurrence involving death or serious physical or psychological injury, or the risk thereof. Serious injury specifically includes loss of limb or function. The phrase "or the risk thereof" includes any process variation for which a recurrence would carry a significant chance of a serious adverse outcome.

sexual abuse *See* abuse.

Shared Visions–New Pathways® (SVNP) An initiative to progressively sharpen the focus of the accreditation process on care systems critical to the safety and quality of patient care.

staff Individuals, such as employees, contractors, or temporary agency personnel, who provide services in the organization.

staffing effectiveness The number, competence, and skill mix of staff as related to the provision of needed services.

standard A statement that defines the performance expectations, structures, or processes that must be in place for an organization to provide safe and high quality care, treatment, and service.

Statement of Conditions™ (SOC) A proactive document that helps an organization to do a critical self-assessment of its current level of compliance and describe how to resolve any *Life Safety Code®* (*LSC*) deficiencies. The SOC was created to be a "living, ongoing" management tool that should be used in a management process that continually identifies, assesses, and resolves *LSC* deficiencies.

sterilization The use of a physical or chemical procedure to destroy all microbial life, including highly resistant bacterial endospores.

structured text *See* information management.

subacute care Care that is rendered immediately after, or instead of, acute hospitalization to treat one or more specific, active, complex medical conditions or to administer one or more technically complex treatments in the context of an individual's underlying long-term conditions and overall situation. Subacute care requires the coordinated services of an interdisciplinary team.

Subacute care is generally more intensive than traditional nursing facility care and less intensive than acute inpatient care. It requires frequent (daily to weekly) patient assessment and review of the clinical course and treatment plan for a limited time period (several days to several months), until a condition is stabilized or a predetermined treatment course is completed.

This definition addresses the following seven factors the Joint Commission considers integral to the provision of subacute care:

Time: Subacute care is rendered immediately after, or instead of, acute hospitalization.

Reason: It treats one or more specific, active, complex, or unstable medical conditions or administers one or more technically complex treatments in the context of a person's underlying long-term conditions and overall situations.

Caregivers: It requires the services of an interdisciplinary team who is trained and knowledgeable to assess and manage the specific conditions and to perform the necessary procedures.

Site: It is provided as an inpatient program.

Frequency: It requires frequent patient assessment and review of the clinical course and treatment plan.

Intensity: It provides care at a level generally more intensive than provided in a traditional nursing facility and less intensive than provided in acute inpatient care.

Duration: It lasts for a limited time or until a condition is stabilized or a predetermined treatment course is completed.

supplemental finding A recommendation that is not required to be addressed in an organization's Evidence of Standards Compliance (*see* definition), but should be addressed by the organization internally. A supplemental finding will also be factored into an organization's Priority Focus Process at its next survey.

surrogate decision maker Someone appointed to act on behalf of another. Surrogates make decisions only when an individual is without capacity or has given permission to involve others. *See also* advocate; family.

survey A key component in the accreditation process, whereby a surveyor(s) conducts an on-site evaluation of an organization's compliance with Joint Commission standards.

full survey A survey that assesses an organization's compliance with all applicable Joint Commission standards.

initial survey A survey of a health care organization not previously accredited by the Joint Commission, or a survey of an organization performed without reference to any prior survey findings.

surveyor For purposes of Joint Commission accreditation, a physician, nurse, administrator, laboratorian, or any other health care professional who meets the Joint Commission's surveyor selection criteria, evaluates standards compliance, and provides education and consultation regarding standards compliance to surveyed organizations or networks.

suspension, automatic Suspensions that are automatically enacted whenever the defined indication occurs, and not requiring discussion or investigation. Examples are loss of licensure, or exceeding the allowed medical record delinquency rate. Privileges are automatically suspended until the license is renewed, or the records are completed or the delinquency rate falls to an accceptable level.

suspension, summary While enacted automatically whenever the defined indication occurs, summary suspensions also require a subsequent evaluation or investigation of the reason the indication occurred and a decision as to whether the suspension should be continued and for what length of time. Examples are the occurrence of a sentinel event that might be related to the licensed independent practitioner's performance, or a significant complaint against the licensed independent practitioner such as misconduct or assault. The summary suspension is enacted while the incident is under investigation.

system A set of interrelated parts that work together toward a common goal.

system tracer A session during the on-site survey devoted to evaluating high-priority safety and quality of care issues on a systemwide basis throughout the organization. Examples of such issues may include infection control, medication management, staffing effectiveness and the use of data.

systems analysis The evaluation of how well a health care organization's systems function.

telemedicine The use of medical information exchanged from one site to another via electronic communications for the health and education of the patient or health care provider, and for the purpose of improving patient care.

threshold for Conditional Accreditation At least two but not more than three standard deviations above the mean number of not compliant standards; the threshold for Conditional Accreditation is one rule for receiving Conditional Accreditation.

threshold for Preliminary Denial of Accreditation At least three standard deviations above the mean number of not compliant standards; the threshold for Preliminary Denial of Accreditation is one rule for receiving Preliminary Denial of Accreditation.

timeliness *See* information management.

titrating orders Orders in which the dose is either progressively increased or decreased in response to the individual's status.

total parenteral nutrition *See* nutrition, parenteral.

tracer methodology A process surveyors use during the on-site survey to analyze an organization's systems, with particular attention to identified priority focus areas, by following individual patients through the organization's health care process in the sequence experienced by the patients. Depending on the health care setting, this may require surveyors to visit multiple care units, departments or areas within an organization or a single care unit to "trace" the care rendered to a patient.

transfer The formal shifting of responsibility for the care of an individual (1) from one care unit to another, (2) from one clinical service to another, (3) from one licensed independent practitioner to another, or (4) from one organization to another organization.

transmission *See* information management.

urgent/immediate care services Those services sought for conditions that are considered less critical than those that need to be seen in an emergency center, but are not scheduled with the individual's primary care provider or the provider's designee.

utilities management Activities selected and implemented by the organization to assess and control the risks of utility systems of buildings that support the provision of care, treatment, and services. Included are those activities that ensure the operational reliability of such systems and those activities for responding to a failure of such systems.

utility systems Building systems for life support; surveillance, prevention, and control of infection; environment support; and equipment support. May include electrical distribution; emergency power; vertical and horizontal transport; heating, ventilating, and air conditioning; plumbing, boiler, and steam; piped gases; vacuum systems; or communication systems including data-exchange systems.

utilization management The examination and evaluation of the appropriateness of the utilization of an organization's resources. Also referred to as a utilization review.

waived testing Tests that meet the Clinical Laboratory Improvement Act of 1988 (CLIA '88) requirements for waived tests; are cleared by the Food and Drug Administration for home use; employ methodologies that are so simple and accurate as to render the likelihood of erroneous results negligible; or pose no risk of harm to the patient if the test is performed incorrectly. *See also* CLIA '88.

Index

A

Abuse. *See also* Abused or neglected patients
  protection of patients from (RI.2.150) RI-19
Abused or neglected patients, assessment of
  (PC.3.10) PC-18–PC-19
Academic education (PC.6.50) PC-27;
  (LD.3.130) LD-20
Account representative, HB-24; APP-19, APP-20
Accountability, IM-15
Accreditation. *See also* Accreditation decision
  process; Accreditation survey; Appeal
  procedures
  appeals, APP-32, APP-40–APP-50
  award, APP-3, APP-35–APP-36
  award display, APP-35–APP-36
  award duration, APP-37
  certificate, APP-35–APP-36
  Conditional, APP-8, APP-10, APP-14, APP-16,
    APP-17, APP-31, APP-32, APP-33
  continuing, APP-37
  continuous compliance, APP-37
  decision categories, APP-33–APP-34
  decisions, APP-33–APP-34
  Denial of, APP-8, APP-13, APP-14, APP-16,
    APP-32, APP-34
  Preliminary, APP-7–APP-8, APP-32, APP-33,
    APP-34
  Preliminary Denial of, APP-8, APP-11, APP-13,
    APP-16, APP-17, APP-30, APP-31, APP-32,
    APP-33; SE-13
  Provisional, ACC-3; APP-31, APP-32, APP-33
  renewal process, APP-37–APP-38
  Report, ACC-3; APP-16, APP-30–APP-31
Accreditation Committee, APP-30, APP-31
Accreditation decision process. *See also*
  Accreditation decision rules
  decision categories
    Accredited, ACC-3, APP-32, APP-33
    Conditional Accreditation, APP-32, APP-33
    Denial of Accreditation, APP-32, APP-34
    Preliminary Accreditation, APP-7–APP-8,
      APP-32, APP-34
    Preliminary Denial of Accreditation, APP-32,
      APP-33
    Provisional Accreditation, ACC-3, APP-32,
      APP-33
    Evidence of Standards Compliance (ESC),
      ACC-3, ACC-31
    Quality Report, ACC-3, ACC-19; APP-13–APP-14

Accreditation decision rules
  Accredited, APP-33
  Conditional Accreditation, APP-33
  Preliminary Accreditation, APP-33
  Preliminary Denial of Accreditation, APP-36
  Provisional Accreditation, APP-33
  weighted, APP-34, APP-35
Accreditation manuals, APP-2. *See also*
  Accreditation survey
Accreditation participation requirements,
  HB-3; APP-6; APR-1–APR-10. *See also*
  Accreditation survey
  acceptance of survey (Requirement 3),
    APR-2–APR-3
  permitting unannounced survey,
    APR-2–APR-3
  permitting unscheduled survey, APR-2–
    APR-3
  Application for Accreditation, APR-2
    providing records and reports
      (Requirement 1), APR-2
    reporting information changes
      (Requirement 2), APR-2
  misrepresentation of information, APR-6–APR-8
    in accreditation process (Requirement 10),
      APR-6–APR-7
    and consulting services (Requirement 12),
      APR-7–APR-8
    falsification, definition of, APR-7
    public (Requirement 11), APR-7
  performance measurement, APR-3–APR-4
    aggregate data (Requirement 6), APR-4
    selection and use of performance measures
      (Requirement 5), APR-3–APR-4
  Periodic Performance Review (PPR)
    (Requirement 14), APR-8–APR-10
  public information interviews, APP-6, APP-23;
    APR-5–APR-6
    notification of Joint Commission about
      requests (Requirement 9), APR-6
    providing notice of (Requirement 8), APR-6
  survey observers (Requirement 13), APR-8
Accreditation Report, ACC-3; APP-16,
  APP-30–APP-31
Accreditation standards. *See* Standards
Accreditation survey. *See also* Accreditation
  participation requirements
  account representative, HB-24; APP-19, APP-20
  Accreditation Report, ACC-3; APP-30–APP-31
  agenda for, ACC-15–ACC-16; APP-22, APP-27

IX

IX – 1

application for, APP-19–APP-20
clinical/service groups, ACC-8, ACC-14–ACC-15
closing conference, APP-28
competence assessment process, ACC-16
complex organization survey process, APP-5
contracted services, APP-5
daily briefing, ACC-16; APP-28
deposit, APP-21–APP-22
Early Survey Policy, APP-7–APP-10
eligibility criteria, APP-1–APP-2
environment of care session, ACC-17
Evidence of Standards Compliance (ESC) report, ACC-3; APP-31
exit briefing, ACC-17
extension, APP-6–APP-7, APP-38–APP-39
extranet site, ACC-2, ACC-3; APP-18
falsification of information, APP-11
feedback session, APP-29
fees for, APP-17
functional integration, APP-3–APP-4
general eligibility criteria, APP-1–APP-2
general survey categories, APP-2
immediate threat to life, APP-30
information accuracy and truthfulness, APP-10–APP-12
initial surveys, APP-10
and laboratory function, APP-34
leadership session, ACC-15–ACC-16; APP-27
Life Safety Code® building tour, ACC-17
manuals, APP-2
measure of success (MOS) report, APP-32
medical staff credentialing and privileging, ACC-16–ACC-17
mergers, consolidations, and acquisitions, APP-38
multiorganization option, APP-6–APP-7
National Patient Safety Goals, HB-3; APP-2–APP-3, APP-13
notification of changes, APP-38–APP-39
notification of public, APP-22–APP-23
observers, APR-8
opening conference, ACC-15; APP-27
organizational integration, APP-3–APP-4
overview, APP-27
Periodic Performance Review (PPR), ACC-1, ACC-5–ACC-7; APP-18–APP-19
physician practices, APP-5
plan of action, ACC-2, ACC-7; APP-18
planning session, ACC-15
policies and procedures, HB-3; APP-1–APP-40
postponement of, APP-21–APP-22
  fees for, APP-21
presurvey activities, ACC-5–ACC-15
Priority Focus Process (PFP), ACC-1, ACC-3, ACC-7–ACC-15; APP-26
  tool, APP-26

process for, HB-1–HB-2; ACC-1–ACC-20; APP-27–APP-30
public information interview, APP-6, APP-22–APP-26
  advance notice of, APP-23
  compliance with, APP-24–APP-25
  conduct of, APP-25–APP-26
  eligibility, APP-25
  handling requests, APP-25
  informing community of, APP-22–APP-25
  process, APP-26
  public posting, APP-22–APP-23, APP-24
  scheduling, APP-25
public information policy, APP-13–APP-17
  complaint information, APP-14–APP-15
  confidential information, APP-16–APP-17
  and public disclosure, APP-14
  Quality Reports, APP-13–APP-14
  release to government agencies, APP-15–APP-16
Public Notice form, APP-24
Quality Reports, ACC-3; APP-13–APP-14
random unannounced, APP-40
re-entering process, APP-36–APP-37
report preparation, ACC-18
schedule for, APP-21–APP-22
scope of, APP-2
scoring compliance and track record achievements, APP-29
scoring format, ACC-3–ACC-5
sentinel events, SE-2–SE-3
single awards, APP-3
special issue resolution, ACC-16
system tracers, ACC-17; APP-28
tailored surveys, APP-3–APP-4
team for, APP-28
team meeting, ACC-17–ACC-18
time line for, ACC-1–ACC-3
tracer methodology, ACC-3, ACC-16, ACC-18–ACC-20; APP-28
unannounced, APP-5–APP-6, APP-39–APP-40; APR-2–APR-3
unscheduled, APP-39–APP-40; APR-2–APR-3
weighted decision rules, APP-34, APP-35
Accreditation Watch, APP-16
and sentinel events, SE-6, SE-7–SE-8, SE-10–SE-11, SE-13
Accredited, ACC-3; APP-8, APP-9, APP-31, APP-32, APP-33
Action plan, SE-2, SE-6, SE-13
follow-up activity, SE-13
review of, SE-7
submission of, SE-11–SE-12
Admissions (PC.1.10) PC-14. *See also* Provision of care, treatment, and services

assessment of patient in (PC.2.20) PC-16
  time frame for (PC.2.120) PC-17
  organization ethics in (RI.1.10) RI-9
  written process for (PC.1.10) PC-14
Advance directives
  patient rights and (RI.2.20; RI.2.80) RI-12,
    RI-15–RI-16
  and restraint or seclusion use (PC.12.40)
    PC-44–PC-45
Adverse drug reaction (MM.6.20) MM-21–MM-22
  data analysis on (PI.2.20) PI-10
Advocacy services (RI.2.170) RI-20
Alcohol/drug dependencies
  assessment of patients for (PC.3.120) PC-19–
    PC-20
Ambulatory care
  and medical record documentation (IM.6.40)
    IM-24
**American Board of Medical Specialties
  (ABMS),** MS-24
American Medical Association (AMA), MS-24
**American Osteopathic Association (AOA)
  Physician Database,** MS-24
Americans with Disabilities Act (ADA), HR-9
  medical staff credentialing and (MS.4.20)
    MS-26–MS-28
  and physician health (MS.4.80) MS-34–MS-35
Analyzing, IM-2
Anesthesia, PC-54. *See also* Sedation
  assessment of patients for (PC.13.20) PC-54–
    PC-55
  data analysis on adverse events (PI.2.20) PI-10
  definition of, PC-54
  discharge from care (PC.13.40) PC-56
  documentation of (PC.13.30) PC-55–PC-56;
    (IM.6.30) IM-23–IM-24
  monitoring physiological status during
    (PC.13.30–PC.13.40) PC-55–PC-56
  plan for (PC.13.20) PC-54–PC-55
  postprocedure assessment (PC.13.40) PC-56
  provision by qualified staff (PC.13.20)
    PC-54–PC-55
Annual operating budget (LD.2.50) LD-12–
  LD-13
Anxiolysis, PC-54. *See also* Sedation
Appeal procedures, APP-32, APP-40–APP-50.
  See also Review and appeal procedures
  conditional accreditation, APP-44–APP-45
    action by Accreditation Committee, APP-45
    charges to organization, APP-45
    review and determination by Joint Commis-
      sion staff, APP-44–APP-45
    survey to determine implementation of ESC,
      APP-44
  evaluation by Joint Commission staff,
    APP-41–APP-43

  decisions by president of Joint Commission,
    APP-43
  determination to recommend conditional
    accreditation, APP-41–APP-42
  determination to recommend that accredita-
    tion be preliminarily denied,
    APP-42–APP-43
  review and determination by Joint Commis-
    sion staff, APP-49–APP-50
  final accreditation decision, APP-50
  notice, APP-50
  procedure relating to not compliant standards,
    APP-48–APP-49
  review by Accreditation Committee,
    APP-43–APP-44
    decision, APP-43–APP-44
    deferred consideration, APP-44
    scope of review, APP-43
  review by board appeal review committee,
    APP-47–APP-48
    participation, APP-48
    procedure for review, APP-47
    review request, APP-47
  Review Hearing Panels, APP-45–APP-46
    charges to organization, APP-46
    notice of time and place, APP-46
    procedure for conduct, APP-46
    report of, APP-46
    right to, APP-45–APP-46
    second consideration by Accreditation
      Committee, APP-46–APP-47
    decision, APP-46–APP-47
    scope of review, APP-46
  status after appeal, APP-50
Application for accreditation, APP-19–APP-20
  account representative, APP-19, APP-20
  accuracy of information, APP-20
  electronic version (e-App), ACC-2; APP-19
  handling changes, APP-20
  participation requirements, APR-2
  renewal process, APP-37–APP-38
Assessment, ACC-9; (PC.2.20–PC.3.130)
  PC-14–PC-21. *See also* Provision of care,
    treatment, and services
  of abuse or neglect (PC.3.10) PC-18–PC-19
  and anesthesia/sedation use (PC.13.20;
    PC.13.40) PC-54–PC-55, PC-56
  for emotional or behavioral disorders
    (PC.3.130) PC-20–PC-21
  goal of, PC-14
  initial (PC.2.130) PC-17
    time frame (PC.2.120) PC-17
  medical staff involvement in (MS.3.10)
    MS-20–MS-21
  nutritional plan criteria (PC.2.20) PC-16
  of pain (PC.8.10) PC-28–PC-29

of patients in restraint or seclusion (PC.12.130) PC-48–PC-49
psychosocial (PC.3.120) PC-19–PC-20
reassessment (PC.2.150) PC-18
written information of (PC.2.20) PC-16
Assessment of staff. *See* Management of human resources
Audit (LD.2.50) LD-12–LD-13
Auditability, IM-13
Authenticate, IM-13. *See also* Medical records
Autopsies
collection of data on (PI.1.10) PI-8–PI-9
and medical staff role (MS.3.10) MS-20–MS-21
Award, APR-7
display, APP-35–APP-36
duration, APP-37
single, APP-3

B

Barber/beautician services (PC.8.60) PC-30
Behavior-management (PC.13.70) PC-57–PC-59. *See also* Emotional/behavioral disorders; Restraint; Seclusion
collection of data on (PI.1.10) PI-8–PI-9
nonphysical techniques for (PC.12.50) PC-44
and restraint and seclusion use (PC.12.10–PC.12.190) PC-38–PC-52
Bioterrorism. *See also* Emergency management
Blood
data collection for (PI.1.10) PI-8–PI-9
medical staff role in use of (MS.3.10) MS-20–MS-21
patient identification, NPSG-2; (PC.5.10) PC-24
Board Appeal Review Committee, APP-47–APP-48. *See also* Appeal procedures
Building design (EC.8.30) EC-34–EC-35. *See also* Management of the environment of care
Building tour, ACC-17
Bylaws (MS.1.20) MS-12–MS-15. *See also* Medical staff

C

Capture, IM-2
Care of the dying (PC.8.70) PC-31
and patient rights (RI.2.80) RI-15–RI-16
Certificate for accreditation, APP-35–APP-36
Chief executive officer (CEO) (MS.1.40) MS-15–MS-16
and executive committee of medical staff (MS.1.40) MS-15–MS-16
exit briefing, ACC-17
medical staff and (MS.1.40) MS-15–MS-16
and temporary clinical privileges, granting of (MS.4.100) MS-36–MS-37
during disasters (MS.4.110) MS-38–MS-39

CLIA '88, PC-61–PC-62
Clinical practice guidelines (LD.5.10–LD.5.40) LD-24–LD-25
approval of (LD.5.30) LD-24–LD-25
criteria for (LD.5.20) LD-24
evaluation of outcomes (LD.5.40) LD-25
Clinical privileges. *See also* Medical staff
bylaws and regulations for (MS.4.20) MS-26–MS-28
continuing education and (MS.5.10) MS-41–MS-42
corrective actions (MS.1.20) MS-12–MS-15
credentialing for (MS.1.20) MS-12–MS-15
fair-hearing and appellate review mechanism (MS.1.20) MS-12–MS-15
focused review process (MS.4.90) MS-35–MS-36
and graduate education programs (MS.2.30) MS-19–MS-20
granting and renewal or revision of (MS.4.20) MS-26–MS-28
application processing (MS.4.20) MS-26–MS-28
chairperson participation (MS.4.20) MS-26–MS-28
criteria for (MS.4.20) MS-26–MS-28
duration of (MS.4.20) MS-26–MS-28
during a disaster (MS.4.110) MS-38–MS-39
mechanisms for (MS.4.20) MS-26–MS-28
provisional (MS.4.20) MS-26–MS-29
queries of NPDB (MS.4.20) MS-26–MS-29
reappraisal for (MS.4.20) MS-26–MS-29
in multiple departments or specific areas (MS.1.20) MS-12–MS-15
renewal, revocation, or revision of (MS.1.20) MS-12–MS-15
scope of (MS.4.20) MS-26–MS-28
setting-specific (MS.4.20) MS-26–MS-28
surveillance of performance (MS.1.20) MS-12–MS-15
suspension of (MS.1.20) MS-12–MS-15
temporary (MS.4.100) MS-36–MS-37
Clinical/service group (CSG), ACC-8, ACC-14–ACC-15
Clinical trials, patient rights in (RI.2.180) RI-20–RI-21
consent forms (RI.2.180) RI-20–RI-21
Closing conference, APP-28, APP-30
Communication, ACC-9–ACC-10. *See also* Leadership
back-up systems (EC.4.10) EC-15–EC-18
emergency procedures (EC.4.10) EC-15–EC-18
effectiveness, NPSG-3; (LD.3.60) LD-17
standardization of abbreviations, NPSG-3
timeliness of reporting, NPSG-3
verification of verbal orders, NPSG-3
and infection control (IC.1.10) IC-9–IC-10

Index

in medical staff organization (MS.2.20) MS-18
patient rights and (RI.2.100) RI-16–RI-17
of restraint and seclusion philosophy
 (PC.12.10) PC-40–PC-41
Compartmentalization, EC-25
Competence
 assessment of, ACC-16; (HR.3.10–HR.3.20)
  HR-13–HR-14. *See also* Management of
  human resources
 time frame for (HR.3.10) HR-13–HR-14
 and waived testing (PC.16.30) PC-63–PC-64
 defining of (HR.1.20) HR-8–HR-9
 and performance evaluations (HR.3.20) HR-14
 of staff (LD.3.70) LD-17
Complaint information, public release of,
 APP-14–APP-15
 hotline, APP-15
Complaint resolution process (RI.2.120)
 RI-17–RI-18
Complex organization survey process, APP-5
*Comprehensive Accreditation Manual for
 Hospitals: The Official Handbook
 (CAMH)*
 update service, HB-23
Conditional Accreditation, decision rule,
 APP-8, APP-10, APP-14, APP-16, APP-17,
 APP-31, APP-32, APP-33
Confidential information, and public informa-
 tion policy, APP-16–APP-17
Confidentiality (IM.2.10) IM-11–IM-12. *See also*
 Ethics, rights, and responsibilities; Manage-
 ment of information
 patient's rights to (RI.2.130) RI-18
Conflict of interest (RI.1.20) RI-9–RI-10
Conflict resolution (RI.1.10) RI-9
 and leadership (LD.1.20) LD-10–LD-11
Consent forms (RI.2.180) RI-20–RI-21. *See also*
 Informed consent
Consulting services, APR-7–APR-8; (LD.3.10;
 LD.3.50) LD-13, LD-16
Continuing accreditation, APP-37
Continuing education. *See also* Management
 of human resources
 of medical staff (LD.3.10) LD-13, LD-16;
  (HR.2.30) HR-10–HR-11; (MS.5.10)
  MS-41–MS-42
 about restraint and seclusion (PC.11.10)
  PC-33–PC-34
Continuous standards compliance, APP-37
Contracted services, APP-5
 within or under control of hospital (LD.3.50)
  LD-13–LD-14
Control chart. *See* Management of information
Credentialing, ACC-10, ACC-16–ACC-17;
 (LD.3.70) LD-17. *See also* Management of
 human resources; Medical staff

challenges to licensure (MS.4.30–MS.4.40)
 MS-29–MS-31
clinical privileges (MS.4.20) MS-26–MS-28
criteria for clinical privileges (MS.4.30) MS-29
and disaster privileges (MS.1.20; MS.4.110)
 MS-12–MS-15, MS-38–MS-39
fair hearing and appeal process (MS.1.20;
 MS.4.50) MS-12–MS-15, MS-31–MS-32
focused review process (MS.4.90) MS-35–MS-36
peer recommendations (MS.4.70) MS-33
primary source verification (MS.4.10)
 MS-23–MS-26
process (MS.4.10) MS-23–MS-26
renewal, revocation, or revision of clinical privileges (MS.4.40) MS-29–MS-31
setting-specific clinical privileges (MS.4.20)
 MS-26–MS-28
staff appointments (MS.4.60) MS-32
telemedicine link care (MS.4.120–MS.4.130)
 MS-39–MS-41
temporary privileging (MS.4.100) MS-36–MS-37
verification of information (MS.4.10)
 MS-23–MS-26
Credentials verification organization (CVO)
 (MS.4.10) MS-23–MS-26
Crosswalks of standards, HB-7
 for ethics, rights, and responsibilities,
  CW-1–CW-4
 for improving organization performance,
  CW-18–CW-19
 for leadership, CW-20–CW-25
 for management of the environment of care,
  CW-26–CW-28
 for management of human resources,
  CW-29–CW-30
 for management of information, CW-31–CW-33
 for medical staff, CW-34–CW-50
 for medication management, CW-15–CW-16
 for nursing, CW-51
 for provision of care, treatment, and services,
  CW-5–CW-14
 for surveillance, prevention, and control of
  infection, CW-17

D
Daily briefing, ACC-16; APP-28
Data, IM-2
Data analysis (PI.2.10) PI-9–PI-10
 undesirable patterns or trends (PI.2.20) PI-10
Data and information
 assessment
  on adverse anesthesia events (PI.2.20) PI-10
  on adverse drug reactions (PI.2.20) PI-10
  on discrepancies in diagnoses (PI.2.20) PI-10
  medication errors (PI.2.20) PI-10
  staffing effectiveness (PI.2.20) PI-10

IX – 5

on transfusion reactions (PI.2.20) PI-10
on variations in performance (PI.2.20) PI-10
bias minimization in (IM.3.10) IM-15–IM-17
capture (IM.3.10) IM-15–IM-17
confidentiality of (IM.2.10) IM-11–IM-12
integrity of (IM.2.20) IM-12–IM-13
methods of capturing (IM.3.10) IM-15–IM-17
security of (IM.2.10–IM.2.20) IM-11–IM-13
Data collection (PI.1.10) PI-8–PI-9. *See also*
  Management of information
  and performance improvement (PI.1.10)
    PI-8–PI-9
  on autopsy services (PI.1.10) PI-8–PI-9
  on behavior management (PI.1.10) PI-8–PI-9
  on blood and blood product use (PI.1.10)
    PI-8–PI-9
  on infection control (PI.1.10) PI-8–PI-9
  on medication management (PI.1.10)
    PI-8–PI-9
  on operative and other procedures (PI.1.10)
    PI-8–PI-9
  on pain management (PI.1.10) PI-8–PI-9
  on quality control (PI.1.10) PI-8–PI-9
  on restraint and seclusion use (PI.1.10)
    PI-8–PI-9
  on resuscitation (PI.1.10) PI-8–PI-9
  on risk management (PI.1.10) PI-8–PI-9
  on utilization management (PI.1.10) PI-8–
    PI-9
  on restraint and seclusion use (PC.12.180)
    PC-51–PC-52
Decision making (IM.3.10–IM.4.10) IM-14–IM-18
  on patient care (RI.1.30) RI-10
Decision categories. *See* Accreditation decision
Decision rules. *See* Accreditation decision rules
Deep sedation, PC-54. *See also* Sedation
Denial of Accreditation, APP-8, APP-13, APP-14,
    APP-16, APP-32, APP-34
Denial-of-care conflicts (RI.1.40) RI-10–RI-11
Diagnostic radiology (LD.3.30) LD-15
Diagnostic testing (PC.3.230) PC-22
Diet. *See* Nutrition care
Dietetic services (LD.3.30) LD-15
Disaster
  clinical privileging during (MS.1.20; MS.4.110)
    MS-12–MS-15, MS-38–MS-39
  obtaining medication during (MM.2.10) MM-11
  recovery plan (IM.2.30) IM-13–IM-14
Discharge
  from anesthesia care (PC.13.40) PC-56
  assessment of patient for (PC.15.20) PC-69
  and continuum of care (PC.15.10) PC-59
  exchange of information during (PC.15.30)
    PC-61
  organizational ethics in (RI.1.10) RI-9
  and patient needs (PC.15.20) PC-60

patient-specific information about (IM.6.10)
  IM-19–IM-22
from postanesthesia care area (PC.13.40) PC-56
process for, PC-59
from sedation care (PC.13.40) PC-56
summary (IM.6.10) IM-19–IM-22
Documentation. *See* Management of information; Medical records; Patient-specific data
Drugs. *See* Alcohol/drug dependencies;
  Medication
Dying patient
  care of, patient's rights (RI.2.80) RI-15–RI-16
  end-of-life care (PC.8.70) PC-31

E

e-App. *See* Application for accreditation
Early Survey Policy Options, APP-7–APP-10.
  See also Accreditation survey
  Option 1 (Preliminary Accreditation),
    APP-7–APP-8, APP-9
    eligibility, APP-7
    first survey, APP-7
    Preliminary Accreditation, APP-7–APP-8
    second survey, APP-8
  Option 2, APP-8–APP-10
    eligibility, APP-8–APP-9
    first survey, APP-9
    second survey, APP-9–APP-10
Education of patient and family. *See also*
  Provision of care, treatment, and services
  academic (PC.6.50) PC-27; (LD.3.130) LD-20
  on care, treatment, and services (PC.6.10)
    PC-26
  appropriateness of (PC.6.30) PC-27
  on grooming activities (PC.8.60) PC-30
  on health practices (PC.6.10) PC-26
  on medical equipment use (PC.6.10) PC-26
  on medication use (PC.6.10) PC-26
  on nutrition (PC.6.10) PC-26
  on oral health (PC.6.10) PC-26
  on pain management (PC.6.10) PC-26
  on rehabilitation techniques (PC.6.10) PC-26
  on restraint use (PC.11.10) PC-33–PC-34
  and leadership coordination of (LD.3.120)
    LD-19
  and medical staff participation (MS.3.20)
    MS-21–MS-22
  on patient rights (RI.3.10) RI-22–RI-23
Education of staff
  on abuse or neglect (PC.3.10) PC-18–PC-19
  on anesthesia and sedation (PC.13.20)
    PC-54–PC-55
  on medication management (MM.2.10) MM-11
  on needs of dying patient and family (PC.8.70)
    PC-31
  on patient rights and ethics (HR.2.10) HR-11

Index

on performance and safety improvement (LD.4.60) LD-23
on restraint and seclusion (PC.11.10; PC.12.30) PC-33–PC-34, PC-41–PC-43
on resuscitation services (PC.9.30) PC-31–PC-32
on waived testing (PC.16.30) PC-63–PC-64
Educational assessment (PC.3.120; PC.3.130) PC-19–PC-21
Educational Commission for Foreign Medical Graduates (ECFMG), MS-24
Electroconvulsive therapy (PC.13.50) PC-56–PC-57
Element(s) of performance (EPs), HB-22; ACC-2, ACC-4; APP-2; NPSG-1
Eligibility requirements
for accreditation survey, APP-1–APP-2
for Early Survey Policy, Option 1, APP-7
for Early Survey Policy, Option 2, APP-8–APP-9
Emergency care
documentation of (IM.6.10) IM-19–IM-22
Emergency department
patient flow efficiency (LD.3.15) LD-13–LD-15
Emergency drills (EC.4.20) EC-18–EC-19
critiquing of (EC.4.20) EC-18–EC-19
fire drills (EC.5.30) EC-21–EC-22
Emergency management (EC.4.10) EC-15–EC-18. *See also* Disaster
alternative utility systems (EC.4.10) EC-15–EC-18
back-up communication systems (EC.4.10) EC-15–EC-18
communitywide organization (EC.4.10) EC-15–EC-18
conduct of hazard vulnerability analysis (EC.4.10) EC-15–EC-18
cooperative planning (EC.4.10) EC-15–EC-18
drills for (EC.4.20) EC-18–EC-19
establishment of alternative care sites (EC.4.10) EC-15–EC-18
evacuation procedures (EC.4.10) EC-15–EC-18
identification and assignment of staff (EC.4.10) EC-15–EC-18
infection control (IC.6.10) IC-13–IC-14
leadership involvement in (LD.3.30) LD-15; (EC.4.10) EC-15–EC-18
and medical equipment (EC.6.10) EC-26–EC-27
and notification of external authorities (EC.4.10) EC-15–EC-18
organization and community command structure (EC.4.10) EC-15–EC-18
radioactive, biological, and chemical isolation and decontamination (EC.4.10) EC-15–EC-18
written plan for (EC.4.10) EC-15–EC-18
Emergency medication systems (MM.2.30) MM-13
Emergency power source (EC.7.20) EC-29–EC-30
Emergency planning. *See* Emergency management
Emergency preparedness. *See* Emergency management
Emotional/behavioral disorders
assessment of patients for (PC.3.130) PC-20–PC-21
Employees. *See* Management of human resources; Staff
Encryption, IM-13
End-of-life care (PC.8.70) PC-31. *See also* Dying patient
Environment of care. *See* Management of environment of care
Environment of care sessions, ACC-17
Environmental tours (EC.1.20) EC-12
Epidemiology. *See* Surveillance, prevention, and control of infection
Equipment. *See* Medical equipment
Equipment maintenance. *See also* Management of environment of care
Equipment management program, ACC-19
Equipment use, ACC-10
Ethical issues. *See* Ethics, rights, and responsibilities
Ethics, rights, and responsibilities (RI), ACC-13–ACC-14; RI-1–RI-23
education of staff on (HR.2.10) HR-11
individual responsibilities (RI.3.10) RI-22–RI-23
statement of responsibilities (RI.3.10) RI-22–RI-23
individual rights (RI.2.10–RI.2.190) RI-11–RI-21
advance directives (RI.2.20; RI.2.80) RI-12, RI-15–RI-16
care at the end of life (RI.2.80) RI-15–RI-16
to care involvement (RI.2.30) RI-12
communication needs (RI.2.100) RI-16–RI-17
complaint resolution (RI.2.120) RI-17–RI-18
to confidentiality (RI.2.130) RI-18
to consent for recording or filming (RI.2.50) RI-13–RI-14
to disclosure of health information (RI.2.20) RI-12
family involvement (RI.2.30) RI-12
to forgo or withdraw life-sustaining treatment (RI.2.80) RI-15–RI-16
to freedom from abuse or neglect (RI.2.150) RI-19
to information on caregiver (RI.2.60) RI-14–RI-15
to informed consent (RI.2.40) RI-13
and organ donation (RI.2.80) RI-15–RI-16
to pain management (RI.2.160) RI-19–RI-20

to pastoral and spiritual services (RI.2.10) RI-11
to personal dignity (RI.2.10) RI-11
to personal possessions (RI.2.140) RI-18–RI-19
to privacy (RI.2.130) RI-18
to protective and advocacy services (RI.2.170) RI-20
to refuse care, treatment and services (RI.2.70) RI-15
in research projects (RI.2.180) RI-20–RI-21
  benefits (RI.2.180) RI-20–RI-21
  consent forms (RI.2.180) RI-20–RI-21
  information confidentiality (RI.2.180) RI-20–RI-21
  investigation in research-related injuries (RI.2.180) RI-20–RI-21
  refusal to participate (RI.2.180) RI-20–RI-21
  risks (RI.2.180) RI-20–RI-21
to security (RI.2.130) RI-18
to a supportive environment (RI.2.140) RI-18–RI-19
to a surrogate decision maker (RI.2.30) RI-12
unanticipated outcomes of care (RI.2.90) RI-16
to visitors (RI.2.100) RI-16–RI-17
in withholding resuscitative services (RI.2.80) RI-15
to work opportunities (RI.2.190) RI-21
organization ethics (RI.1.10–RI.1.40) RI-9–RI-11
  and conflict resolution (RI.1.10) RI-9
  conflicts of interest (RI.1.20) RI-9–RI-10
  and decision-making integrity (RI.1.30) RI-10
  and denial-of-care issues (RI.1.40) RI-10–RI-11
  for marketing, admission, transfer, discharge, and billing (RI.1.10) RI-9

Ethics, rights, and responsibilities function
chapter descriptions, RI-4–RI-8
crosswalk of standards, CW-1–CW-4
goal of, RI-1
overview of, RI-1
revisions in, HB-3
scoring changes, HB-8
standards, RI-2–RI-3

Evaluation. *See* Credentialing; Management of human resources; Performance

Evidence of Standards Compliance (ESC), ACC-3, ACC-5; APP-31; APR-1
and National Patient Safety Goals, NPSG-1
process, APP-31

Evidence of Standards Compliance report (ESC report), ACC-3; APP-31–APP-32

Exit conference, ACC-17; APP-28

Extension survey, APP-5, APP-6, APP-38–APP-39

Extranet site, Joint Commission, ACC-2, ACC-3; APP-18

and application for accreditation, APP-19–APP-20

F

Fair-hearing and appeal process (MS.4.50) MS-31–MS-32
Fall prevention, NPSG-4–NPSG-5
Falsification of information, APP-11; APR-1, APR-7
Family. *See also* Education of patient and family; Surrogate decision maker
and care decisions (RI.1.40; RI.2.30) RI-10–RI-11, RI-12
and care plan involvement (PC.4.10) PC-22–PC-23
and nonformulary medication (MM.2.40) MM-13–MM-14
and organ donation requests (LD.3.110) LD-18–LD-19
and restraint and seclusion use (PC.12.40; PC.12.80) PC-40, PC-43–PC-44, PC-45
and unanticipated outcomes of care (RI.2.90) RI-16
FDA. *See* Food and Drug Administration
Feedback sessions, APP-29
Fees, for survey, APP-17
Fire drills (EC.5.30) EC-21–EC-22
Fire safety risk management (EC.5.10) EC-19–EC-20
development and implementation of fire response plan (EC.5.10) EC-19–EC-20
documentation of alarm and extinguishing systems (EC.5.40) EC-22–EC-24
fire drills conduct (EC.5.30) EC-21–EC-22
implementation of fire safety processes (EC.5.10) EC-19–EC-20
inspection, testing, and maintenance of systems (EC.5.10) EC-19–EC-20
interim life safety measures (ILSM) policy (EC.5.50) EC-24–EC-25
Life Safety Code® compliance (EC.5.20) EC-20–EC-21
maintenance of fire-safety equipment (EC.5.40) EC-22–EC-24
organizational review of furnishing acquisitions (EC.5.10) EC-19–EC-20
protection during building construction (EC.5.50) EC-24–EC-25
written plan for (EC.5.10) EC-19–EC-20
Focused review (MS.4.90) MS-35–MS-36
Food and Drug Administration (FDA). *See* Simplifying compliance activities
medication dispensing (MM.4.70) MM-19
Forensics
education and orientation of staff on (HR.2.10) HR-11

Free text, IM-1
Functional integration, APP-3–APP-4
Functional status screening (PC.2.20; PC.2.120) PC-16, PC-17

G

Governance (LD.1.10) LD-10. *See also* Leadership; Medical staff
 compliance with law and regulation (LD.1.30) LD-11
 and conflicts of interest (RI.1.20) RI-9–RI-10
 responsibilities (LD.1.20) LD-10–LD-11
 operational (LD.2.10) LD-11
Government agencies, release of data to, APP-15–APP-16
Graduate Medical Education Committee (GMEC) (MS.2.30) MS-19–MS-20
Guidelines for Design and Construction of Hospitals and Health Care Facilities (EC.8.30) EC-34–EC-35

H

Hand hygiene, NPSG-4; (IC.3.10, IC.4.10) IC-10–IC-12
Hazard vulnerability analysis (EC.4.10) EC-15–EC-18
Hazardous materials and waste risk management (EC.3.10) EC-14–EC-15
 appropriate space and equipment for (EC.3.10) EC-14–EC-15
 documentation for use of (EC.3.10) EC-14–EC-15
 emergency procedures (EC.3.10) EC-14–EC-15
 hazardous gas and vapor monitoring and disposal (EC.3.10) EC-14–EC-15
 identification of materials (EC.3.10) EC-14–EC-15
 inventory maintenance for (EC.3.10) EC-14–EC-15
 labeling of (EC.3.10) EC-14–EC-15
 manifests for handling of (EC.3.10) EC-14–EC-15
 selection, handling, storage, transport, use, and disposal procedures (EC.3.10) EC-14–EC-15
 separate storage areas for (EC.3.10) EC-14–EC-15
 written plan for (EC.3.10) EC-14–EC-15
HAZMAT. *See* Hazardous materials and waste risk management
Health care–associated infection (HAI) (IC.1.10) IC-9. *See also* Surveillance, prevention, and control of infection
 hand hygiene guidelines, NPSG-4
 prevention priorities and goals (IC.3.10) IC-10–IC-11
 risk reduction of, NPSG-4
 and sentinel events, NPSG-4

Health Insurance Portability and Accountability Act of 1996 (HIPAA), APP-13
High-risk medications (MM.7.10; MM.7.40) MM-22–MM-23
 investigational (MM.7.40) MM-23
Hospital Accreditation Standards (HAS)
 accreditation and, HB-1
 element of performance, HB-22
 purpose, HB-1
 rationale, HB-22
 reformatting of functional chapters, HB-21–HB-22
 revisions in, HB-1–HB-7
 scoring category and MOS designation changes, HB-8–HB-20
 standard, HB-22
Hospital leaders. *See* Leadership
Housekeeping activities (PC.8.60) PC-30
Human resources management. *See* Management of human resources
Hydration status (PC.2.20) PC-16
Hygiene and grooming (PC.8.60) PC-30

I

Identification
 of medical record entries' authors (IM.6.10) IM-19–IM-22
 in medical record (IM.6.10) IM-19–IM-22
 before medication administration (MM.5.10) MM-20
Immediate threat to life, APP-30, APP-34
Improving organization performance (PI), PI-1–PI-12. *See also* Medical staff
 adverse drug reaction (PI.2.20) PI-10
 aggregation of data (PI.2.10) PI-9–PI-10
 analysis of data (PI.2.10) PI-9–PI-10
 anesthesia, adverse events (PI.2.20) PI-10
 data collection for (PI.1.10) PI-8–PI-9
 leadership role in (LD.4.10; LD.4.50; LD.4.70) LD-21, LD-23
 medical staff role in (MS.3.10–MS.3.20) MS-20–MS-22. *See also* Medical staff
 medication errors (PI.2.20) PI-10
 and patient safety (PI.3.10) PI-11
 proactive program (PI.3.20) PI-12
 restraint and seclusion use (PC.11.20) PC-34
 and safety (LD.4.60) LD-23
 sentinel events, SE-1; (PI.2.30–PI.3.20) PI-10–PI-12
 staffing effectiveness (PI.2.20) PI-10
 with statistical techniques (PI.2.10) PI-9–PI-10
 transfusion reactions (PI.2.20) PI-10
 undesirable variation in performance (PI.2.20) PI-10

Improving organization performance function. *See also* Improving organization performance; Management of information; Measurement; Performance
    chapter description, PI-3–PI-7
    crosswalk of standards, CW-18–CW-19
    overview of, PI-1
    revisions in, HB-5
    scoring changes in, HB-13–HB-14
    standards, PI-2
Incontinence (PC.8.60) PC-30
Indicator screening (HR.1.30) HR-9–HR-11
    Joint Commission list (HR.1.30) HR-10–HR-11
Individual tracer activity, ACC-16, ACC-18
Infant abduction (EC.2.10) EC-13–EC-14
Infection. *See also* Surveillance, prevention, and control of infection
    identification of risks (IC.2.10) IC-10
    risk reduction of health care–associated (IC.1.10) IC-9–IC-10
Infection control, ACC-10
Infection control program, ACC-10. *See also* Surveillance, prevention, and control of infection
    collaboration of staff (IC.8.10) IC-15
    data collection on (PI.1.10) PI-8–PI-9
    effectiveness evaluation (IC.5.10) IC-12–IC-13
    management (IC.7.10) IC-14
Information Accuracy and Truthfulness Policy, in accreditation survey, APP-10–APP-12, APP-34, APP-40
Information Collection and Evaluation System (ICES), EC-1
Information management, ACC-11. *See also* Management of information
Informed consent (RI.2.40) RI-13
    in research projects (RI.2.180) RI-20–RI-21
    benefits (RI.2.180) RI-20–RI-21
    refusal to participate (RI.2.180) RI-20–RI-21
    risks (RI.2.180) RI-20–RI-21
Infusion pump safety, NPSG-4
Initial assessment, of patients (PC.2.20–PC.2.130) PC-16–PC-17
    for minimization of restraint or seclusion use (PC.12.40) PC-43–PC-44
    time frame for (PC.2.120) PC-17
        functional status (PC.2.120) PC-17
        for history and physical examination (PC.2.120) PC-17
        per hospital policy (PC.2.130) PC-17
        nursing (PC.2.120) PC-17
        nutritional (PC.2.120) PC-17
Initial surveys, ACC-8; APP-10, APP-27
In-service training (HR.2.30) HR-12–HR-13. *See also* Continuing education

Institute for Safe Medication Practices (ISMP), MM-22
Integrity, IM-12
Interactive text, IM-1
Interim life safety measures (ILSM) (EC.5.50) EC-24–EC-25
Invasive procedures. *See* Operative and other procedures
Investigational medication (MM.7.40) MM-23
    orders for (MM.3.20) MM-14–MM-15

J

Joint Commission on Accreditation of Healthcare Organizations
    account representative, HB-24; APP-19, APP-20
    complaint hotline, APP-15
    Customer Service, HB-24; EC-21
    Department of Communications, APP-36
    display of logo of, APP-36
    extranet site, ACC-5; APP-18
    information resources, HB-24–HB-25
    logo, APP-36
    manuals, APP-2
    National Patient Safety Goals, HB-3; APP-2, APP-13; NPSG-1–NPSG-6
    Office of Quality Monitoring, ACC-8; APP-25; SE-9
    Perspectives®, HB-22; APP-37, APP-40
    Pricing Unit, APP-17, APP-21, APP-39; SE-12
    Quality Check®, ACC-3; APP-14
    Quality Report, ACC-3, APP-13–APP-14
    Satellite Network, HB-25
    screening indicator list, HR-10–HR-11
    sentinel event database, SE-9
    Sentinel Event Hotline, SE-9, SE-11, SE-14
    sentinel event reporting, SE-4, SE-6
    Standards Interpretation Group, HB-22, HB-24
    Standards Review Task Force, HB-21
    Web site, HB-23, HB-24; APP-14, APP-38; SE-9, SE-11, SE-14; EC-21
Joint Commission Resources (JCR), HB-25
    Web site, HB-25

K

Knowledge-based information
    assessment of need for (IM.1.10) IM-10–IM-11
    as resource (IM.5.10) IM-18–IM-19

L

Laboratory services. *See* Pathology and clinical laboratory services
Latex allergies. *See* Food and Drug Administration (FDA)
Leadership (LD), LD-1–LD-25. *See also* Improving organization performance; Medical Staff

clinical practice guidelines (LD.5.10) LD-24
   approval of (LD.5.30) LD-24–LD-25
   criteria for (LD.5.20) LD-24
   evaluation of outcomes (LD.5.40) LD-25
conference, APP-27
and conflict resolution (LD.1.20) LD-10–LD-11
contracted services (LD.3.50) LD-16
governance (LD.1.10–LD.1.20) LD-10–LD-11
   compliance with law and regulation (LD.1.30) LD-11
   effectiveness of (LD.2.20) LD-12
   and hospital operation (LD.2.10) LD-11
   responsibilities of (LD.1.20) LD-10–LD-11
management
   annual audit (LD.2.50) LD-12–LD-13
   annual operating budget (LD.2.50) LD-12–LD-13
   long-term capital expenditure plan (LD.2.50) LD-12–LD-13
performance improvement and safety
   allocation of adequate resources (LD.4.60) LD-23
   effectiveness measurement (LD.4.70) LD-23
   and environment of care (EC.9.20–EC.9.30) EC-36–EC-37
   integration of patient safety program (LD.4.40) LD-21–LD-22
   new or modified services or processes design (LD.4.20) LD-21
   performance improvement expectations (LD.4.10) LD-21
   priorities for unusual/urgent events (LD.4.50) LD-23
planning
   academic education (LD.3.130) LD-20
   for care, treatment, and services (LD.3.10) LD-13
   competency and qualifications of staff (LD.3.70) LD-17
   consistency with mission, vision, and goals (LD.3.20) LD-14–LD-15
   consultation or contractual arrangements (LD.3.50) LD-16
   effective communication (LD.3.60) LD-17
   implementation of policies and procedures (LD.3.90) LD-18
   organ donation and procurement policies and procedures (LD.3.110) LD-18–LD-19
   patient flow efficiency (LD.3.15) LD-13–LD-14
   and patient legal or correctional restrictions (LD.3.150) LD-20
   provision of patient education activities (LD.3.120) LD-19
   provision of space allocation (LD.3.80) LD-17–LD-18
   psychiatric or substance abuse services referrals (LD.3.140) LD-20
   short- and long-term planning (LD.3.10) LD-13
   standard of care, treatment, and services (LD.3.20) LD-14–LD-15
   timeliness of services (LD.3.30) LD-15
   transplant services (LD.3.110) LD-18–LD-19
restraint and seclusion role (PC.11.10) PC-33–PC-34, PC-40

Leadership conference, APP-27
Leadership function. *See also* Chief executive officer; Leadership
   chapter description, LD-5–LD-9
   crosswalk of 2003 to 2004 standards, CW-20–CW-25
   overview of, LD-1
   revisions in, HB-5
   scoring changes in, HB-14–HB-15
   standards, LD-2–LD-4
Leadership session, ACC-15–ACC-16
Legal assessment (PC.3.120; PC.3.130) PC-19–PC-21
Licensed independent practitioner. *See also* Medical staff
   and clinical privileges (MS.4.20) MS-26–MS-28
   and contracted services (LD.3.50) LD-16
   and decision making for patient care (RI.1.30) RI-10
   health of (MS.4.80) MS-34–MS-35
   management of patient care by (LD.3.70) LD-17
   and use of restraint or seclusion (PC.11.10; PC.11.40; PC.12.70; PC.12.90; PC.12.110) PC-33–PC-36, PC-45–PC-48
Licensure verification (HR.1.20) HR-8–HR-9
Life safety. *See* Fire safety risk management
Life Safety Code® (LSC) (EC.5.20) EC-20–EC-21
   building tour, ACC-17
   and changes between surveys, APP-38
   and construction (EC.5.50) EC-24–EC-25
Life support equipment, EC-27
Life sustaining treatment
   conflict in, patients' rights (RI.2.80) RI-15–RI-16
   decision to forgo or withdraw, patients' rights (RI.2.80) RI-15–RI-16
Long-term capital expenditure plan (LD.2.50) LD-12–LD-13

M

Management of the environment of care (EC), EC-1–EC-37
   emergency drills (EC.4.20) EC-18–EC-19
   critiquing of (EC.4.20) EC-18–EC-19
   fire drills (EC.5.30) EC-21–EC-22

emergency management (EC.4.10) EC-15–EC-18. *See also* Disaster
  alternative utility systems (EC.4.10) EC-15–EC-18
  back-up communication systems (EC.4.10) EC-15–EC-18
  communitywide organization (EC.4.10) EC-15–EC-18
  conduct of hazard vulnerability analysis (EC.4.10) EC-15–EC-18
  cooperative planning (EC.4.10) EC-15–EC-18
  drills for (EC.4.20) EC-18–EC-19
  establishment of alternate care sites (EC.4.10) EC-15–EC-18
  evacuation procedures (EC.4.10) EC-15–EC-18
  identification and assignment of staff (EC.4.10) EC-15–EC-18
  leadership involvement in (EC.4.10) EC-15–EC-18
  and notification of external authorities (EC.4.10) EC-15–EC-18
  organization and community command structure (EC.4.10) EC-15–EC-18
  radioactive, biological, and chemical isolation and decontamination (EC.4.10) EC-15–EC-18
  written plan for (EC.4.10) EC-15–EC-18
fire safety risk management (EC.5.10) EC-19–EC-20
  development and implementation of fire response plan (EC.5.10) EC-19–EC-20
  documentation of alarm and extinguishing systems (EC.5.40) EC-22–EC-24
  fire drills conduct (EC.5.30) EC-21–EC-22
  implementation of fire safety processes (EC.5.10) EC-19–EC-20
  inspection, testing, and maintenance of systems (EC.5.10) EC-19–EC-20
  interim life safety measures (ILSM) policy (EC.5.50) EC-24–EC-25
  Life Safety Code® compliance (EC.5.20) EC-20–EC-21
  maintenance of fire-safety equipment (EC.5.40) EC-22–EC-24
  organizational review of furnishing acquisitions (EC.5.10) EC-19–EC-20
  protection during building construction (EC.5.50) EC-24–EC-25
  written plan for (EC.5.10) EC-19–EC-20
hazardous materials and waste risk management (EC.3.10) EC-14–EC-15
  appropriate space and equipment for (EC.3.10) EC-14–EC-15
  documentation for use of (EC.3.10) EC-14–EC-15
  emergency procedures (EC.3.10) EC-14–EC-15
  hazardous gas and vapor monitoring and disposal (EC.3.10) EC-14–EC-15
  identification of materials (EC.3.10) EC-14–EC-15
  inventory maintenance for (EC.3.10) EC-14–EC-15
  labeling of (EC.3.10) EC-14–EC-15
  manifests for handling of (EC.3.10) EC-14–EC-15
  selection, handling, storage, transport, use, and disposal procedures (EC.3.10) EC-14–EC-15
  separate storage areas for (EC.3.10) EC-14–EC-15
  written plan for (EC.3.10) EC-14–EC-15
measuring and improving activities (EC.9.10–EC.9.30) EC-35–EC-37
  analysis and resolution of issues (EC.9.20) EC-36–EC-37
  monitoring of environment conditions (EC.9.10) EC-35–EC-36
  staff involvement (EC.9.30) EC-37
medical equipment risk management (EC.6.10) EC-26–EC-27
  emergency procedures (EC.6.10) EC-26–EC-27
  equipment hazard notices and recalls (EC.6.10) EC-26–EC-27
  incident reporting per Safe Medical Devices Act of 1990 (EC.6.10) EC-26–EC-27
  intervals for inspection, testing, and maintenance (EC.6.10) EC-26–EC-27
  inventory criteria (EC.6.10) EC-26–EC-27
  maintenance, testing, and inspection of (EC.6.20) EC-27
  operation strategies (EC.6.10) EC-26–EC-27
  selection and acquiring process (EC.6.10) EC-26–EC-27
  written plan for (EC.6.10) EC-26–EC-27
nonsmoking policy (EC.1.30) EC-12–EC-13
physical environment elements (EC.8.10) EC-33–EC-34
  appropriate storage space for patients (EC.8.10) EC-33–EC-34
  building design (EC.8.30) EC-34–EC-35
  door locks (EC.8.10) EC-33–EC-34
  equipment accommodations (EC.8.10) EC-33–EC-34
  furnishings and equipment standards (EC.8.10) EC-33–EC-34
  lighting (EC.8.10) EC-33–EC-34
  provision of space (LD.3.80) LD-17–LD-18
  ventilation (EC.8.10) EC-33–EC-34
safety risk management (EC.1.10) EC-11–EC-12

conduct of environmental tours (EC.1.20) EC-12
and conduct of proactive risk assessments (EC.1.10) EC-11–EC-12
leadership for coordination of (EC.1.10) EC-11–EC-12
maintenance of grounds and equipment (EC.1.10) EC-11–EC-12
policies and procedures for (EC.1.10) EC-11–EC-12
product safety recall responses (EC.1.10) EC-11–EC-12
for safe environment (EC.1.20) EC-12
smoking policy (EC.1.30) EC-12–EC-13
written plan for (EC.1.10) EC-11–EC-12
security risk management (EC.2.10) EC-13–EC-14
and conduct of risk assessments (EC.2.10) EC-13–EC-14
emergency care vehicular access (EC.2.10) EC-13–EC-14
identification of staff, patients, and visitors (EC.2.10) EC-13–EC-14
implementation of security procedures (EC.2.10) EC-13–EC-14
infant or pediatric abduction prevention (EC.2.10) EC-13–EC-14
leadership for coordination of (EC.2.10) EC-13–EC-14
media or VIP procedures (EC.2.10) EC-13–EC-14
and workplace violence (EC.2.10) EC-13–EC-14
written plan for (EC.2.10) EC-13–EC-14
smoking policy (EC.1.30) EC-12–EC-13
utility risk management (EC.7.10) EC-27–EC-29
documentation of maintenance (EC.7.30) EC-30–EC-31
emergency power source provision (EC.7.20) EC-29–EC-30
maintenance, testing, and inspection of (EC.7.40) EC-31–EC-32
emergency procedures (EC.7.10) EC-27–EC-29
intervals for inspection, testing, and maintenance (EC.7.10) EC-27–EC-29
inventory risk criteria (EC.7.10) EC-27–EC-29
labeling for emergency shutdown (EC.7.10) EC-27–EC-29
maintenance, testing, and inspection of (EC.7.30) EC-30–EC-31
medical gas and vacuum systems maintenance, testing, and inspection (EC.7.50) EC-32–EC-33
operation strategies (EC.7.10) EC-27–EC-29

process to minimize pathogenic biological agents in water systems (EC.7.10) EC-27–EC-29
system design and installation (EC.7.10) EC-27–EC-29
ventilation equipment (EC.7.10) EC-27–EC-29
written plan for (EC.7.10) EC-27–EC-29

Management of the environment of care function. *See also* Management of environment of care; Planning
chapter description, EC-6–EC-10
crosswalk of standards, CW-26–CW-28
goal of, EC-1
overview of, EC-1–EC-3
revisions in, HB-5–HB-6
scoring changes in, HB-16–HB-17
standards for, EC-4–EC-5

Management of human resources (HR), HR-1–HR-14. *See also* Continuing education; Leadership; Medical staff; Staff
assessing competence (HR.3.10–HR.3.20) HR-13–HR-14
performance evaluations (HR.3.20) HR-14
time frame for (HR.3.10) HR-13–HR-14
orienting, training, and educating staff (HR.2.10–HR.2.30) HR-11–HR-13
forensic staff (HR.2.10) HR-11
on infection control (HR.2.10) HR-11
in-service education and training (HR.2.30) HR-12–HR-13
orientation process (HR.2.10) HR-11
on patient rights (HR.2.10) HR-11
and patient safety (HR.2.10–HR.2.20) HR-11–HR-12
on policies and procedures (HR.2.10) HR-11
on restraint and seclusion use (HR.2.10) HR-11
planning (HR.1.10–HR.1.30) HR-8–HR-11
adequate number of staff members (HR.1.10) HR-8
assessment of staff effectiveness (HR.1.30) HR-9–HR-11
clinical/service screening indicators (HR.1.30) HR-9–HR-11
licensure verification (HR.1.20) HR-8–HR-9
screening indicators list (HR.1.30) HR-10–HR-11

Management of human resources function. *See also* Continuing education; Leadership; Management of human resources; Planning; Staff
chapter description, HR-3–HR-7
crosswalk of standards, CW-29–CW-30
overview, HR-1
revisions in, HB-6

2005 Hospital Accreditation Standards

scoring changes in, HB-18
standards, HR-2
Management of information (IM), IM-1–IM-25.
  See also Measurement; Medical record
  confidentiality and security (IM.2.10–IM.2.30)
    IM-11–IM-14
    communication of policy to staff (IM.2.10)
      IM-11–IM-12
    confidentiality of information (IM.2.10)
      IM-11–IM-12
    continuity plan (IM.2.30) IM-13–IM-14
    data integrity (IM.2.20) IM-12–IM-13
    disaster recovery plan (IM.2.30) IM-13–IM-14
    monitoring of policy (IM.2.10) IM-11–IM-12
    privacy of information (IM.2.10) IM-11–IM-12
    security of information (IM.2.20) IM-12–IM-13
    written process for (IM.2.10) IM-11–IM-12
  data collection
    timeliness, accuracy, and efficiency of
      (IM.3.10) IM-15–IM-17
  data and information
    confidentiality of (IM.2.10) IM-11–IM-12
    integrity of (IM.2.20) IM-12–IM-13
    privacy of (IM.2.10) IM-11–IM-12
  information-based decision making (IM.4.10)
    IM-17–IM-18
    accessibility of record information (IM.4.10)
      IM-17–IM-18
    and comparative performance data
      (IM.4.10) IM-17–IM-18
    data collection and aggregation (IM.4.10)
      IM-17–IM-18
  information management processes (IM.3.10)
    IM-15–IM-17
    data capture methods (IM.3.10) IM-15–IM-17
    quality control systems (IM.3.10) IM-15–IM-17
    retention of data and information (IM.3.10)
      IM-15–IM-17
    standardization of abbreviations, acronyms,
      and symbols (IM.3.10) IM-15–IM-17
    storage and retrieval systems (IM.3.10)
      IM-15–IM-17
    timely and accurate dissemination (IM.3.10)
      IM-15–IM-17
    tool availability (IM.3.10) IM-15–IM-17
    uniform data definitions (IM.3.10) IM-15–IM-17
  knowledge-based information (IM.5.10)
    IM-18–IM-19
    assessment of need for (IM.1.10) IM-10–IM-11
    as resource (IM.5.10) IM-18–IM-19
  medical records
    ambulatory care visits (IM.6.40) IM-24
    assembly of components (IM.6.60) IM-25

    contents of (IM.6.20) IM-22–IM-23
    and discharge (IM.6.30) IM-23–IM-24
    emergency care visits (IM.6.10) IM-19–IM-22
    postoperative documentation in (IM.6.30)
      IM-23–IM-24
    retention time (IM.6.10) IM-19–IM-22
    retrieval of (IM.6.60) IM-25
    review of (IM.6.10) IM-19–IM-22
    verbal orders in (IM.6.50) IM-24–IM-25
  patient-specific information (IM.6.10–IM.6.60)
    IM-19–IM-25
    anesthesia and sedation use, documentation
      of (PC.13.30) PC-55–PC-56; (IM.6.30)
      IM-23–IM-24
    authentication of medical records (IM.6.10)
      IM-19–IM-22
    content of medical record (IM.6.20)
      IM-22–IM-23
    documentation of operative or other procedures (IM.6.30) IM-23–IM-24
    quick assembly of patient's record (IM.6.60)
      IM-25
    summary lists (IM.6.40) IM-24
    verbal orders (IM.6.50) IM-24–IM-25
  planning (IM.1.10) IM-10–IM-11
    assessment of information needs (IM.1.10)
      IM-10–IM-11
    information management processes
      (IM.1.10) IM-10–IM-11
    knowledge-based information (IM.1.10)
      IM-10–IM-11
    scope and complexity of services (IM.1.10)
      IM-10–IM-11
    selecting, integrating, and using information-
      management technology (IM.1.10)
      IM-10–IM-11
Management of information function.
  See also Management of information;
    Measurement
  chapter description, IM-5–IM-9
  crosswalk of standards, CW-31–CW-33
  goal of, IM-1
  overview of, IM-1–IM-2
  revisions in, HB-6–HB-7
  scoring changes in, HB-18–HB-19
  standards of, IM-3–IM-4
Marketing
  organization ethics in (RI.1.10) RI-9
Measure(s) of success (MOS), HB-8–HB-20;
  ACC-2; APP-18–APP-19, APP-27, APP-31; SE-9;
  APR-9
  report, APP-32
Measurement. *See also* Data colllection;
  Management of information
  and environment of care (EC.9.10–EC.9.30)
    EC-35–EC-37

IX – 14

Index

Media, and environmental security (EC.2.10) EC-13–EC-14
and patient rights (RI.2.50) RI-13–RI-14
Medical equipment, IC-11
patient education on use of (PC.6.10) PC-26
Medical equipment risk management (EC.6.10) EC-26–EC-27
emergency procedures (EC.6.10) EC-26–EC-27
equipment hazard notices and recalls (EC.6.10) EC-26–EC-27
incident reporting per Safe Medical Devices Act of 1990 (EC.6.10) EC-26–EC-27
and infection control program (IC.3.10) IC-10–IC-11
intervals for inspection, testing, and maintenance (EC.6.10) EC-26–EC-27
inventory criteria (EC.6.10) EC-26–EC-27
maintenance, testing, and inspection of (EC.6.20) EC-27
operation strategies (EC.6.10) EC-26–EC-27
selection and acquiring process (EC.6.10) EC-26–EC-27
written plan for (EC.6.10) EC-26–EC-27
Medical history and physical (PC.2.120; MS.2.10) PC-17, MS-16–MS-18
by non-licensed independent practioners (MS.2.10) MS-16–MS-18
Medical records. *See also* Management of information
for ambulatory care, requirements for (IM.6.40) IM-24
delinquent (IM.6.10) IM-19–IM-22
documentation of
  anesthesia use (PC.13.30) PC-55–PC-56; (IM.6.30) IM-23–IM-24
  behavior management procedures (PC.13.70) PC-57–PC-59
  electroconvulsive therapy (PC.13.50) PC-56–PC-57
  operative and other procedures (IM.6.30) IM-23–IM-24
  psychosurgery (PC.13.60) PC-57
  restraint and seclusion use (PC.11.30; PC.11.100; PC.12.170) PC-35, PC-38, PC-50
  sedation use (IM.6.30) IM-23–IM-24
electronic health information (IM.6.10) IM-19–IM-22
for emergency care, requirements of (IM.6.10) IM-19–IM-22
entries in (IM.6.10) IM-19–IM-22
  authors, identification of (IM.6.10) IM-19–IM-22
  dating and authentication of (IM.6.10) IM-19–IM-22

information in (IM.6.20) IM-22–IM-23
  timely management of (IM.6.10) IM-19–IM-22
information retention time (IM.6.10) IM-19–IM-22
medical staff role in completion of (MS.3.20) MS-21–MS-22
medication monitoring information in (IM.6.40) IM-24
retention of (IM.6.10) IM-19–IM-22
review of (IM.6.10) IM-19–IM-22
verbal orders in (IM.6.50) IM-24–IM-25
Medical staff (MS), MS-1–MS-42. *See also* Clinical privileges; Licensed independent practitioner
accountability to governing body (MS.1.10) MS-12
appointment and reapointment to (MS.4.40) MS-29–MS-31
  adverse decision (MS.4.50) MS-31–MS-32
  continuing education and (MS.2.30) MS-19–MS-20
  criteria for (MS.1.20; MS.4.60) MS-12–MS-15, MS-32
  duration of (MS.4.60) MS-32
  peer recommendations in (MS.4.40) MS-29–MS-31
  reappraisal for (MS.4.40) MS-29–MS-31
autopsy performance, criteria, and staff notification (MS.3.10) MS-20–MS-21
bylaws (MS.1.20) MS-12–MS-15
  adoption (MS.1.20) MS-12–MS-15
  amendment (MS.1.20–MS.1.30) MS-12–MS-15
  appointment criteria and qualifications (MS.1.20) MS-12–MS-15
  approval and compliance by governing body (MS.1.20) MS-12–MS-15
  corrective actions (MS.1.20) MS-12–MS-15
  credentialing, privileging, and appointment (MS.1.20; MS.4.10) MS-12–MS-15, MS-23–MS-26
  department chair qualifications, roles, and responsibilities (MS.1.20) MS-12–MS-15
  development of (MS.1.20) MS-12–MS-15
  executive committee provisions (MS.1.20) MS-12–MS-15
  fair hearing (MS.1.20) MS-12–MS-15
  temporary privileging (MS.4.100) MS-36–MS-37
care of patients (MS.2.10–MS.2.20) MS-16–MS-18
  communication and (MS.2.20) MS-18
  consultations (MS.2.20) MS-18
  coordination of (MS.2.20) MS-18
  management of (MS.2.20) MS-18
  medical history (MS.2.10) MS-16–MS-18
  non-inpatient services (MS.2.10) MS-16–MS-18

and patient safety (MS.2.10) MS-16–MS-18
and patient satisfaction (MS.2.10) MS-16–MS-18
quality of (MS.2.10) MS-16–MS-18
service providers (MS.1.20) MS-12–MS-15
clinical privileges of. *See* Clinical privileges
communication among Graduate Medical Education Committee (MS.2.30) MS-19–MS-20
competence of (LD.3.70) LD-17; (HR.1.20) HR-8–HR-9
continuing medical education (MS.5.10) MS-41–MS-42
contracted services. *See* Contracted services
credentialing, privileging, and appointment (MS.4.10–MS.4.130) MS-22–MS-41
 challenges to licensure (MS.4.30) MS-29
 clinical privileges (MS.4.20) MS-26–MS-28
 criteria for clinical privileges (MS.4.20) MS-26–MS-28
 and disaster privileges (MS.4.110) MS-38–MS-39
 fair hearing and appeal process (MS.4.50) MS-31–MS-32
 focused review process (MS.4.90) MS-35–MS-36
 peer recommendations (MS.4.70) MS-33
 primary source verification (MS.4.10) MS-23–MS-26
 process (MS.4.10) MS-23–MS-26
 renewal, revocation, or revision of clinical privileges (MS.4.40) MS-29–MS-31
 setting-specific clinical privileging (MS.4.20) MS-26–MS-28
 staff appointments (MS.4.60) MS-32
 telemedicine link care (MS.4.120–MS.4.130) MS-39–MS-41
 temporary privileging (MS.4.100) MS-36–MS-37
 verification of information (MS.4.10) MS-23–MS-26
department chair qualifications, roles, and responsibilities (MS.1.20) MS-12–MS-15
disaster privileges (MS.4.110) MS-38–MS-39
executive committee (MS.1.40) MS-15–MS-16
 and chief executive officer (MS.1.40) MS-15–MS-16
 composition of (MS.1.20) MS-12–MS-15
 functions of (MS.1.40) MS-15–MS-16
 medical department chair (MS.1.20) MS-12–MS-15
 meetings (MS.1.40) MS-15–MS-16
 membership (MS.1.40) MS-15–MS-16
 participation in governance (MS.1.40) MS-15–MS-16
 recommendations to governing body (MS.1.40) MS-15–MS-16
 selection of members (MS.1.20) MS-12–MS-15
fair hearing and appeal (MS.4.50) MS-31–MS-32
and governance (LD.1.10) LD-10
graduate education programs (MS.2.30) MS-19–MS-20
 communication and (MS.2.30) MS-19–MS-20
 compliance with residency review (MS.2.30) MS-19–MS-20
 defined process (MS.2.30) MS-19–MS-20
 delineation of participants (MS.2.30) MS-19–MS-20
 written description of patient care activities (MS.2.30) MS-19–MS-20
participation in governance (LD.1.10) LD-10
peer recommendation (MS.4.70) MS-33
performance improvement (MS.3.10–MS.3.20) MS-20–MS-22
 adverse privileging decisions (MS.3.10) MS-20–MS-21
 assessment of patients (MS.3.10) MS-20–MS-21
 autopsies (MS.3.10) MS-20–MS-21
 blood and blood components (MS.3.10) MS-20–MS-21
 clinical practice patterns (MS.3.10) MS-20–MS-21
 communication among staff (MS.3.20) MS-21–MS-22
 completion of medical records (MS.3.20) MS-21–MS-22
 coordination of care (MS.3.20) MS-21–MS-22
 departures from established practice (MS.3.10) MS-20–MS-21
 education of patients and families (MS.3.20) MS-21–MS-22
 and leadership role (MS.3.10) MS-20–MS-21
 medications (MS.3.10) MS-20–MS-21
 operative and other procedures (MS.3.10) MS-20–MS-21
 patient safety data (MS.3.10) MS-20–MS-21
 sentinel event data (MS.3.10) MS-20–MS-21
physician health (MS.4.80) MS-34–MS-35
staff structure (MS.1.10–MS.1.30) MS-11–MS-15
 accountability to governing body (MS.1.10) MS-12
 bylaws (MS.1.20) MS-12–MS-15
 organization of (MS.1.10) MS-12
 primary function, MS-11
 principles for (MS.1.10) MS-12
 self governance of (MS.1.10) MS-12
 uniform quality of care, treatment, and services (MS.1.10) MS-12
telemedicine (MS.4.120–MS.4.130) MS-39–MS-41

temporary privileging (MS.4.100) MS-36–MS-37
waived testing (PC.16.20) PC-48
Medical staff function. *See also* Medical staff
  chapter description, MS-6–MS-10
  crosswalk of standards, CW-34–CW-50
  overview, MS-1–MS-2
  revisions in, HB-7
  scoring changes in, HB-19–HB-20
  standards, MS-3–MS-5
Medication errors (MM.6.20) MM-21–MM-22
  data analysis on (PI.2.20) PI-10
  and order transcription (MM.3.20) MM-14–MM-15
Medication management (MM), ACC-11; MM-1–MM-23
  administering (MM.5.10–MM.5.20) MM-20–MM-21
    safety and accuracy of (MM.5.10) MM-20
    self-administered (MM.5.20) MM-20–MM-21
    verification of orders (MM.5.10) MM-20
  and care continuum, NPSG-4
  data collection on (PI.1.10) PI-8–PI-9
  evaluation of management system (MM.8.10) MM-23
  high-risk medications (MM.7.10; MM.7.40) MM-22–MM-23
    investigational (MM.7.40) MM-23
    management process for (MM.7.10) MM-22
  and medical staff involvement (MS.3.10) MS-20–MS-21
  monitoring (MM.6.10–MM.6.20) MM-21–MM-22
    and adverse drug events and medication errors (MM.6.20) MM-21–MM-22
  ordering and transcribing (MM.3.10–MM.3.20) MM-14–MM-15
    errors during (MM.3.20) MM-14–MM-15
  and patient care continuum, NPSG-4
  patient education about use of (PC.6.10) PC-26
  patient-specific information (MM.1.10) MM-10–MM-11
    accessible to staff (MM.1.10) MM-10–MM-11
  preparing and dispensing (MM.4.10–MM.4.80) MM-15–MM-19
    availability after hours (MM.4.10; MM.4.50) MM-15–MM-16, MM-18
    labeling method (MM.4.30) MM-17
    recalled system (MM.4.70) MM-19
    returned medication (MM.4.80) MM-19
    review for appropriateness (MM.4.10) MM-15–MM-16
    review of prescriptions (MM.4.10) MM-15–MM-16
    safe dispensing (MM.4.40) MM-17–MM-18
    safe preparation of (MM.4.20) MM-16
  safety of, NPSG-3
    limitation of drug concentrations, NPSG-3
    removal of concentrated electrolytes, NPSG-3
    review of look-alike/sound-alike drugs, NPSG-3
  selection and procurement (MM.2.10) MM-11
    availability of dispensing list (MM.2.10) MM-11
    procurement for unavailable (MM.2.10) MM-11
    review for safety and efficacy (MM.2.10) MM-11
    shortages and outages process (MM.2.10) MM-11
    written criteria for (MM.2.10) MM-11
  storage (MM.2.20–MM.2.40) MM-12–MM-14
    area inspection (MM.2.20) MM-12–MM-13
    emergency medications (MM.2.30) MM-13
    of expired, damaged, or contaminated (MM.2.20) MM-12–MM-13
    labeling accuracy (MM.2.20) MM-12–MM-13
    process for nonformulary medications (MM.2.40) MM-13–MM-14
    removal of electrolytes from care area (MM.2.20) MM-12–MM-13
Medication management function. *See also* Medication management
  chapter description, MM-5–MM-9
  crosswalk of standards, CW-15–CW-16
  overview, MM-1–MM-2
  revisions in, HB-4
  scoring changes in, HB-12–HB-13
  standards, MM-3–MM-4
Mergers, consolidations, and acquisitions, APP-38; APR-2
Minimal sedation, PC-54
Misrepresentation of information, APR-6–APR-8
Mitigation activities, EC-16
Moderate sedation, PC-54
Multiorganization option, APP-6–APP-7

N

National Patient Safety Goals, HB-3; APP-2; APP-13; NPSG-1–NPSG-6
  communication effectiveness (Goal 2), NPSG-3
    confirmation of verbal orders, NPSG-3
    standardization of abbreviations, NPSG-3
  compliance, NPSG-1
  fall prevention (Goal 9), NPSG-4–NPSG-5
  infusion pump safety (Goal 5) NPSG-4
  medication use safety (Goal 3), NPSG-3
    annual review of look-alike/sound-alike drugs, NPSG-3
    limiting of drug concentrations, NPSG-3
    removal of electrolytes, NPSG-3
  and patient identification accuracy (Goal 1), NPSG-2

patient medication continuum (Goal 8), NPSG-4
  communication with providers, NPSG-4
  purpose of, NPSG-2
  risk reduction of health care–associated infections (Goal 7), NPSG-4
    hand hygiene guidelines, NPSG-4
    and sentinel events, NPSG-4
  and *Sentinel Event Alert,* NPSG-2
  Universal Protocol, NPSG-5–NPSG-6
    wrong site, wrong procedure, wrong person surgery, NPSG-5–NPSG-6
National Practitioner Data Bank (NPDB) (MS.4.20) MS-26–MS-28
Near miss, SE-3
Neglect (PC.3.10) PC-18–PC-19. *See also* Abused or neglected patients
Neglected patients. *See* Abused or neglected patients
Nonformulary medication (MM.2.40) MM-13–MM-14
Nonrepudiation, IM-13
Nonsmoking policy (EC.1.30) EC-12–EC-13
Nuclear medicine (LD.3.30) LD-15
Nurse executive (NR.1.10) NR-8
  appointment of (NR.2.10) NR-9
  authority of (NR.1.10) NR-8
  functions of (NR.1.10) NR-8
  qualifications of (NR.2.10) NR-9
  responsibilities and authority (NR.1.10) NR-8
    approval of policies and procedures (NR.1.10; NR.3.10) NR-8–NR-10
    for directing nursing services (NR.1.10) NR-8
    for establishing standards of nursing practice (NR.3.10) NR-9–NR-10
    selection or appointment process (NR.2.10) NR-9
Nursing (NR), NR-1–NR-10. *See also* Nurse executive; Provision of care, treatment, and services
  assessment of patient for (PC.2.120) PC-17
  care (LD.3.30) LD-15
  policies and procedures (NR.3.10) NR-9–NR-10
  services (NR.1.10; NR.3.10) NR-8–NR-10
  standards of patient care (NR.3.10) NR-9–NR-10
  standards of practice (NR.3.10) NR-9–NR-10
Nursing function. *See also* Nurse executive; Nursing
  chapter description, NR-3–NR-7
  crosswalk of standards, CW-51
  overview of, NR-1
  revisions in, HB-7
  scoring changes in, HB-20
  standards, NR-2
Nutrition care (PC.7.10) PC-28
  altered diet schedules (PC.7.10) PC-28
  assessment of patient for (PC.2.20) PC-16
  cultural preferences (PC.7.10) PC-28

  distribution and administration (PC.7.10) PC-28
  patient education on (PC.6.10) PC-26
  preparation, storage, and distribution (PC.7.10) PC-28
  safe and accurate provision of (PC.7.10) PC-28
  special diets (PC.7.10) PC-28
  substitutions (PC.7.10) PC-28
Nutrition screening (PC.2.120) PC-17

O

Occupational Safety and Health Administration (OSHA). *See* Management of human resources;
Omnibus Budget Reconciliation Act of 1980, APP-15
Opening conference, ACC-15; APP-27
Operative and other procedures (PC.13.20) PC-54–PC-55
  additional diagnostic data needed (IM.6.30) IM-23–IM-24
  assessment of patient for (PC.13.20) PC-54–PC-55
  blood and blood components in (PC.13.20) PC-54–PC-55
  data collection on (PI.1.10) PI-8–PI-9
  medical staff role in (MS.3.10) MS-20–MS-21
  mental assessment for (IM.6.30) IM-23–IM-24
  monitoring in (PC.13.40) PC-56
  plan of care for (PC.13.20) PC-54–PC-55
  postprocedure care for (IM.6.30) IM-23–IM-24
    mental status (PC.13.40) PC-54–PC-55
    monitoring in (PC.13.40) PC-54–PC-55
    physiological assessment (PC.13.40) PC-54–PC-55
Oral health
  education of patient on (PC.6.10) PC-26
  program implementation (PC.8.60) PC-30
Organ donation and procurement (LD.3.110) LD-18–LD-19
  family notification (LD.3.110) LD-18–LD-19
  hospital death (LD.3.110) LD-18–LD-19
  maintenance of potential donors (LD.3.110) LD-18–LD-19
  patient rights (RI.2.80) RI-15–RI-16
  policies and procedures (LD.3.110) LD-18–LD-19
  state laws regulation (LD.3.110) LD-18–LD-19
  tissue/eye banks and hospital agreements (LD.3.110) LD-18–LD-19
Organization ethics (RI.1.10–RI.1.40) RI-9–RI-11. *See also* Ethics, rights, and responsibilities
Organization performance. *See* Improving organization performance
Organizational integration, APP-3–APP-4
Organizational structure, ACC-11–ACC-12

Index

Orientation, ACC-12; (HR.2.10) HR-11. *See also* Continuing education; Management of human resources
OSHA. *See* Occupational Safety and Health Administration
Outdoor recreation (PC.8.50) PC-29–PC-30
Overview, APP-27

P

Pain management
    data collection on (PI.1.10) PI-8–PI-9
    education of patient on (PC.6.10) PC-26
    and patient assessment (PC.8.10) PC-28–PC-29
    patient's right to (RI.2.160) RI-19–RI-20
Pastoral care (RI.2.10) RI-11
Pathology and clinical laboratory services
    and accreditation survey process, APP-34
    contracted services (LD.3.50) LD-15
    and leadership (LD.3.30) LD-15
    waived testing (PC.16.10–PC.16.40) PC-61–PC-65
    staff responsible for (PC.16.20) PC-62–PC-63
Patient care services. *See* Provision of care, treatment and services
Patient identification, NPSG-2
Patient flow management (LD.3.15) LD-13–LD-14
Patient rights. *See* Ethics, rights, and responsibilities; Provision of care, treatment and services
Patient safety, ACC-12–ACC-13; APP-30. *See also* Safety; National Patient Safety Goals
Patient-specific data and information
    (IM.6.10–IM.6.60) IM-19–IM-25
    for ambulatory care services (IM..40) IM-24
    anesthesia use, documentation of (PC.13.30) PC-55–PC-56; (IM.6.30) IM-23–IM-24
    authentication of medical records (IM.6.10) IM-19–IM-22
    content of medical record (IM.6.20) IM-22–IM-23
    documentation of operative or other procedures (IM.6.30) IM-23–IM-24
    in medication management system (MM.1.10) MM-10–MM-11
    quick assembly of patient's record (IM.6.60) IM-25
    sedation use, documentation of (PC.13.30) PC-55–PC-56; (IM.6.30) IM-23–IM-24
    verbal orders (IM.6.50) IM-24–IM-25
Peer recommendation (LD.3.70) LD-17; (MS.4.70) MS-33
Performance
    evaluations (HR.3.20) HR-14
    measure, APR-3–APR-4
    measurement systems, APR-3–APR-4
Performance improvement. *See* Improving organization performance

Periodic Performance Review (PPR), ACC-1, ACC-5–ACC-7; APP-18–APP-19; APR-1
    accreditation participation requirement, APR-8–APR-10
    full, ACC-6; APR-9
    option 1, ACC-6; APR-9
    option 2, ACC-6; APR-9
    option 3, ACC-7; APR-9–APR-10
    and National Patient Safety Goals, NPSG-1
Personal care and support services (RI.2.140) RI-18–RI-19; (PC.8.60) PC-30
Perspectives®, HB-22; APP-37, APP-40; APR-3
Pharmacy compounding. *See* Food and Drug Administration
Pharmacy services
    after hours (MM.4.10; MM.4.50) MM-15–MM-16, MM-18
    contract services (LD.3.50) LD-16
    and leadership (LD.3.30) LD-15
    medication returns (MM.4.80) MM-19
Physical assessment (PC.2.20) PC-16
Physical environment, ACC-13; (EC.8.10) EC-33–EC-34
Physician practices, APP-5
Plan for improvement. *See* Interim life safety measures; *Life Safety Code®*
Plan of action, ACC-2, ACC-7; APP-18
Plan of care (PC.4.10) PC-22–PC-23. *See also* Provision of care, treatment, and services
Plan of correction. *See* Conditional accreditation
Planning
    for environment of care
        emergency management (EC.4.10) EC-15–EC-18
        for emergency power system (EC.7.20) EC-29–EC-30
        for fire prevention (EC.5.10) EC-19–EC-20
        for hazardous materials and waste management (EC.3.10) EC-14–EC-15
        use of interim life safety measures (ILSM) (EC.5.50) EC-24–EC-25
        for *Life Safety Code®* compliance (EC.5.20) EC-20–EC-21
        for medical equipment management (EC.6.10) EC-26–EC-27
        for safe environment (EC.1.10) EC-11–EC-12
        for secure environment (EC.2.10) EC-13–EC-14
        smoking policy (EC.1.30) EC-12–EC-13
        for utility systems management (EC.7.10) EC-27–EC-29
    hospital planning
        budget development, approval and review (LD.2.50) LD-12–LD-13
        financial audit (LD.2.50) LD-12–LD-13

missions (LD.3.10) LD-13
patient care services (LD.3.90) LD-18
patient overflow (LD.3.15) LD-13–LD-14
scope of services (LD.3.10) LD-13
sources of patient care (LD.3.10) LD-13
timeliness of services (LD.3.30) LD-15
for human resources (HR.1.10–HR.1.30)
  HR-8–HR-11
of information management (IM.1.10)
  IM-10–IM-11
assessment of information needs (IM.1.10)
  IM-10–IM-11
information management processes
  (IM.1.10) IM-10–IM-11
knowledge-based information (IM.1.10)
  IM-10–IM-11
scope and complexity of services (IM.1.10)
  IM-10–IM-11
Policies and procedures. *See also* Accreditation
  survey
for behavior management techniques
  (PC.13.70) PC-57–PC-59
for denial-of-care conflicts (RI.1.40) RI-10–RI-11
development by leadership for care, treatment,
  and services (LD.3.90) LD-18
for infection control program (IC.1.10) IC-9–
  IC-10
for information security (IM.2.20) IM-12–IM-13
for medications (MM.3.20; MM.5.10)
  MM-14–MM-15, MM-20
for nonformulary medication (MM.2.40)
  MM-13–MM-14
for nursing (NR.1.10; NR.3.10) NR-8–NR-10
for restraint and seclusion (PC.11.30; PC.11.50;
  PC.12.190) PC-34–PC-35, PC-36, PC-52
for resuscitation services (PC.9.30) PC-31–PC-32
for safety (EC.1.10) EC-11–EC-12
staff orientation on (HR.2.10) HR-11
for waived testing (PC.16.10; PC.16.40) PC-62,
  PC-64
Postponement of survey, APP-21–APP-22
fees for, APP-21
Practice guidelines (LD.5.10–LD.5.40) LD-24–
  LD-25. *See also* Clinical practice guidelines
criteria (LD.5.20) LD-24
Preliminary Accreditation, APP-7–APP-8,
  APP-32, APP-33, APP-34
Preliminary Denial of Accreditation, decision
  rule, APP-8, APP-11, APP-13, APP-16, APP-17,
  APP-30, APP-31, APP-32, APP-33; SE-13; APR-1
Preparedness activities, EC-16
Prescribing or ordering. *See* Medications
Presurvey activities, ACC-5–ACC-15
Primary source verification (MS.4.10)
  MS-23–MS-26

Priority focus area (PFA), ACC-8–ACC-14; APP-26
assessment and care/services, ACC-9
communication, ACC-9–ACC-10
credentialed practitioners, ACC-10
equipment use, ACC-10
infection control, ACC-10
information management, ACC-11
medication management, ACC-11
organizational structure, ACC-11–ACC-12
orientation and training, ACC-12
patient safety, ACC-12–ACC-13
physical environment, ACC-13
quality improvement, ACC-13
rights and ethics, ACC-13–ACC-14
staffing, ACC-14
Priority Focus Process (PFP), ACC-1, ACC-3,
  ACC-7–ACC-15; APP-11, APP-26
priority focus areas (PFA), ACC-8–ACC-14;
  APP-26
priority focus tool (PFT), APP-26
Priority Focus Tool (PFT), APP-26
Privacy
of information (IM.2.10) IM-11–IM-12
patient's right to (RI.2.130) RI-18
Privileging, ACC-16–ACC-17; (LD.3.70) LD-17.
  See also Clinical privileging
during disasters (MS.4.110) MS-38–MS-39
Processing, IM-2
Protected health information, IM-12
Protective services (RI.2.170) RI-20
Provision of care, treatment, and services
  (PC), PC-1–PC-65. *See also* Assessment; Education of patients and family; Initial assessment; Nutritional care; Restraint; Seclusion
admissions criteria (PC.1.10) PC-14
assessment (PC.2.20–PC.3.130) PC-14–PC-21
of criteria for abuse or neglect victims
  (PC.3.10) PC-18–PC-19
educational (PC.3.120) PC-19–PC-20
for emotional or behavioral disorders
  (PC.3.130) PC-20–PC-21
goal of, PC-14
initial assessment (PC.2.130) PC-17
time frames (PC.2.120) PC-17
legal (PC.3.120) PC-19–PC-20
nursing (PC.2.120) PC-17
nutritional plan screening (PC.2.120) PC-17
psychosocial (PC.3.120) PC-19–PC-20
reassessments (PC.2.20; PC.2.150) PC-16,
  PC-18
for substance abuse disorders (PC.3.120)
  PC-19–PC-20
vocational (PC.3.120) PC-19–PC-20
written data and information from (PC.2.20)
  PC-16
data collection on patient needs (PI.1.10)
  PI-8–PI-9

and denial of care (RI.1.40) RI-10–RI-11
diagnostic services (PC.3.230) PC-22
discharge or transfer (PC.15.10–PC.15.30)
    PC-59–PC-61
    continuum of care process (PC.15.10) PC-59
    exchange of patient information (PC.15.30)
        PC-61
    and needs assessment (PC.15.20) PC-60
education (PC.6.10–PC.6.50) PC-26–PC-27
    academic (PC.6.50) PC-27
    appropriateness of (PC.6.10) PC-26
    and barriers to (PC.6.10) PC-26
    on care plan (PC.6.10) PC-26
    on health practices (PC.6.10) PC-26
    learning styles (PC.6.30) PC-27
    on medical equipment use (PC.6.10) PC-26
    on medication use (PC.6.10) PC-26
    on nutrition, diets, and oral health (PC.6.10)
        PC-26
    on pain management (PC.6.10) PC-26
    on rehabilitation and habilitation techniques
        (PC.6.10) PC-26
end-of-life care (PC.8.70) PC-31
entry to care, treatment, and services (PC.1.10)
    PC-14
and leadership planning (LD.3.10) LD-13
and medical staff competence (LD.3.70) LD-17
and medication use, NPSG-4
nutritional care (PC.7.10) PC-28
    diet schedules (PC.7.10) PC-28
    food preferences (PC.7.10) PC-28
    food substitutes (PC.7.10) PC-28
    storage and preparation conditions
        (PC.7.10) PC-28
organizational ethics in (RI.1.10) RI-9
outdoor recreation (PC.8.50) PC-29–PC-30
pain management (PC.8.10) PC-28–PC-29
    assessment of (PC.8.10) PC-28–PC-29
patient and family involvement in (RI.2.30)
    RI-12
and patient/family responsibilities (RI.3.10)
    RI-22–RI-23
and patient rights (RI.2.10) RI-11
personal hygiene and grooming (PC.8.60) PC-30
    education on (PC.8.60) PC-30
    housekeeping activities (PC.8.60) PC-30
    incontinence (PC.8.60) PC-30
    oral health care (PC.8.60) PC-30
planning (PC.4.10) PC-22–PC-23
provision of (PC.5.10–PC.5.60) PC-23–PC-26
    coordination of care (PC.5.60) PC-25–PC-26
    goal of, PC-23–PC-24
    interdisciplinary and collaborative (PC.5.50)
        PC-25
    internal and external resources for (PC.5.60)
        PC-25–PC-26

and refusal of (RI.2.70) RI-15
restraint and seclusion (PC.11.10–PC.12.190)
    PC-32–PC-52
resuscitation services (PC.9.30) PC-31–PC-32
    appropriateness of equipment (PC.9.30)
        PC-31–PC-32
    availability of (PC.9.30) PC-31–PC-32
    staff training for (PC.9.30) PC-31–PC-32
special procedures (PC.13.20–PC.13.70)
    PC-53–PC-59
    behavior management procedures
        (PC.13.70) PC-57–PC-59
    electroconvulsive therapy use (PC.13.50)
        PC-56–PC-57
    monitoring during (PC.13.30–PC.13.40)
        PC-55–PC-56
    operative or other procedures (PC.13.20)
        PC-54–PC-55
    psychosurgery (PC.13.60) PC-57
    sedation or anesthesia administration
        (PC.13.20) PC-54–PC-55
and unanticipated outcomes (RI.2.90) RI-16
waived testing (PC.16.10–PC.16.60) PC-61–PC-65
    assessment of staff competence (PC.16.30)
        PC-63–PC-64
    identification of staff (PC.16.20) PC-62–PC-63
    maintenance of test records (PC.16.60) PC-65
    policies and procedures for (PC.16.10;
        PC.16.40) PC-62, PC-64–PC-65
    quality control checks (PC.16.50) PC-65
    staff training and competence (PC.16.30)
        PC-63–PC-64
Web sites, PC-61
**Provision of care, treatment, and services
    function.** *See also* Provision of care, treat-
    ment, and services
    chapter descriptions, PC-9–PC-13
    crosswalk of standards, CW-5–CW-14
    overview, PC-1
    revisions in, HB-4
    scoring changes in, HB-8–HB-11
    standards, PC-2–PC-8
Provisional Accreditation, ACC-3; APP-31,
    APP-32, APP-33
Psychological assessment (PC.2.20) PC-16
Psychosocial status, assessment of (PC.3.120)
    PC-19–PC-20
Psychosurgery (PC.13.60) PC-57
Public information interview, APP-6;
    APP-22–APP-26, APP-27. *See also*
    Accreditation survey
    participation requirements, APP-2; APR-5–APR-6
Public Information Policy, APP-13–APP-17. *See
    also* Accreditation survey
Public Notice form, APP-24

Q

Quality Check®, ACC-3; APP-14
Quality control
    checks (PC.16.50) PC-65
    collection of data on (PI.1.10) PI-8–PI-9
    and data monitoring (IM.3.10) IM-15–IM-17
    maintenance of records (PC.16.60) PC-65
    and medication management (MM.4.50) MM-18
Quality improvement, ACC-13
Quality Reports, ACC-3; APP-13–APP-14
    commentary for, APP-13
    and Quality Check®, APP-14

R

Random unannounced surveys, APP-40
Rationale, HB-22
Reassessment (PC.2.150) PC-18
    written information of (PC.2.20) PC-16
Referrals
    for abuse or neglect victims (PC.3.10) PC-18–PC-19
Rehabilitation care and services
    and leadership (LD.3.30) LD-15
    patient education about (PC.6.10) PC-26
Report generation, IM-15
Requirements for improvement, ACC-3; APP-13, APP-14, APP-15, APP-30, APP-31; NPSG-1; APR-1
Research
    and patient rights (RI.2.180) RI-20–RI-21
Respiratory care services
    and leadership (LD.3.30) LD-15
Restraint (PC.11.10–PC.12.190) PC-32–PC-52. *See also* Seclusion
    assessment and assistance of patients (PC.12.40; PC.12.130) PC-43–PC-44, PC-48–PC-49
    for behavioral health care (PC.12.10–PC.12.190) PC-38–PC-52
    exceptions to, PC-39–PC-40
    communication of philosophy to staff (PC.12.10) PC-40–PC-41
    data collection on use of (PC.12.180) PC-51–PC-52; (PI.1.10) PI-8–PI-9
    debriefing of practices (PC.12.160) PC-49–PC-50
    definition of, PC-33
    discontinuation of (PC.12.150) PC-49
    documentation in medical record (PC.11.100; PC.12.170) PC-38, PC-50–PC-51
    and emergency medical services (PC.12.30) PC-41–PC-43
    and emergency use (PC.12.60) PC-44
    evaluation of patient (PC.12.90) PC-45–PC-46
    extended or multiple use of (PC.12.120) PC-48
    family role, PC-40
    leadership role, PC-40
    licensed independent practitioner orders (PC.11.40; PC.12.70) PC-35–PC-36, PC-45
    limitations of use (PC.11.10) PC-33–PC-34
    care plan for (PC.4.10) PC-22–PC-23
    emergency use (PC.12.60) PC-44
    nonphysical techniques (PC.12.50) PC-44
    monitoring of patients in (PC.11.70; PC.12.140) PC-37–PC-38, PC-49
    nonclinical purposes (LD.3.150) LD-20
    notification of family (PC.12.80) PC-45
    orders for (PC.12.100) PC-46–PC-47
    age time limitations (PC.12.100) PC-46–PC-47
    performance improvement processes (PC.11.20) PC-34
    policies and procedures (PC.11.30; PC.11.50; PC.12.190) PC-34–PC-35, PC-36, PC-52
    protocols for (PC.11.60) PC-37
    reduction of use, PC-40
    reevaluation of patient (PC.12.110) PC-47–PC-48
    staff training and competence (PC.12.30) PC-41–PC-43; (HR.2.10) HR-11
    for direct care staff (PC.12.30) PC-41–PC-43
    for initiation and evaluations of (PC.12.30) PC-41–PC-43
    for performing 15-minute assessments (PC.12.30) PC-41–PC-43
    staffing levels (PC.12.20) PC-41
    time limitations of (PC.12.100) PC-46–PC-47
    use of, PC-40
Resuscitative care
    availability of (PC.9.30) PC-31–PC-32
    data collection on (PI.1.10) PI-8–PI-9
    and patient rights (RI.2.80) RI-15–RI-16
Retrievability, IM-15
Review and appeal procedures, APP-32, APP-40–APP-50. *See also* Appeal procedures
    Accreditation Committee
    review by, APP-43–APP-44
    second consideration by, APP-46–APP-47
    Board Appeal Review Committee, review by, APP-47–APP-48
    conditional accreditation, APP-44–APP-45
    evaluation by Joint Commission staff, APP-41–APP-43
    final accreditation decision, APP-49–APP-50
    notice, APP-50
    procedure relating to not compliant standards, APP-48–APP-49
    Review Hearing Panels, APP-45–APP-46
    status of organization pending a final decision and effective date of final decision, APP-50
Review Hearing Panel, APP-40, APP-45–APP-46. *See also* Review and appeal procedures

Index

Risk management activities
  collection of data on (PI.1.10) PI-8–PI-9
Root cause analysis, SE-2, SE-3, SE-8, SE-13; (PI.2.30) PI-10–PI-11
  minimum scope of, SE-8
  review of, SE-7
  submission of, SE-11–SE-12

S

Safe Medical Devices Act (EC.6.10) EC-26–EC-27
Safety. *See also* Management of environment of care
  data collection on (PI.1.10) PI-8–PI-9
  identification of risks (PI.3.20) PI-12
  implementation of patient safety program (LD.4.40) LD-21–LD-22
  and leadership activities (MS.2.10) MS-16–MS-18
  and medical staff role (MS.3.10) MS-20–MS-21
  and medication preparation (MM.4.20) MM-16
  and minimization of risks (HR.2.20) HR-12
  orientation process for (HR.2.10) HR-11
  and performance improvement (PI.3.10) PI-11; (LD.4.60) LD-23
  risk management plan (EC.1.10) EC-11–EC-12
    conduct of environmental tours (EC.1.20) EC-12
    and conduct of risk assessments (EC.1.10) EC-11–EC-12
    leadership for coordination of (EC.1.10) EC-11–EC-12
    maintenance of grounds and equipment (EC.1.10) EC-11–EC-12
    policies and procedures for (EC.1.10) EC-11–EC-12
    product safety recall responses (EC.1.10) EC-11–EC-12
    for safe environment (EC.1.20) EC-12
    smoking policy (EC.1.30) EC-12–EC-13
    written plan for (EC.1.10) EC-11–EC-12
Scheduling survey, APP-21–APP-22
Scope of care or services, APP-2–APP-5
Scoring, HB-8–HB-20; ACC-3–ACC-5; APP-29
Seclusion (PC.11.10–PC.12.190) PC-32–PC-52. *See also* Restraint
  assessment and assistance of patients (PC.12.130) PC-48–PC-49
  for behavioral health care (PC.12.10–PC.12.190) PC-38–PC-52
    exceptions, PC-39–PC-40
  communication of philosophy to staff (PC.12.10) PC-40–PC-41
  data collection on use of (PC.12.180) PC-51–PC-52; (PI.1.10) PI-8–PI-9
  debriefing of practices (PC.12.160) PC-49–PC-50
  discontinuation of (PC.12.150) PC-49
  documentation in medical record (PC.12.170) PC-50–PC-51
  and emergency use (PC.12.60) PC-44
  evaluation of patient (PC.12.90) PC-45–PC-46
  extended or multiple use (PC.12.120) PC-48
  family role, PC-40
  initial assessment of patient (PC.12.40) PC-43–PC-44
  leadership role, PC-40
  licensed independent practitioner orders (PC.12.70) PC-45
  monitoring of patients in (PC.12.140) PC-49
  nonclinical purposes (LD.3.150) LD-20
  notification of family (PC.12.80) PC-45
  orders for (PC.12.100) PC-46–PC-47
    age time limitations (PC.12.100) PC-46–PC-47
  policies and procedures (PC.12.190) PC-52
  reduction of use, PC-40
  reevaluation of patient (PC.12.110) PC-47–PC-48
  staff training and competence (PC.12.30) PC-41–PC-43; (HR.2.10) HR-11
    for direct care staff (PC.12.30) PC-41–PC-43
    for initiation and evaluations of (PC.12.30) PC-41–PC-43
    for performing 15-minute assessments (PC.12.30) PC-41–PC-43
  staffing levels (PC.12.20) PC-41
  use of, PC-40
Security, IM-2
  of information (IM.2.10–IM.2.20) IM-11–IM-13
  patient's right to (RI.2.130) RI-18
  risk management plan (EC.2.10) EC-13–EC-14
    and conduct of risk assessments (EC.2.10) EC-13–EC-14
    emergency care vehicular access (EC.2.10) EC-13–EC-14
    identification of staff, patients, and visitors (EC.2.10) EC-13–EC-14
    implementation of security procedures (EC.2.10) EC-13–EC-14
    infant or pediatric abduction prevention (EC.2.10) EC-13–EC-14
    leadership for coordination of (EC.2.10) EC-13–EC-14
    media or VIP procedures (EC.2.10) EC-13–EC-14
    and workplace violence (EC.2.10) EC-13–EC-14
    written plan for (EC.2.10) EC-13–EC-14
Sedation. *See also* Anesthesia
  assessment for (PC.13.20) PC-54–PC-55
  data analysis on adverse events (PI.2.20) PI-10
  definitions of, PC-54
  discharge from care (PC.13.40) PC-56
  documentation in medical record (IM.6.30) IM-23–IM-24

monitoring physiological status during (PC.13.30–PC.13.40) PC-55–PC-56
plan for (PC.13.20) PC-54–PC-55
provisions by qualified individuals (PC.13.20) PC-54–PC-55
Sentinel Event Alert, SE-9
National Patient Safety Goals, NPSG-2
Sentinel events, HB-3; APP-14; SE-1–SE-14.
See also Accreditation survey
Accreditation Watch, SE-6, SE-7–SE-8, SE-10–SE-11, SE-13
database, SE-9
definition of, SE-1
organization-specific, SE-1–SE-2
and health care–associated infection, NPSG-4
Hotline, SE-9, SE-11, SE-14
implementation procedures of policy, SE-9–SE-14
disclosable information, SE-10
events not reported, SE-9–SE-10
follow-up activity, SE-13
handling of documents, SE-13
initial on-site review, SE-10
initiation of Accreditation Watch, SE-10–SE-11
Joint Commission response, SE-12–SE-13
oversight of policy, SE-13–SE-14
submission of action plan, SE-11–SE-12
submission of root cause analysis, SE-11–SE-12
voluntary reporting, SE-9
and leadership (LD.4.20) LD-21
and patient safety (PI.3.10) PI-11
policy goals, SE-1
process for managing (PI.2.30) PI-10–PI-11
related standards, SE-1–SE-3
action plan, SE-2
expectations, SE-2
organization-specific definition, SE-1–SE-2
root cause analysis, SE-2
survey process, SE-2–SE-3
reporting of unanticipated adverse events (HR.2.30) HR-12–HR-13
reviewable, SE-3–SE-9
Accreditation Watch, SE-7–SE-8
awareness of, SE-4
criteria, SE-3–SE-4
follow-up activities, SE-8–SE-9
minimum scope of root cause analysis, SE-8
reporting to Joint Commission, SE-4, SE-6
required response, SE-6
review of action plan, SE-7
review of root cause analysis, SE-7
reviewable and nonreviewable examples, SE-5–SE-6
root cause analysis (PI.2.30) PI-10–PI-11
Sentinel Event Alert, SE-9

Shared Visions–New Pathways, HB-1, HB-3.
See also Accreditation survey
time line, ACC-2
Smoking (EC.1.30) EC-12–EC-13
Social assessment (PC.2.20) PC-16
Social work services
and leadership (LD.3.30) LD-15
Special interventions. *See also* Behavior management; Restraint; Seclusion
behavior-management procedures (PC.13.70) PC-57–PC-59
electroconvulsive therapy (PC.13.50) PC-56–PC-57
psychosurgery (PC.13.60) PC-57
restraint (PC.11.10–PC.12.190) PC-32–PC-53
seclusion (PC.11.10–PC.12.190) PC-32–PC-53
Special issue resolution, ACC-16
Spiritual service. *See* Pastoral care
Staff. *See also* Management of human resources; Medical staff
adequate number of (HR.1.10) HR-8
education and training of (HR.2.30) HR-12–HR-13; (MS.5.10) MS-41–MS-42. *See also* Continuing education
on restraint and seclusion use (PC.12.30) PC-41–PC-43
and tracer methodology, ACC-19–ACC-20
and waived testing (PC.16.20–PC.16.30) PC-62–PC-64
Staffing, ACC-14
Staffing effectiveness, ACC-14; (HR.1.30) HR-9–HR-11
data analysis on (PI.2.20) PI-10
Standards, HB-22. *See also* specific standards
revisions in, ACC-3–ACC-5
Statement of Conditions™ (SOC) compliance document (EC.5.20) EC-20–EC-21
and changes between surveys, APP-38
Statement of Fire Safety (SFS)
and changes between surveys, APP-38
Stored Emergency Power Supply Systems (SEPSS) (EC.7.40) EC-31–EC-32
Structured text, IM-1
Substance abuse (PC.3.120) PC-19–PC-20
assessment of patient needs (PC.3.120) PC-19–PC-20
care referrals (LD.3.140) LD-20
Sufficient progress, EC-21
Summary of major revisions, HB-4–HB-7
Surrogate decision maker (RI.2.30) RI-12
and informed consent (RI.2.40) RI-13
Surveillance, prevention, and control of infection (IC), ACC-10; IC-1–IC-16
data collection in (PI.1.10) PI-8–PI-9
infection control program (IC.1.10–IC.6.10) IC-9–IC-14

Index

communication systems (IC.1.10) IC-9–IC-10
emergency management plan (IC.6.10) IC-13–IC-14
establishment of priorities and goals (IC.3.10) IC-10–IC-11
evaluation of effectiveness (IC.5.10) IC-12–IC-13
hand hygiene (IC.3.10–IC.4.10) IC-10–IC-12
implementation of interventions (IC.4.10) IC-11–IC-12
implementation of program (IC.1.10) IC-9–IC-10
minimization of risk (IC.1.10) IC-9–IC-10
outbreak investigation systems (IC.1.10) IC-9–IC-10
reporting systems (IC.1.10) IC-9–IC-10
review of risk analysis (IC.2.10) IC-10
risk assessment for (IC.2.10) IC-10
use of surveillance activities (IC.2.10) IC-10
written plan for (IC.1.10) IC-9–IC-10
and staff training and education (HR.2.30) HR-12–HR-13
structures and resources (IC.7.10–IC.9.10) IC-14–IC-16
allocation of adequate resources (IC.9.10) IC-15–IC-16
collaboration of staff (IC.8.10) IC-15
effective program management (IC.7.10) IC-14
Surveillance, prevention, and control of infection function. *See also* Surveillance, prevention, and control of infection
chapter description, IC-4–IC-8
crosswalk of 2004 to 2005 standards, CW-17
overview of, IC-1–IC-2
revisions in, HB-4–HB-5
scoring changes in, HB-13
standards, IC-3
Survey. *See* Accreditation survey
Survey agenda, APP-22
Survey fees, APP-17
Survey observers, APR-8
Survey planning session, ACC-15
Survey process, ACC-1–ACC-20; APP-27–APP-30
Survey team, APP-28
leadership, APP-28–APP-29
meeting, ACC-17–ACC-18
Surveyor report preparation, ACC-18
System tracer, ACC-19; APP-28
data use, ACC-19
infection control, ACC-19
medication management, ACC-19

T

Tailored surveys, APP-3–APP-4. *See also* Accreditation survey
complex organization survey process, APP-5
Telemedicine
and credentialing and privileging processes (MS.4.120–MS.4.130) MS-39–MS-41
Timeliness, IM-15
Tracer methodology, ACC-3, ACC-16, ACC-18–ACC-20; APP-28
individual tracer activity, ACC-18
and staff role, ACC-19–ACC-20
system tracer activity, ACC-19
Training, ACC-12. *See also* Continuing education; Education; Management of human resources
Transfers
exchange of information during (PC.15.30) PC-61
and medication continuum process, NPSG-4
organization ethics in (RI.1.10) RI-9
and patient needs (PC.15.10–PC.15.20) PC-59–PC-60
Transfusion reactions, data analysis (PI.2.20) PI-10
Transmission, IM-1
Transplant services (LD.3.110) LD-18–LD-19. *See also* Organ donation and procurement

U

Unannounced survey, APP-5–APP-6, APP-27, APP-39–APP-40; APR-1
United States Pharmacopoeia (USP), MM-22
Universal Protocol, NPSG-5–NPSG-6
wrong site, wrong procedure, wrong person, NPSG-5–NPSG-6
Unscheduled and unannounced surveys, APP-5–APP-6, APP-27, APP-39–APP-40; APR-1
accreditation participation requirements, APR-2–APR-3
Utility systems risk management (EC.7.10) EC-27–EC-29. *See also* Management of environment of care
documentation of maintenance (EC.7.30) EC-30–EC-31
emergency power source provision (EC.7.20) EC-29–EC-30
maintenance, testing, and inspection of (EC.7.40) EC-31–EC-32
emergency procedures (EC.4.10; EC.7.10) EC-15–EC-18, EC-27–EC-29
intervals for inspection, testing, and maintenance (EC.7.10) EC-27–EC-29
inventory risk criteria (EC.7.10) EC-27–EC-29
labeling for emergency shutdown (EC.7.10) EC-27–EC-29

maintenance, testing, and inspection of (EC.7.30) EC-30–EC-31
medical gas and vacuum systems maintenance, testing, and inspection (EC.7.50) EC-32–EC-33
operation strategies (EC.7.10) EC-27–EC-29
process to minimize pathogenic biological agents in water systems (EC.7.10) EC-27–EC-29
system design and installation (EC.7.10) EC-27–EC-29
ventilation equipment (EC.7.10) EC-27–EC-29
written plan for (EC.7.10) EC-27–EC-29
Utilization management
data collection on (PI.1.10) PI-8–PI-9

V

Verbal orders, documentation of (IM.6.50) IM-24–IM-25
for medications (MM.3.20) MM-14–MM-15
for restraint or seclusion (PC.12.90–PC.12.100) PC-45–PC-47
verifcation of, NPSG-3
Visitors, patients' rights to (RI.2.100) RI-16–RI-17
Vocational assessment (PC.3.120; PC.3.130) PC-16–PC-17

W

Waived testing (PC.16.10–PC.16.60) PC-61–PC-65. *See also* Pathology and clinical laboratory services
competence of staff responsible for (PC.16.30) PC-63–PC-64
identification of responsible staff (PC.16.20) PC-62–PC-63
maintenance of test records (PC.16.60) PC-65
policies and procedures for (PC.16.10; PC.16.40) PC-62, PC-64–PC-65
quality control of (PC.16.50) PC-65
Web sites, PC-61
Web sites
Family Violence Prevention Fund, PC-18
Frequently Asked Questions, HB-23
Joint Commission, HB-23, HB-24; APP-14, APP-38; SE-9, SE-11, SE-14; EC-21
Joint Commission Resources, HB-25
performance measurement, APR-3
for *Perspectives*®, HB-23
Quality Check®, APP-14
waived tests, PC-61
Weighted decision rules, APP-34
Whom Do I Call, HB-24–HB-25
Work programs (RI.2.190) RI-21
Wrong-site surgery, NPSG-5–NPSG-6
preoperative verification process, NPSG-5
site marking, NPSG-5–NPSG-6
"time-out," NPSG-6

This volume may ~~~~~ late for 2 weeks.
Renewals ma~
X6-6050; fr